Whole Body Healing

Natural Healing with Movement,
Exercise, Massage and Other Drug-Free Methods

Whole Body Healing

By CARL LOWE, JAMES W. NECHAS
and the Editors of <u>Prevention</u>® Magazine

 Rodale Press, Emmaus, Pa.

Library of Congress Cataloging in Publication Data
Lowe, Carl.
    Whole body healing.

    Includes index.
    1. Therapeutics, Physiological. 2. Physical
fitness. 3. Health. 4. Healing. I. Nechas,
James William. II. Prevention (Emmaus, Pa.)
III. Title.
RM701.L68 1983   613.7   82-16577
ISBN 0-87857-441-7 hardcover

    4 6 8 10 9 7 5 3   hardcover

Notice

The therapies discussed in this book are strictly adjunctive or complementary to medical treatment. Self-treatment can be hazardous with a serious ailment. We therefore urge you to seek out the best medical assistance you can find whenever it is needed.

Editor: William Gottlieb

Research Chief: Carol Baldwin

Assistant Research Chief: Carol Matthews

Research Project Coordinator: Joann Williams

Research Associates: Martha Capwell, Holly Clemson, Takla Gardey, Sue Ann Gursky, Christy Kohler, Susan Nastasee, Susan Zarrow

Copy Editors: Robert Warmkessel, Jan Barckley

Assistant Editor: Marian Wolbers

Office Personnel: Diana Gottshall, Sue Lagler

Book Design: Joan Peckolick

Art Direction: Karen A. Schell

Illustrations by: Michael Radomski

Project Photographer: Margaret Smyser

    Supplementary Photography:
    Photo on page 153 by Alice Bissell
    Photo on page 92 by Paul Boyer
    Photo on page 373 by T. L. Gettings
    Photo on page 94 by Mitchell T. Mandel
    Photo on page 351 ©Karsh Ottowa, courtesy of the Rolf
      Institute
    Photos on pages 12-13, 189, 223, 470-73 and 476-77 by
      Christie Tito
    Photos on pages 89 and 91 by Sally Ann Ullman

We thank the following for advice on various parts of this book:
    Irmgard Bartenieff, André Bernard, Deborah Caplan, Dianne
    Dulicai, Sharon Holmes, Anna Hyder, Judith Lasater, Ph.D., Norma
    Leistiko, William Newman, Ph.D., James Pursey, Ph.D.

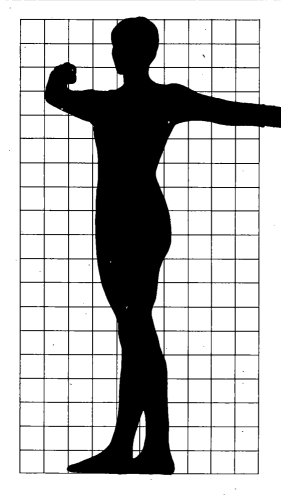

Contents

INTRODUCTION

Most of us probably don't think of the body as our ally in the quest for good health. That's because most of us don't usually think about the body at all. We take it for granted. At least while we're healthy.

But the truth is, the body constantly works to keep our system balanced and strong. That work is called healing. And healing is a process as never-ending as your breathing or heartbeat. Every time you cut yourself, the body heals, mending damaged skin and tissue. Every time a virus takes hold, the body heals (or tries to), as white blood cells rush to repel the invader. A cough in a smoky room. A pain that alerts you to a medical problem. A good night's sleep after a tough day. All are healing.

In *Whole Body Healing,* the editors of *Prevention* magazine offer natural healing through physical activities: exercise (like walking), movement (like yoga), and massage (like acupressure). Yet even though these methods don't contact your cells directly like a vitamin supplement or food, they still nourish and help every part of your body. How?

It's like the relationship between TV broadcasters and the images on your television set. You watch shows without the broadcasters coming into your house. They just sit at the station with their controls, and the picture appears on your TV. The methods in *Whole Body Healing* work the same way. What you do to your body on the outside broadcasts messages to the organs and systems on the inside. For instance, when you exercise, your body sends a set of signals to your inner organs that tell your circulatory system to increase the blood flow to your muscles. Your body raises your metabolic rate, burning more calories than if you just sat around. Your body tells your glands to release endorphins, hormones that relieve pain and put you in a good mood.

In short, the methods in this book help your body send healing messages. (That's why we included the "Special Index of Conditions and Diseases" – so you can quickly find which methods work best for your health problem.) But *Whole Body Healing* doesn't only help you *get* well. It helps you to *stay* well – to prevent sickness by keeping your body flexible and strong. And that's natural healing at its best.

ACUPUNCTURE AND ACUPRESSURE

Whenever I feel a headache coming on, I purposely make it worse. I put both of my thumb knuckles into the middle of my eyebrows and dig in as hard as I can. The pain is crushing. I rotate each knuckle clockwise and I slowly count to 30. My forehead feels as though bright sheets of metal just under the skin are pressing into my brain. I usually have to close my eyes in order to stand it. At the count of 30 I let go, but for the first few seconds afterward, the pain persists just as though I was still pushing.

"Am I a berserk masochist? Not really, because after that first moment of residual pain when I stop torturing my

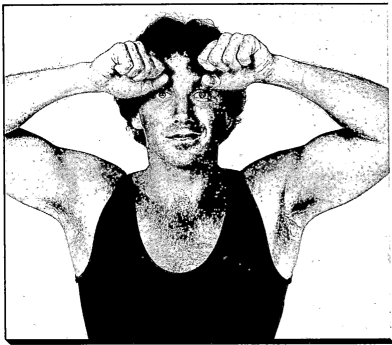

The thumbs are used to press the Yuyao points. These points can cure headaches.

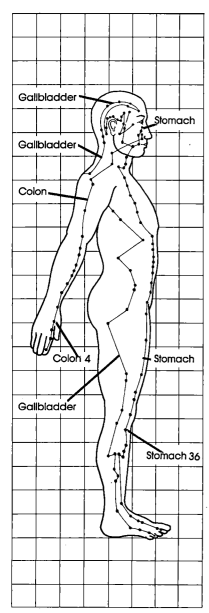

These are the stomach, gall-bladder, and colon acupuncture meridians. Each meridian point controls a different part of the body. Two particularly important points are stomach 36 and colon 4 (also known as the Hegu point).

brow, all of my head pain usually disappears, including the dull throb of my developing headache."

What one of our authors, Carl Lowe, has been doing is stopping his headaches through the use of acupressure. Acupressure, acupuncture and electro-acupuncture are meridian therapies – methods of treating physical problems through manipulation of points on the skin. The name "meridian therapy" is derived from the positioning of the points along lines, or meridians, that travel along the body. Acupressure manipulates these points through pressure on the surface of the body, electro-acupuncture through electrical stimulation, and acupuncture through needle insertion.

Why MDs Rejected Acupuncture

Meridian therapies, originally Chinese treatments, have been known to American medicine since the 1890s but were mostly ignored by the American medical establishment until the 1970s. The reason for their long disuse? First of all, the philosophy of these therapies doesn't mesh well with the principles American MDs usually apply. The traditional Western medical approach to remedying disease or discomfort is to apply a drug or therapy that directly attacks the problem. For example, when confronted by a patient suffering from an infection, a doctor will prescribe an antibiotic known to be effective against the ailment. Chinese methods, on the other hand, work indirectly by encouraging the body to rectify the problem itself. The emphasis is on preventing disease and giving the body the tools to preserve health. To the inexperienced observer, the manipulation of certain meridian points to remedy functional problems can seem like hocus-pocus. The point that gets stimulated often has no obvious connection to the bodily area where the problem exists. You can successfully treat a stiff neck, for instance, through manipulation of the Hegu point, a point on the hand near the thumb.

The Headache Point

Our intrepid author, Carl Lowe, uses pressure on the mid-points of his eyebrows to treat all of his headaches, no matter where the pain originates. The Chinese name for this point is Yuyao. It is an unusual point because, unlike most acupuncture points, it is not associated with any particular internal organ in the body. Howard Kurland, M.D., who originated the acupressure technique Carl uses, identifies this point in his book *Quick Headache Relief Without Drugs* (William Morrow, 1977). This point on the eyebrow lies in a small depression right above the pupil of the eye where the brow narrows. If you think of the eyebrow as a fish, this point would be its waistline. This is where the supraorbital nerve emerges, and it is very tender to the touch, much more sensitive than most meridian points. Like the Yuyao point, most meridian points are associated with a nerve ending near the skin surface.

The proximity of meridian points to emerging nerves on the skin or just under it, and meridian therapy's ability to cure many kinds of pain, have suggested the "gate theory" explanation of how the therapy works. According to this theory, pain is a slow neural signal that travels from a problem area to the spinal column and then up the spinal column to the brain. The point at which these impulses enter the spinal cord is a kind of "nerve gate." The sense of touch, which meridian therapy stimulates, travels four times as fast as pain impulses. Therefore, these faster impulses reach the nerve gate first and block the entrance of pain signals, preventing the brain from registering them. Many dentists, for instance, use electro-acupuncture as a painkiller during dental work. If the gate theory is correct, then acupuncture sets up a "nerve block" that prevents the pain of tooth drilling or extraction from reaching the patient's brain.

Good Nutrition Helps

Several studies have suggested that meridian therapies also relieve pain and cure dysfunction by stimulating the release of neurotransmitters. These chemicals, which include serotonin, norepinephrine and the endorphins, are normally secreted by the body in order to deal with stressful situations. They are antidepressants, and they can have a morphinelike effect on the brain.

According to Ronald Lawrence, M.D., a Los Angeles neurologist with extensive experience practicing and teaching meridian therapy, the therapy's relationship to the neurotransmitters makes good nutritional practices a must for those undergoing treatment. "When you put the acupuncture needle in, you generate more serotonin or more endorphins, but you will not be able to increase the level of these neuro-

Good Sources of Vitamin B6

Food	Portion	Amount (milligrams)
Bananas	1 medium	0.892
Salmon	3 ounces	0.633
Mackerel, Atlantic	3 ounces	0.597
Chicken, light meat	3 ounces	0.510
Beef liver	3 ounces	0.465
Sunflower seeds	¼ cup	0.453
Halibut	3 ounces	0.389
Tuna, canned	3 ounces	0.361
Lentils, dry	¼ cup	0.285
Rice, brown, raw	¼ cup	0.275
Kidney, beef	3 ounces	0.238
Brewer's yeast, debittered	1 tablespoon	0.200
Filberts, whole	¼ cup	0.184
Buckwheat flour, dark	¼ cup	0.142

The Recommended Dietary Allowance is 2-2.2 milligrams.

SOURCES: Adapted from

Pantothenic Acid, Vitamin B6 and Vitamin B12 in Foods, Home Economics Research Report No. 36, by Martha Louise Orr (Washington, D.C.: Agricultural Research Service, U.S. Department of Agriculture, 1969).

U.S. Department of Agriculture Handbooks No. 8-5 and 456.

Information obtained from Nutrient Data Research Group, U.S. Department of Agriculture, 1981.

transmitters unless the basic nutritional material is there. For instance, to develop serotonin, the body needs tryptophan, a basic amino acid, as well as vitamin B_6 and B_{12}."

Good sources of B_6 are bananas, organ meats, fish and whole grain products. B_{12} is found in meat, milk and eggs. Meat, milk and cheese are high in tryptophan.

Eliminate Painkillers

Meridian therapy often eliminates the need for painkilling drugs. Carl has used acupressure for his headaches for the past six months and has almost completely stopped taking aspirin or acetaminophen. "I find that acupressure works better and faster than aspirin," he says. "It's cheaper than aspirin, too. Pressing on my head doesn't cost a thing.

Good Sources of Vitamin B12

Food	Portion	Amount (milligrams)
Beef liver	3 ounces	49.0
Tuna, canned	3 ounces	1.9
Lamb	3 ounces	1.7
Beef, lean	3 ounces	1.5
Haddock	3 ounces	0.95
Swiss cheese	2 ounces	0.95
Milk, whole	1 cup	0.87
Cottage cheese, low-fat	½ cup	0.80
Egg	1 large	0.66
Cheddar cheese	2 ounces	0.47
Chicken, light meat	3 ounces	0.29

The Recommended Dietary Allowance is 3 micrograms.

SOURCES: Adapted from
Pantothenic Acid, Vitamin B6 and Vitamin B12 in Foods, Home Economics Research Report No. 36, by Martha Louise Orr (Washington, D.C.: Agricultural Research Service, U.S. Department of Agriculture, 1969).
U.S. Department of Agriculture Handbooks No. 8-1 and 8-5.
Information obtained from Nutrient Data Research Group, U.S. Department of Agriculture, 1981.

Good Sources of Tryptophan

Food	Portion	Amount (milligrams)
Beef liver	3 ounces	334
Calf liver	3 ounces	323
Chicken, light meat	3 ounces	307
Chicken liver	3 ounces	292
Veal, round	3 ounces	289
Beef, round	3 ounces	258
Bluefish	3 ounces	229
Swiss cheese	2 ounces	228
Cheddar cheese	2 ounces	182
Milk, whole	1 cup	113
Peanut butter	2 tablespoons	106

SOURCES: Adapted from
Amino Acid Content of Foods, Home Economics Research Report No. 4, by M. L. Orr and B. K. Watt (Washington, D.C.: Agricultural Research Service, U.S. Department of Agriculture, 1968).
U.S. Department of Agriculture Handbooks No. 8-1, 8-5 and 456.
Information obtained from Nutrient Data Research Group, U.S. Department of Agriculture, 1981.

"But I don't want to sound like a commercial for acupressure. It's not perfect – you don't get full relief all of the time. And pressing on the Yuyao points hurts like the devil. My wife is unable to use these points because she finds the pain of pushing down on them too intense. But I find the pain bearable because I know that when I stop, my headache will usually be gone. If it isn't all gone, I'll press some more. That's another advantage acupressure has over drugs – you can do it as often as you like, and you can't overdose. Anyway, the next time my wife has a headache, I'm going to help her find another point she can press that won't hurt so much."

Using different points for the same problem is another advantage of the meridian therapies: they can be individualized. Some points will work better for you than for others. If you use acupressure for a particular problem, it is perfectly safe to experiment with several points to see which works best for you. According to Dr. Lawrence, relying on *standard* points to treat problems rather than finding the *best* points for an individual is "cookbook therapy," which is never as effective as exploring the meridians to see where the problem is.

"Cookbook acupuncture is popular because Americans are always in a hurry," says Dr. Lawrence. "And let's face it, we doctors are sometimes to blame. We'll be treating a patient, and we have others out in the waiting room, and we don't always feel we can take the time to find the best points when we know the standard points that usually solve a particular problem. But the best way to do this therapy is take your time and find the points that will have the most effect on the individual," he says.

"One way to find the right meridian point to use is by its soreness. The tenderness of a point is a good sign that you're in the right place."

Wonderful for Asthma

Dr. Lawrence continued, "Another good sign when using acupuncture – and I think acupuncture is the most effective of the meridian therapies – is a red histamine flare that is generated by the insertion of the needle. You might say, 'Isn't that histamine reaction bad for the body?' No. Because it causes the body to generate its own antihistamines, which can then fight against things like bronchial asthma. That's why acupuncture is a wonderful treatment for asthma.

"Just yesterday I had a mother come in with a ten-year-old who had asthma, and I could tell when I put the needle in and we got a strong red flare reaction that we were going to get good results. You can also feel a temperature rise on the skin around the point where you have the needle insert-ed, when you're in a good spot. Feeling this heat on the skin requires some sensitivity. I've developed the sensitivity of my fingers using my hands a lot in this work. This is one of the great lacks, by the way, in American medicine. Not in chiropractic or osteopathic but in medicine. It's that MDs don't learn to use their hands or their fingers to feel. It's a common medical shortcoming. It's important. They don't touch people enough. That's hopefully going to be chang-ing. People that manipulate, people that do acupuncture, learn to feel – and it's all in the feel.

"As a matter of fact, once you have enough practice, you can hold your hand above a person, over the acupunc-ture points, and you can feel the change in temperature."

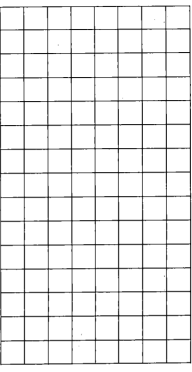

Try a Little Tenderness

When doing self-applied acupressure, tenderness of a merid-ian point is the easiest way to be sure you are in the right place once the approximate anatomical location has been found. A runner we talked to used this method to treat a shin splint in his left leg that caused him pain in the front of his calf. His story illustrates some of the right and wrong ways to use acupressure.

When doing self-applied acu-pressure, tenderness of a meridian point is the easiest way to be sure you are prob-ing in the right place once the approximate anatomical location has been found.

"I got my shin splint from running too much on con-crete and then twisting my leg coming off a curb. The pain was just below the knee, and I decided to treat it by press-ing the standard points for shin splints.

"The first point I used was stomach 36 (point 36 on the stomach meridian: see photo) on the outside of my leg. I also rubbed spleen 9 on the inside of the leg around the knee level. But these points only seemed to make the pain worse, so I stopped acupressure treatments for a while.

"But my shins kept hurting, even when I wasn't run-ning. I thought about going to the doctor to have an X-ray to see if I had a small stress fracture, but I just didn't want to be bothered. Also, I figured the only thing the doctor could do would be to tell me to stop running for six weeks.

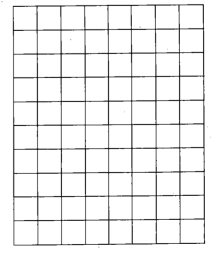

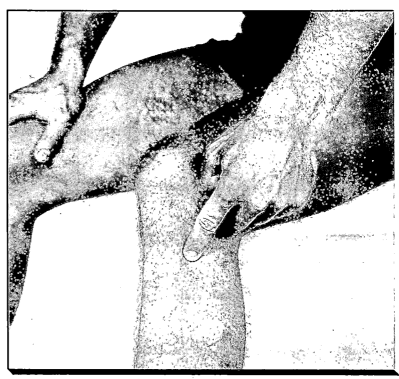

Rubbing stomach 36 can relieve leg pain.

So I decided to try to find other points that might help. I traced the spleen meridian up my left leg, and when I came to where I thought spleen 10 was I found a small knot of pain. I pressed this point on both legs and the pain went away. I still haven't started running again, because the pain in my shin keeps coming back. But when it does, I just rub spleen 10 again to relieve it.

"But one great thing happened that I never expected – in using spleen 10 for my leg, I also relieved lower back pain that has bothered me for a long time. Since I had been concentrating so much on my leg, I didn't realize the pain was gone until I got up off my soft couch one day and noticed that the stiffness I usually feel in my back when I first stand up had vanished. When I thought about it, it dawned on me that my back hadn't bothered me since I started pressing spleen 10."

Diagnose First, Press Second

Our runner made two mistakes. First, he treated what could have been a serious problem (a suspected stress fracture)

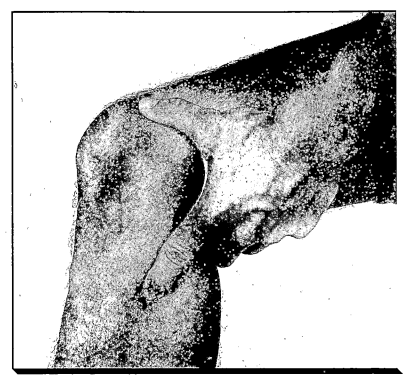

Spleen 9 is on the lower leg.

without seeking medical advice. Pain that persists even after the activity that caused it has been stopped should be taken seriously. If his injury had been a stress fracture and acupressure had relieved the pain enough to allow the resumption of running, a more serious injury could have resulted (such as multiple fractures).

"The meridian therapies should only be used when there is a sure diagnosis," says Todor Gencheff, M.D., a Wisconsin physician who teaches acupuncture to other doctors. "Otherwise, by relieving the pain you may mask the symptoms of a serious problem."

So, before you treat any problem, make sure that you know what you are treating. For instance, if you suddenly develop chronic, blinding headaches, see a doctor before trying to treat them yourself.

The second mistake our runner made was stopping the treatments when the shin pain became worse.

"Very often meridian therapy will make the problem seem worse before it begins to help," says Dr. Lawrence. "I caution patients that the pain may become more intense

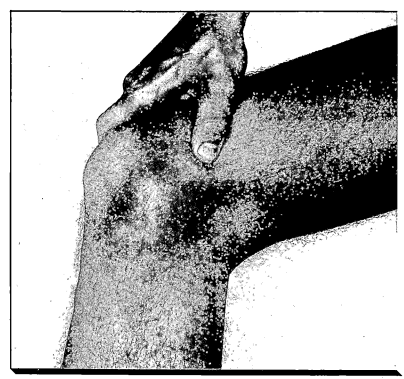

Spleen 10 is on the thigh.

during the first 24 hours after the first treatment. That's a *good* signal, and usually indicates the treatment is going to be beneficial."

Acupressure: Do It Yourself

For best results with acupressure, you'll have to get used to pressing hard with your fingers on your skin, sometimes as hard as you can. Needles are used in acupuncture because the points for treatment lie a little below the skin, sometimes as deep as an inch and a half. With acupressure, you're not substituting your fingers for needles; you're substituting pressure for direct stimulation, and that pressure travels down to the treatment points.

For most treatments, the thumb seems to work best.

Dr. Kurland recommends bending the thumb so that it forms a right angle; this position, he says, enables you to apply the most force. Our experience, however, shows that the position you should use depends on the part of the body you treat. If you press a point on the top of your thigh, for example, you can probably get sufficient force if you make a fist with your thumb straight out alongside it and press down using your arm and shoulder muscles. For this point – and many others – you need maximum leverage and force. But if you press a point on the back of the neck or on the back of the head, then follow Dr. Kurland's advice.

For Best Results, Relax

Now that we've told you how to press hard – don't. Not right away, at least. When you first start, you have to accustom yourself to finding and pressing the points. During this learning period you should be relaxed and comfortable, so don't jab yourself too hard in the beginning. There will be plenty of time for that later.

Lying and sitting down are the best positions for acupressure; they're more relaxing than standing. Unfortunately, it's not always possible to sit or lie down when you need pain relief. One man we interviewed who uses acupressure for his backaches often has pain while shopping in supermarkets; shopping involves standing for a long time and pushing a heavy cart. The man uses points around his knees for his pain. To massage them in the supermarket, he finds a relatively untraveled aisle, bends over and pretends to scratch his knees.

It's also a good idea not to eat before using acupressure. No one's sure why, but it may be that the process of digestion interferes with acupressure's antipain signals. At a minimum, wait an hour after you eat to use the technique. Another caution is from the Chinese: traditionally, they forbid the use of meridian therapies on pregnant women. They believe the manipulation of a pregnant woman's bodily energy by these techniques can harm the fetus. Modern research has neither proven nor disproven that belief, but, to be on the safe side, it is best *not* to use acupressure, acupuncture or electro-acupuncture on a pregnant woman.

As we said before, the technique you use to apply pressure can vary. Experience will show which technique works best for you. To apply pressure on a small, specific point, use the tip of your finger and your fingernail (see photo). Keep your fingernails short to avoid cutting your-

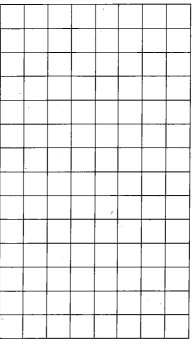

For best results with acupressure, you have to get used to pressing hard with your fingers on your skin. The treatment points lie below the skin, sometimes as deep as an inch and a half.

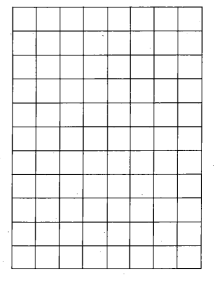

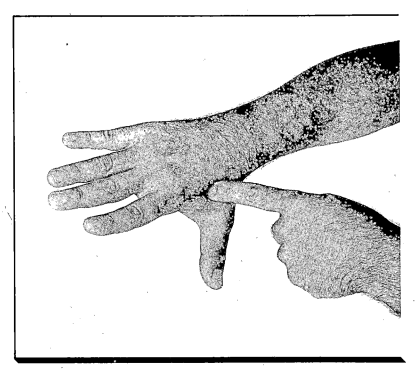

Pressing straight in on an acupoint.

self. For general stimulation over a wider portion of your body, use the meaty section of your fingertip away from the fingernail. If you're a beginner, the second method is preferable until you gain more accuracy in finding the points. Stimulating a wider area increases the possibility of hitting the right spot and not letting inaccuracy deprive you of results.

You can press a point in four main ways:

- Pushing straight down in a series of pulses, alternately pushing and releasing pressure;
- Moving your finger in shrinking concentric circles on the skin, starting the motion in an orbit around the point and gradually closing in on the point;
- Spiraling your finger outward from a point (the reverse of the previous motion); or
- Making a steady circular motion in and around the point.

As a beginner, use this last motion – in and around the point. When you use this motion, pressing the meat of your finger against your skin, you'll have the best chance of finding your acupressure points.

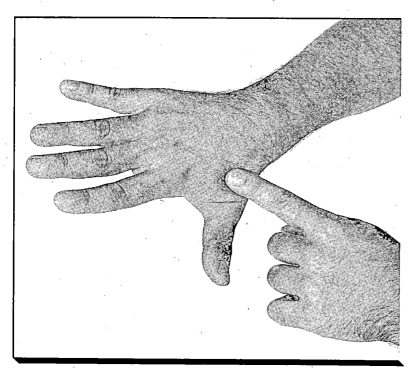

Rubbing a circle around the Hegu point.

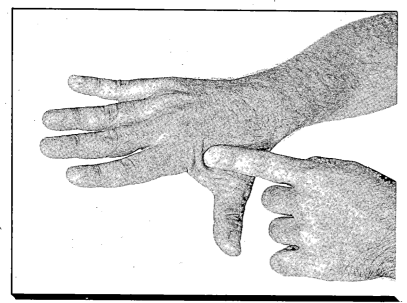

The circular motion stimulates the hidden point.

Heading Off Pain

In our experience, the most effective point to use for headache relief is the Yuyao point, the point we mentioned earlier that lies in the center of the eyebrows. (All meridian points come in pairs, in mirrored locations on both sides of the body.) If you run your finger along your eyebrow, you'll notice a dip in the surface that feels as though two bones are joining under the skin. This is the Yuyao point. It is where the supraorbital nerve comes closest to the surface of your head. This point, in the middle of your eyebrow, is right over the pupil.

Use the knuckles of your thumbs to press on the Yuyao point. In a seated position, place the knuckles against both points in the eyebrows and slowly turn them back and forth, increasing the pressure until you feel pain. If pressing with your knuckles doesn't produce a good deal of pain, then you probably are pressing in the wrong place. This point, so close to a nerve, should be very tender when you apply sufficient force. If you don't feel pain, chances are you're just pressing on the bone behind your eyebrows.

When treating the Yuyao point, press both sides simultaneously – that seems to produce the best results. According to Dr. Kurland, this point is good for relieving headaches caused by sinus problems. We have found that it can clear up other kinds of headaches as well.

Don't be afraid of the pain that arises while pressing on this point. It subsides when you stop. And so will most or all of your headache.

The Hegu Point—Key to the Upper Body

The Hegu point helps relieve any pain in the head and arms. Stiff necks as well as headaches succumb to pressure on it. Dentists use this point to induce analgesia during tooth extractions. In Chinese, Hegu means "meeting of the valleys" – it's an influential point, and stimulating it can affect many important areas of the body.

To locate the Hegu point, lay your left hand on a flat surface. Position the thumb so that it forms a right angle with the index finger. Now feel along the bone that extends back from the knuckle of the index finger. Along the index finger bone is the Hegu point. The point actually lies a little down and under the index finger bone. If you press down right alongside the bone, you have to press sideways, after you reach a sufficient depth, to reach the point under the bone. To make sure you touch the Hegu point and not just a random point on the hand, see if you get a "funny bone" type of feeling when you apply pressure. As you press harder you should feel the pressure radiating along the nerves in your hand. This sensation signals that you are on the Hegu point.

An early-morning stiff neck will usually respond to Hegu stimulation. To get the best results, treat the point before breakfast. In fact, stimulate it before you even get out of bed! Grasp the meaty web of your left hand (the part between the thumb and index finger). Rest the thumb of your right hand on the back of your left hand and the other four fingers on its palm. Probe with your thumb until you locate the Hegu point. Rub the point in slow circles for at least 30 seconds and then switch hands. You should notice an almost immediate improvement in the condition of your neck. If the pain comes back, repeat the procedure.

If you treat someone else's Hegu points, it is easy to treat both points at the same time. Your friend should be sitting and facing you, hands on his or her knees. You simply reach out, grasp both hands and treat the points (see photo).

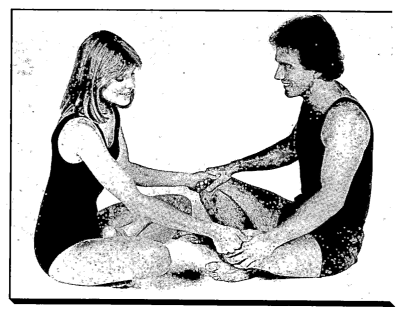

You can easily treat both Hegu points simultaneously.

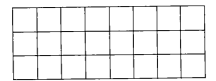

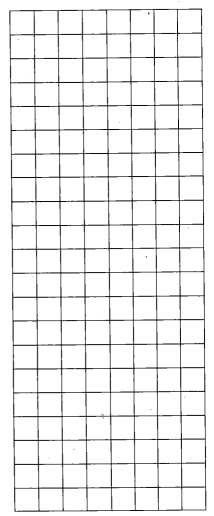

If you have an urgent dental problem, you can use your Hegu point for relief until you see the dentist. But don't substitute acupressure for dental help. Use it until you can see a dentist, not instead of seeing one.

If you have an urgent dental problem, you can use your Hegu point for relief until you see the dentist. But don't substitute acupressure for dental help! Just as it would be foolhardy and dangerous to take a painkiller like morphine for a broken leg and not have a doctor set it, so you should never use acupressure to put off treating a serious medical problem. Use it *until* you can see a doctor or dentist, but don't use it *instead* of seeing one.

You can also use the Hegu point to make pressing the Yuyao point less painful. In fact, since stimulating the Hegu point may relieve a headache entirely, you may not have to use Yuyao at all. But even if it doesn't, the Yuyao point will be less sensitive than if you treated your headache with it alone.

Let Your Headache Out the Back Door

Another good location for dealing with headaches and stiff necks is the two Fengchi points on the back of the head. To find the points, sit down, lean your head forward and look at the floor. Just behind either ear you should feel the mastoid bone. Then, using both hands, locate in the center of your neck a long muscle that connects the base of the neck to the skull. With your head bent forward, this central muscle feels like an upside-down ice cream cone with its point at the skull and its ice cream at the knob at the base of your neck. Next, move your hands along the base of the skull out from this central muscle, toward the mastoid bone; you should come across a depression on either side of your head midway between the central muscle and the mastoid bones (see photo). If you push hard into these depressions, up and into your skull, you are pressing on the Fengchi points.

When you treat headaches or stiff necks, use the Fengchi points either along with or instead of the Hegu or Yuyao points. Remember, it depends on what works for you. If the Fengchi points alone give you immediate relief, stick with them. Or you may find a certain sequence of points that works best. For example, you may have early-morning headaches. One possible remedy is to rub your Hegu points for a few minutes just after you awake. Then, after you sit up in bed, take the same amount of time pressing the Fengchi points. That might end your problem. Later on in the morning, if the headache comes back, treat it again.

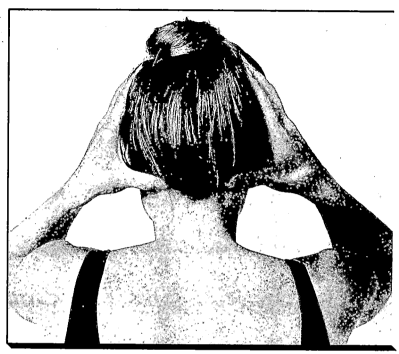

The thumbs are ideal for pressing the Fengchi points.

Leg Points to Ease Your Back Pain

Chronic lower back pain is one of the nemeses of modern medicine. Modern life has produced stress and strain that have outstripped the coping ability of this part of the anatomy. In our chapter on back troubles, we describe techniques to *prevent* an aching back; here we will fill you in on some acupressure points that will ease the pain.

A good point for backache relief is Xuehai. Located on top of the thigh, this point is also effective for relieving shin splint pain, a malady that attacks many runners. As we mentioned earlier in the chapter, a runner who treated his Xuehai point because of shin splints unexpectedly cleared up the pain in his lower back.

To locate this point on your left leg, sit down, then cross your legs by placing your left ankle on your right knee; your right foot should be flat on the floor. Now lean forward and place the palm of your right hand as flat as you can over your left knee. With your palm on your kneecap, put your thumb at a right angle to your hand and bend it so that the joint forms a right angle. Xuehai is underneath your thumb. To be sure you have located this point, apply

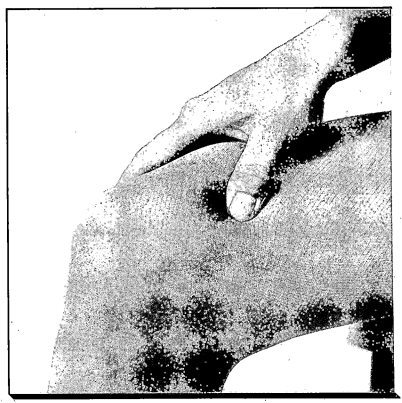

Xuehai is on the thigh.

thumb pressure around your thigh in the area we just described until you feel a sensation radiating out from the pressure. Some low back pain sufferers will also experience a certain amount of pain and tenderness at this point. That's a good sign! The tenderness means that the point is related to your problem and when treated may help alleviate a lot of your pain.

There's another way to find the Xuehai point. Sit with your feet flat on the floor and trace a line with your thumb from the inside border of your kneecap straight back along your thigh. Press down periodically with your thumb as it moves along your leg; when you feel a point that causes pain, or the "funny bone" feeling we described before, you've found the point that you want to treat. If your sensitive point doesn't seem to be in exactly the right place according to our directions, don't let that stop you from using it. The only important criterion for using a point

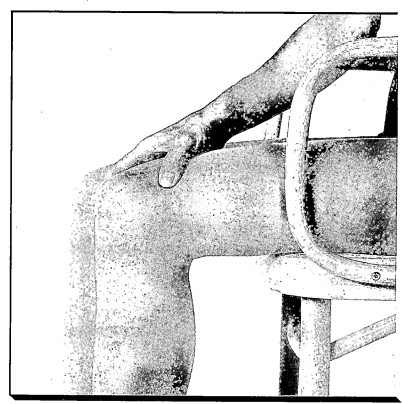

Pressing Liangqiu with the thumb.

in acupressure is that it works.

The Liangqiu point, another good backache treatment point, is also located on the thigh but is along the outside. To find it, sit with your feet flat on the floor. Next, extend one of your legs out straight and lay one of your thumbs alongside the top border of your kneecap. Then place your other thumb along that one, on the side not touching the knee. Next to this second thumb, on a line with the outside border of the kneecap, is the Liangqiu point (see photo).

A woman we talked to who uses the Liangqiu point for backaches always has her husband press the point for her.

"It's too ticklish for me to do it myself," she says. "Even when my husband presses the point, it's almost too much to take. I wouldn't let him do it if it didn't help my back so much." You, too, may find both the Liangqiu and the Xuehai points very ticklish. That kind of sensitivity is a good sign of a point's effectiveness.

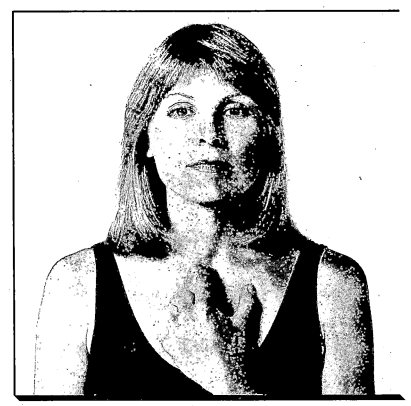

The Tiantu point can help asthma.

Acupressure against Asthma

The Tiantu point at the base of the throat is useful for combating colds, coughs and asthma. To locate it (unlike the other points, Tiantu is at one spot rather than two), run your finger along your neck toward your chest. As you reach the place where the throat meets the chest, you'll discover an indentation bordered by a round, bony structure called the suprasternal notch. To reach the Tiantu point, press your index finger into the depression above the suprasternal notch, and then put pressure downward toward the chest cavity (see photo). A word of caution: be careful if you massage a young child's Tiantu point. As you press the point on your own chest, you'll notice a slight choking sensation; many children find it frightening. If your child suffers from asthma, this point will help only if he doesn't mind the discomfort.

Push-Button Relief from Fatigue

According to traditional Chinese philosophy, acupressure points lie on meridians – channels of energy that flow through your body. As a result, it comes as no surprise – to traditionalists, at least – that massaging some of these points can pep you up as well as cure pain and aid healing. Traditional Chinese practitioners would explain this result by saying that acupressure dissolves blockages in the energy channels and lets the energy flow freely. In turn, this flow gives you an increased feeling of alertness and well-being.

The Yuyao point in the middle of the eyebrow is also good for clearing up mental fatigue. Another good point for pulling yourself out of drowsiness is Taichong, which is on the foot. Dr. Lawrence told us that he uses this point to overcome fatigue. "After a long day at the office, when I'm bushed but I want to go out at night or I have something else that I have to do, I'll needle my foot to give myself a boost. It's a great pickup."

Massaging Taichong with your fingers can give you almost

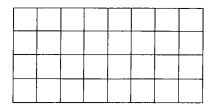

Acupressure points lie on meridians—channels of energy that flow through your body. Massaging these points can pep you up as well as cure pain and aid healing.

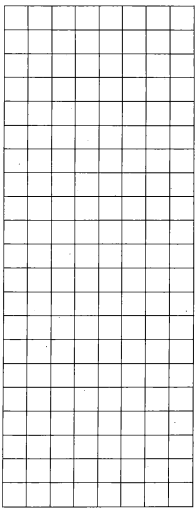

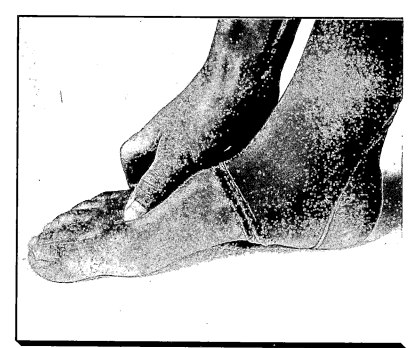

Taichong is located on the foot.

the same results that Dr. Lawrence gets. The point is located on the top of the foot behind the webbing that joins the big toe and the second toe. To find the point, run your finger back from this webbing, in a straight line between the toe bones (the first and second metatarsal bones). It will enter a groove between the bones. This groove lies just behind a firm mound of flesh that, in turn, lies just behind the toe webbing. Probe this groove with your finger until you find a point that is more sensitive than the surrounding area. That is the Taichong point.

Zusanli, a point just below the knee, is also good for getting your juices flowing. Massaging this point can also relieve abdominal pain and motion sickness.

Zusanli is approximately three inches below the knee-cap on the outside edge of the leg (see photo). The point lies between the two bones in the leg, the tibia and the fibula. These bones meet just below the kneecap, and Zusanli is just below that juncture. To find it, sit with your feet on

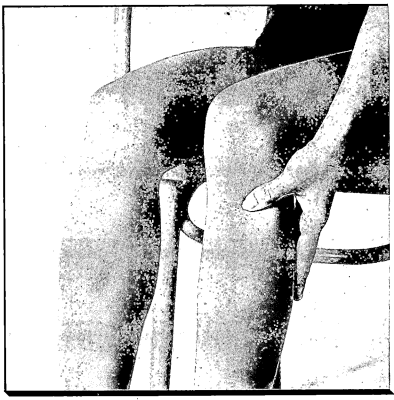

The Zusanli point is just under the knee.

the floor and wrap your left hand around your right knee-cap. Move your hand down your leg until your index finger lies just below the border of your kneecap. The Zusanli point lies just below the tip of your pinkie.

Some doctors recommend Zusanli for shin splints and other pains in the lower leg. If one of your legs is swollen or badly inflamed and you want to use Zusanli, massage it on the leg that doesn't hurt (of course, see a doctor, also, to find out what's wrong with your leg). That's a good general rule for all acupressure: if a point that you want to treat lies right on an injured spot, go to the point on the other side of your body.

The "Smelling Salts" Point

Yongquan means "jumping spring" – for a good reason. Located just behind the ball of the foot, this point helps revive someone who has fainted. It's usually very sensitive, but if you can stand pressing on it, it will also revive your energy and rescue you from fatigue. Just remember, go easy. Yongquan is the acupressure version of smelling salts.

To find this point, first sit down and examine the bottom of one of your feet. You'll notice that the top of the ball of your foot near the big toe has a mound of flesh. Put your finger at the border of this mound, in between the big toe and the second toe, and trace the semicircle that surrounds it. The Yongquan point is along this border at a spot one-third the distance toward the back of the foot. There should be a slight depression here and a *lot* of ten-derness when you push the tip of your finger into it. When you push on the Yongquan point in the right place and with enough pressure, you'll want to pull your foot away (just like a "jumping spring"). That's how sensitive Yongquan is – and how powerful acupressure is in pushing the buttons that turn on your body's healing energies.

Acupuncture: Pinpointing the Cure

As we told you earlier, acupressure is only *one* way to stimulate the points. And, although acupressure works, it's not the most effective method for chronic ailments. Acupuncture – direct stimulation of the points with needles – takes the laurels in that category. And a doctor who thinks it highly deserves them is Arthur Kaslow, M.D., who prac-

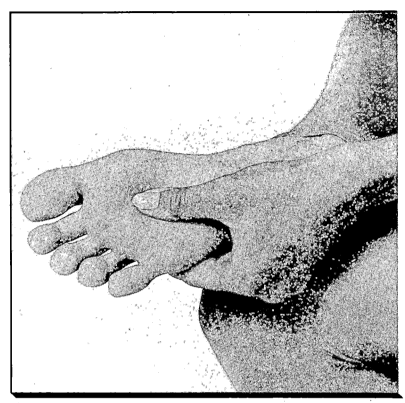

Yongquan is a sensitive point on the bottom of the foot.

tices in California's Santa Ynez Valley.

"For more than 30 years, I practiced conventional medicine, prescribing drugs and, when necessary, recommending surgery," Dr. Kaslow told us. "But about 8 years ago a patient of mine came in and insisted that I do acupuncture on him. He had seen a demonstration on television in which acupuncture needles were used during surgery instead of anesthetic. This man had agonizing pain as a result of a trucking accident that happened more than 25 years ago. I had seen him for 5 or 6 years and had given him medicine to keep him comfortable.

"I begged off. But he insisted. We pulled out an acupuncture chart from a magazine and he said, 'You've got the needles. Do it. If it doesn't work, it doesn't work! Let's see what happens.' So I tried it. He forced me into it, really. When you see a man in agony the way he was – he had severe pain running down his legs – the least you can do is try.

Impressed by Results

"Amazingly, the first treatment worked! He came back a few days later for another treatment and that worked, too. I was deeply impressed. I guess if I hadn't seen such immediate good results I would never have gone into acupuncture. I had never done anything like that before with such quick relief to the patient.

"I looked around to see where I could get some training. I went up to Canada, where Oriental doctors had been doing it for years, and studied with a Japanese doctor. I talked to a lot of his patients with a variety of problems, and they all said the same thing: they had real relief for the first time in years! So I became interested.

"While training in Canada, I learned about electro-acupuncture, came back and tried it on my one acupuncture patient. He was relieved of his agonizing pain after three or four treatments!

"Now this is a small town. Within days, people had found out about my success with this man's pain and were coming to see me in droves; the office was filled, and people sat outside on the patio and in their cars waiting to get in."

Not long after that, Dr. Kaslow started using what he calls "response point therapy."

"It's a modification of acupuncture. We use the principles of acupuncture to find points on the body that will give us a response. But instead of puncturing with a needle to stimulate the points, I developed a dull-tipped, specially designed probe which transmits a very low-intensity, safe amount of electrical current. There's no "shock," but rather a pleasant tingling feeling when the probe is used on the response point.

"And it gives immediate relief. I seldom have a patient who doesn't have some relief. I know of no therapies that are getting better results for pain relief than we are. And as an added benefit, we don't have to use toxic drugs. In the treatment of arthritis, for example, it exceeds any results I've ever been able to get with drugs or physiotherapy. Seventy to 80 percent of my patients have long-term pain relief without drugs.

"I don't know for sure how it works, but I have thought out a possible explanation. I think there is electrical energy continually flowing in the body. We can't measure it precisely, but we know it's there. We can take electrocardio-

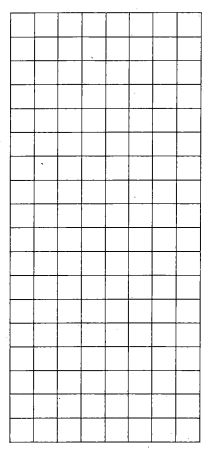

This treatment gives immediate relief. I know of no therapies that are getting better results for pain relief than we are. And we don't have to use toxic drugs.

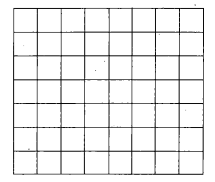

grams and electroencephalograms, which measure a certain kind of electric energy flow in the heart and brain, for instance. But when we zero in on certain points – response points – and apply an electric stimulus, we either speed up or slow down the energy flow. I think this tends to bring the body back into a state of balance – or, as the Chinese refer to it, a state of 'yin-yang.'

"We've been successful with rheumatoid arthritis, migraines, multiple sclerosis, foot drop, and bladder incontinence. Bladder incontinence is one of the most annoying and humiliating problems people can have. We can usually stop incontinence with two or three treatments. One of my multiple sclerosis patients called me to tell me that she was so grateful and wanted to thank me for giving her something she hadn't had in years – a night's sleep in a dry bed.

"Many of the people who come to us are desperate. They consider themselves 'medical rejects.' They've been to a dozen doctors, and they come to us with a bushel basket of drugs. Now, with response point therapy, we do things for many of them that we could never do before. After many years of practice, the satisfaction I get out of this is just unbelievable. We're not all that smart, either. The Chinese have been doing this for 5,000 years!"

Pain Clinics Discover Acupuncture

Since acupuncture is extremely effective in controlling pain, the therapy has become increasingly popular in hospital pain clinics around the country. Medical specialists have found acupuncture to be an effective long-range analgesic that can control chronic pain more safely than repeated doses of addictive drugs.

One such specialist is Philip H. Sechzer, M.D., an anesthesiologist at the Maimonides Medical Center in Brooklyn, who heads a team of pain control experts that includes neurosurgeons, internists, psychologists and oral surgeons. The main goal of this team is to prevent pain during surgery and to relieve it when it accompanies a chronic disease such as arthritis.

An example of the kind of case Dr. Sechzer deals with is that of a man who had been out of work for two years with painful arthritis. "He walked only with difficulty and with the help of a cane," Dr. Sechzer told us. "During the first four acupuncture treatments, the swelling in his feet went down to the point where he was able to get his left shoe on without difficulty."

During the fourth to sixth treatments, the pain in the man's feet subsided completely, but his left knee remained stiff, according to Dr. Sechzer. By the seventh treatment, there was no pain, just some discomfort in the left knee and in the right foot and hand.

Treatment continued, and by the time the man underwent his tenth to sixteenth treatments, he was well enough to return to work part-time.

Another case involved a 55-year-old housewife suffering from tic douloureux, an extremely painful condition that afflicts the muscles of the face and forehead.

Dr. Sechzer says that the woman had been suffering from the condition on the left side of her face for about 11 years. "She came to us and described her condition. We told her that we were extremely pessimistic about any possible results," he says.

But with each of the first six treatments, the facial contractions decreased little by little. The muscles of her face that had been contracted and contorted became more relaxed.

At the end of 9½ months of treatment, the problem was gone, and she had no pain. "And more importantly," says Dr. Sechzer, "her features are normal."

Complete Relief from Arthritis Pain

Dr. Sechzer and a colleague, Soon Jack Leung, M.D., compiled figures on patients who came to the Maimonides Medical Center for treatment. The figures included 223 patients who received a total of 1,271 acupuncture treatments for conditions ranging from arthritis to multiple sclerosis.

The largest group of patients consisted of 109 individuals who suffered from different types of arthritis, such as rheumatoid arthritis and osteoarthritis. Final figures showed that 81 patients classified as having arthritis of one kind or another experienced either complete or partial improvement of their conditions (4 patients experienced complete improvement, 77 exhibited only partial): Of the remaining 28 patients, 27 had no improvement, and 1 became worse.

The greatest improvement was achieved in the group suffering from orthopedic problems, including disc disease, sciatica and lower back pain. Of the 43 patients treated, 36 experienced significant improvement from acupuncture

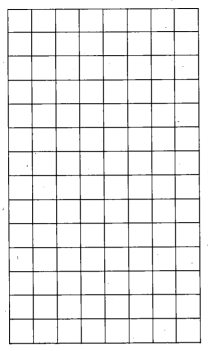

therapy: 6 patients improved completely, and 30 got partial relief. The condition of the remaining 7 was unchanged (*Bulletin of the New York Academy of Medicine,* September, 1975).

According to Dr. Sechzer, acupuncture works best in problems of a "mechanical" type. In this classification he included pain problems brought on by the swelling of arthritic joints or the pain of deep back disease.

Finding a Local Acupuncturist

Unfortunately, if you are looking for an acupuncturist, there's no directory to help you out. Elizabeth Frost, M.D., a doctor at Albert Einstein Hospital in New York City who has had experience reviving comatose patients with acupuncture, suggests contacting your local hospital's pain clinic (if it has one) and asking if it employs an acupuncturist or if it can recommend one. Cher Hsu, M.D., of Flushing, New York, an anesthesiologist affiliated with Flushing Hospital who uses acupuncture in his work with chronic pain patients, says that the best bet is referrals from others who have

Acupuncture has become popular in hospital pain clinics around the country. Medical specialists have found that acupuncture can control pain more safely than strong drugs.

used a local acupuncturist. The alternative, he says, is referral by your family doctor.

Some states, like California and New York, have licensing procedures for acupuncturists. These states test acupuncturists for basic proficiency in their technique. If your state has a similar certification procedure, it could help you find certified acupuncturists nearby.

What to Look For in an Acupuncturist

The first thing to find out about an acupuncturist is where and for how long he or she has studied acupuncture. If the acupuncturist's total amount of learning was a weekend seminar in the Bahamas, you should seek help elsewhere. The more extensive the educational background, the more the acupuncturist probably knows about the technique's benefits and dangers. The chief danger of the technique, when it's done by an inexperienced practitioner, is the puncturing of a lung. According to Dr. Lawrence, needling of the points in and around the chest carries the slight danger of hitting and deflating a lung. Any acupuncturist you consult should be aware of this danger.

You should also make sure that the acupuncturist either

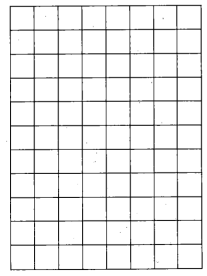

sterilizes his or her needles between treatments or uses sterile, disposable needles. The most commonly used needles are stainless steel, which, among acupuncturists, is considered a "neutral" metal. In other words, when the acupuncturist manipulates the "chi," or bodily energy, the stainless-steel content of the needle has no effect on where the energy goes. Occasionally another metal, such as gold, will be used in order to have a particular effect on the energy. Many excellent acupuncturists, however, use stainless steel exclusively. The sterilizing technique for the needles should conform to the same sterilizing standards as those for surgical instruments. They should be heated and pressurized (the same way you pressure-cook food) in an autoclave or similar device. Although infections from improperly sterilized needles are rare, just dipping needles into a chemical solution between treatments is insufficient to avoid contamination. You shouldn't use an acupuncturist who doesn't clean the needles properly.

Finally, the most important thing to know about an acupuncturist is his or her effectiveness. If you can, talk to former patients helped by the acupuncturist to learn how he or she deals with patients. As we mentioned before, a good acupuncturist should examine each patient carefully to determine which points will be the most effective for the individual. An acupuncturist who is in tune with the needs of the patient will disdain "cookbook" acupuncture – the practice of treating standard points for standard problems. Standard points are not necessarily the best points to treat. Each person has different trigger points that hold the key to better health. A good acupuncturist takes the time to test a patient's reactions and find these points.

There is no guarantee that acupuncture will cure or help everyone; no medicine or treatment can make that claim. But the acupuncture needle, in the hands of a skilled acupuncturist, can tap hidden sources of health energy that many of us never knew existed.

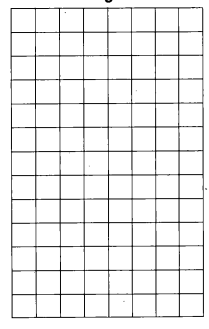

When you take the pulse from your wrist, place your index and second fingers near the arm's outer edge.

AEROBIC EXERCISE AND DANCE

Geez! Isn't that always the way it is? Just when you discover something that's good tasting or good for you or fun, someone turns it into a brand name or a commercial enterprise. Like granola or the London Bridge. Or aerobic dancing. Aerobic dancing used to be a way of doing serious exercise in a deceptively nonserious way – a way of combining walking, jogging and running with rhythmic dancelike movements and setting the whole gumbo to music, a way of working your heart and blood-pumping mechanism by doing fun stuff you might *want* to be doing anyway.

All that's still true, but aerobic dancing is now Aerobic Dancing, Inc., with an address and a chief executive officer. Writing to the address (18907 Nordhoff Street, Box 6600, Northridge, CA 91328) now gets you the name of a carefully trained local instructor who can guide you through some preplanned gyrations to produce limited-guarantee fitness. Of course, he or she will also take some of your money. Buying a book called – appropriately – *Aerobic Dancing* (Rawson, Wade, 1979) by Jacki Sorensen, the chief executive officer we talked about, will get you the same program between hard covers and a leg up (so to speak) on getting in shape at home. Naturally, the book costs money, too. The question we'd like to ask is this: is it necessary to have an incorporated fitness program? Well, maybe yes, and maybe no, but the answer involves a number of other questions. Some of them have to do with aerobic dancing, and some have to do with you. What is aerobic exercise? Is dancing good and safe exercise? Can dancing become an aerobic exercise? On your side of the issue: what kind of person are you – better yet, what kind of exerciser are you? Are you a self-starter? Can you discipline yourself to do something that is difficult and demanding (but fun) on a regular, three-times-a-week basis? Or do you need a taskmaster? Do you know enough dance steps to keep your legs (and heart) moving during several six-minute bursts of the Bee Gees or Chuck Mangione (or even Chubby Checker or the Dovells – remember "The Bristol Stomp")? Or do you need a choreographer? Let's take this inquiry one step at a time.

The Meaning of "Aerobic"

"Aerobic" is not a particularly new word, and it originally had nothing to do with exercise. It means "living or taking place only in the presence of oxygen" (which, of course, includes most of what we do every day), and in Biology 110 classes it is often paired with "anaerobic" to describe germs – aerobic bacteria require oxygen to be germy, and anaerobic ones do not.

Before you assume that we are comparing you all to microbes, let us hasten to say that we are using "aerobic" with one of the sideline meanings it has developed thanks to the work of an Air Force doctor, Kenneth H. Cooper, M.D. Dr. Cooper was entrusted with the health and fitness of the service's hotshot pilots several years ago, and he discovered that in order to please his superiors, he had to have results the day before he started. That meant knowing exactly what fitness *was* and which exercise activities would take his charges there most efficiently. Dr. Cooper once told *Runner's World* magazine (December, 1979) that fitness was the ability to do the things in life you wanted to do "with energy and enthusiasm in a safe and effective manner."

That belief led him to look at the people who are normally thought fit to see which of them do *all* the things they want to do, not just their particular athletic passion, "with energy and enthusiasm." He looked åt a healthy but inactive person, a muscle-blossomed weightlifter, and one guy who rode his bike three miles to work each day. When he got all these folks in the laboratory to measure their "energy and enthusiasm" scientifically, he found that the bike rider's *e* and *e* index was the highest. The rider had the best "endurance fitness," which Dr. Cooper defined as "the ability to do prolonged work without undue fatigue." This kind of fitness "has little to do with pure muscular strength or agility." But it has a lot "to do with the body's *overall* health, the health of the heart, the lungs, the entire cardiovascular [heart, lungs and circulatory] system and the other organs, *as well as* the muscles." Like we said: fitness is being able to do what you want to with "energy and enthusiasm," ease and grace.

Oxygen Is the Fuel of Exercise

All of this led Dr. Cooper to look still more closely at the

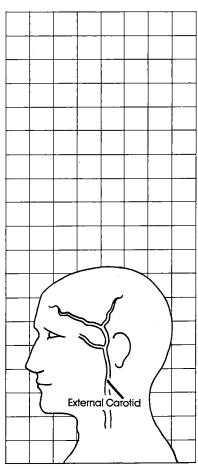

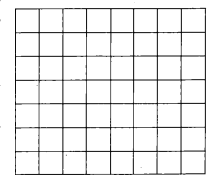

A good place to take your pulse is at the temple. The arteries along the side of the head have a strong, easily felt pulse.

bike pedaler. Why *exactly* was he more fit than the other guys? After some mad-scientist-like tinkering in the lab, he decided that the "key to endurance training is oxygen consumption." The body needs oxygen to produce the energy that fuels all activity. Since it can't store this fuel, it must constantly bring the stuff on board and deliver it to the muscle or organ that's performing. Therefore, the amount of oxygen "that the body can bring in and deliver – your maximum oxygen consumption – is the best measure of fitness." In other words: for most things, our ability to take in and process oxygen is sufficient. But because "most things" usually means watching TV or otherwise sitting these days, as some things become more demanding than these activities, our capacities fall *way* behind. The spread, or difference, between the minimum fuel requirement of a particular task and our maximum ability to supply it, then, is the best measure of our fitness, according to Dr. Cooper. "The most physically fit have the greatest spread" (or reserve); the least fit, the lowest spread. In some, the minimum and maximum are almost identical."

To get crudely scientific about it and to put the problem in still other words, the air we inhale contains 21 percent oxygen. During exhausting work, the percentage of this available oxygen that we exhale (or don't use) decreases and can be used as a rough sign of the exhaler's fitness. A flabby, unconditioned man may puff out air which is still 18 percent oxygen, and that means that he's using only 3 percent of what's around. The average guy who maybe plays racquetball a couple times a week rejects all but 4 percent of the oxygen he brings in, while the serious exerciser in good shape may be able to use 5 percent of the total.

A New Definition of Exercise

Okay. Now what? How does one improve his ability to deliver oxygen to his muscles and use it once it gets there? He does exercises that exercise the body's oxygen delivery system, pump up the lungs (which extract oxygen from the air we breathe and inject it into the blood), beef up the heart (which circulates the blood), and strengthen the blood vessels (which carry the oxygen-rich fuel to muscles that need it). You notice that Dr. Cooper does not suggest that you build big muscles, which may merely provide added body weight to cart around and generate more endurance-robbing lactic acid, the waste product of muscle activity. So what *do* you do? To find out, Dr. Cooper and his staff tested hundreds of activities, from calisthenics to Parcheesi, to determine which ones *best* exercised the lungs, heart and blood-circulation mechanisms. Along the way they (1) created an exercise rating system, (2) developed an accompanying exercise program, (3) came up with a new and very elaborate definition of fitness and exercise, and (4) wrote a book about the whole experience. That book, *Aerobics* (M. Evans, 1968), has now been glossed by *The New Aerobics* (M. Evans, 1970), *Aerobics for Women* (M. Evans, 1972) and *The Aerobics Way* (M. Evans, 1977), but the whole library still contains the same message. It has a view of exercise that says the proper program is "doing a certain amount of specific exercise four or five times a week – walking, jogging, running, swimming, cycling, any number of familiar activities – long enough to push your heart rate up to 130 to 150 beats a minute, depending on your age and the duration of the activity."

This produces what Dr. Cooper calls "the training effect," which is simply the boost to the heart, lungs and blood vessels that he defines as acceptable exercise. How long do you have to work out under the new regime?

> If the exercise is vigorous enough to produce a sustained heart rate of 150 beats per minute or more, the training-effect benefits begin about five minutes after the exercise starts and continue as long as the exercise is performed. If the exercise is not vigorous enough to produce or sustain a heart rate of 150 beats per minute, but is still demanding oxygen, the exercise must be continued considerably longer than five minutes, the total period of time depending on the oxygen consumed *(Aerobics,* M. Evans, 1968).

What kinds of things should you be doing? Anything you want to, actually, as long as the activity has gotten a high grade in Dr. Cooper's scientific tests.

Dr. Cooper's Point System

Most of the space in Dr. Cooper's books is taken up with explanations of his point and rating system. He measured the medical effects of most popular sports and recreations in the lab and gave each a point value according to its ability to produce the training effect. Twenty-eight received passing marks, and his tables, found in his books, will tell you how long a person of *your* age and *your* present con-

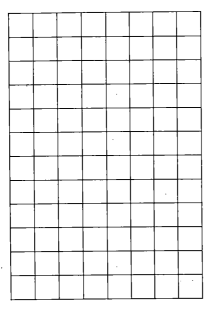

Aerobic training can change your whole outlook on life. You'll learn to relax, develop a better self-image and be able to better tolerate the stress of daily living. You'll sleep better and get more work done with less fatigue.

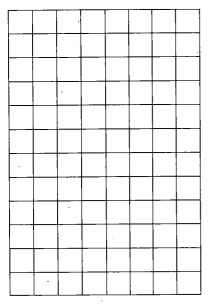

ditioning must do each of them to achieve this desired end. You'll need one of the books to get the whole story, but let it be said here that Dr. Cooper believes running, swimming, cycling, walking, running in place, handball, basketball and squash (in that order) are the best aerobic exercises. These activities give you the best return on your energy investment, a return which your body records as gains in strength in its oxygen-processing equipment and Dr. Cooper records as "points" – the more energy you invest in an activity, the more points Cooper's system awards your sport. For instance, you can earn 5 CooperPoints each for:

- Running one mile in less than 8 minutes;
- Swimming 600 yards in less than 15 minutes;
- Cycling five miles in less than 20 minutes;
- Running in place for 12½ minutes; or
- Playing handball for 35 minutes.

To get in and stay in good aerobic shape, Dr. Cooper says, you must earn at least 30 points (if you are a man) and 24 points (if you are a woman) on your invested energy principle each week. And you'll need to know these point values when, sweat dripping and spirits dropping, you ask yourself, "How much of this is enough?"

Just that answer might make listening to Dr. Cooper worthwhile, but there are other dividends to his investment program, dividends that offer considerable health security at any age. After getting into CooperShape, you'll – but let's let him speak for himself:

- The training effect increases the efficiency of the lungs, conditioning them to process more air with less effort. During exhausting work, a conditioned man may process nearly twice as much air per minute as a deconditioned man, providing his body with more oxygen for the energy-producing process.
- The training effect increases the efficiency of the heart in several ways. It grows stronger and pumps more blood with each stroke, reducing the number of strokes necessary. A conditioned man may have a resting heart rate 20 beats per minute slower than a deconditioned man, saving as many as 10,000 beats in one night's sleep. Even during maximum exertion, a conditioned heart can pump all the blood (and oxygen) the body needs at much lower rates than a deconditioned heart. In contrast, a deconditioned heart may pump dangerously

fast during maximum exertion in its attempt to deliver enough oxygen.

- The training effect increases the number and size of the blood vessels that carry the blood to the body tissue, saturating the tissue throughout the body with energy-producing oxygen.
- The training effect increases the total blood volume, again providing more means for delivering more oxygen to the body tissue.
- The training effect improves the tone of the muscles and blood vessels, changing them from weak and flabby tissue to strong and firm tissue, often reducing blood pressure in the process.
- The training effect changes fat weight to lean weight, often toughening up the body without actual weight loss.
- The training effect increases maximal oxygen consumption by increasing the efficiency of the means of supply and delivery. In the very act of doing so, it is improving the overall condition of the body, especially its most important parts, the lungs, the heart, the blood vessels and the body tissue, building a bulwark against many forms of illness and disease.
- The training effect may change your whole outlook on life. You'll learn to relax, develop a better self-image, be able to tolerate the stress of daily living better. And, what is very important, you'll sleep better and get more work done with less fatigue, including desk work.

Which should bend us back to aerobic dancing.

But Is Dancing Good Exercise?

Of course, you don't have to buy one of Dr. Cooper's books to get in life-extending shape, nor do you have to indulge in one of his certified healthful activities. All you have to do is find some sufficiently vigorous pastime and do it regularly – and nonstop enough. You might, in fact, try aerobic dancing. Most people who have tried it claim that it's more fun than most of the things Dr. Cooper recommends: it's less boring than running around a track or living room, less puckering than swimming, less expensive than bike riding and less Super Bowlish than handball or squash. But if Dr. Cooper doesn't mention it, how good can it be? Well, that depends. Dancing *is* rigorous. William G. Hamilton, M.D., orthopedist to the New York City Ballet and consultant orthopedist to several other dance companies, says dance "requires tremendous strength, endurance and timing, mobility of joints and great flexibility. Unless you have all these factors going for you, you simply cannot, for example, jump in the air, turn twice and land in fifth position, exactly facing the audience." And do it three times in two hours, we might add. Edward Villella, a principal dancer with the City Ballet now semiretired, says that "it takes more strength to get through a six-minute *pas de deux* than to get through four rounds of boxing," and *he* was the welterweight boxing champ of his college.

What's more, the Institute of Sports Medicine and Athletic Trauma at Lenox Hill Hospital in New York City, a medical-school think tank that measures athletic activity the way Dr. Cooper does, claims that ballet is second only to football in the seriousness of its physical demands; that is, it's more demanding than basketball, wrestling or even hockey. But, you say, we're not professional dancers. And, we reply, that's not the problem. The problem here is that when most people dance – in a disco, at a bar mitzvah or wedding reception – they don't do it long enough or continuously enough to achieve the training effect. They stop, start, sit down, have a piece of cake and so on. To be aerobic, dance has to keep you in motion constantly; it must gradually build up your heart rate to about 150 beats per minute, keep the heart rate there for a period of time determined by your age and current conditioning, and then slowly let it down to its normal pace. When dance does all of these things for you, it is very good exercise indeed.

Herb Weber, Ph.D., a member of the physical education department at East Stroudsburg State College in East Stroudsburg, Pennsylvania, has studied the demands of aerobic dancing on ten normally fit (or unfit) young women who were part of a carefully designed research study at the school. The women danced six routines of about 3½ minutes each and alternated them with five nearly 2-minute periods of walking or jogging. They did this three days a week, and the whole business took about a half hour each day. When Dr. Weber hooked the women up to his laboratory equipment, he discovered that the physical cost *and benefits* of this high-intensity dancing were equal to that of either a half-hour jog at 5½ miles per hour or a half hour of basketball, handball or swimming. So dancing *can be* a good aerobic exercise.

Where to Aerobic-Dance

Okay (again). You say you're convinced of the benefits of aerobic dancing but don't know how to get started. You could get professional help at a health club, Y or dance studio offering the service. You might get in touch with one of the corporate dispensers of aerobic dancing information and find one of their franchised teachers in your area. You could even buy a corporate program's book or record and work from it. Or you might do everything on your own. Which of these options you choose depends on who you are. If you put stuff off forever, or if you start a million things you don't finish, try corporate aerobic dancing. Here are some addresses to help you:

> Mary Mayta
> Aerobic Fitness, Inc.
> 1117 Oakwood Court
> Derby, KS 67037
>
> Nancy Kabriel
> Rhythmic Aerobics, Inc.
> 4740 S. Mingo Road
> Tulsa, OK 74145
>
> Judi Sheppard Missett
> Jazzercise, Inc.
> 2808 Roosevelt Street
> Carlsbad, CA 92008

If none of these groups nor Jacki Sorensen's Aerobic Dancing, Inc., has an outlet nearby, try the Y. If it doesn't offer dancing, get Ms. Sorensen's *Aerobic Dancing* or *Jazzercise* (Bantam, 1978) by Judi Sheppard Missett. Both of these books contain all you need to know to get going.

If, however, you finished your macrame project, your adventure in canning, or that dabble in cabinetmaking, you might consider designing your own aerobic dance program. To help, we visited a bunch of the professional ones and offer this description of the best as a guide and a recipe for yours. First, though, how do you know if it's *safe* to proceed? Dr. Ken Cooper's wife, Millie, in *Aerobics for Women* offers this ten-item checklist as a help:

1. My physician is satisfied with my weight.

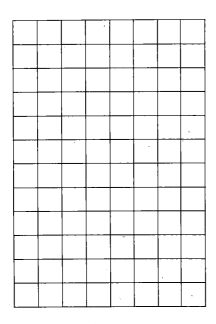

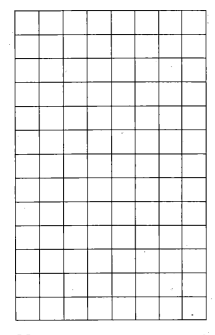

Aerobic dancing requires good foot support. Tennis shoes are better than running shoes, because they offer side-to-side support as well as front-to-back hold.

2. I have adequate control over my eating, smoking and drinking habits.
3. I can run a few blocks or climb a few flights of stairs without becoming short of breath.
4. My resting heart rate is usually in the efficient 55 to 70 beats per minute range. (As a test, sit and relax for five minutes, then check your pulse for a minute against a watch or clock with a second hand.)
5. My doctor says my blood pressure is normal.
6. My heredity gives me nothing to worry about in terms of heart or lung disease or diabetes.
7. My blood vessels seem to be healthy enough – for example, I don't have a problem with varicose veins.
8. I rarely have trouble with acid stomach, heartburn, indigestion and the like.
9. I'm seldom if ever constipated.
10. I have nice firm muscle tone – no flabs or sags.

If your answer to any of these questions is no, Mrs. Cooper suggests that you see a doctor before beginning. Aerobic Dancing, Inc., offers these precautions: if you're under 30, you can start at once if you've had a checkup within the past year and the doctor found nothing to frown about. For people between the ages of 30 and 39, the company recommends a checkup no more than three months before you start and says that the exam should include an EKG (electrocardiogram) look at your heart while you are resting. Between 40 and 59, Aerobic Dancing, Inc., wants the EKG – still in the last three months – done while you are exercising. This is called a "stress test," and it will help determine what heart rate you should aim for while dancing. For people over 59, the group requires a stress test immediately before embarking on the exercise.

Getting Supplied for Aerobic Dance

All clear? Let's go on. What do you need for aerobic dancing? A reasonable amount of space. The goal in aerobic dancing is simply to keep moving in time to peppy music, but it's a lot more fun if you don't have to stay put or dodge furniture while doing it. The living room is okay, we guess, but an empty basement is better, and the backyard (weather and neighbors permitting) is terrific. The more space you have, the less confining your choreography has to be. That's one reason why many people choose professional organizations for aerobic dance. They have gyms and studios to offer. You won't need special clothing for this activity, but you might want to consider these things in choosing what to wear. Your clothes should *not* be confining, and shorts and shirt or a sweat suit are perfect. If you want to be very authentic, you can go for a leotard and tights, but remember this: you might become chilled during a slow period in your routine. With them or with shorts, think about the knitted leg warmers real-life dancers use to combat cold. Don't go barefooted! (Unless you're going to be on a beach.) A lot of aerobic dancing is a second cousin to jogging, and you'll need good foot support. Ms. Sorensen, the executive officer of Aerobic Dancing, Inc., recommends tennis shoes over running shoes, because they offer side-to-side support as well as front-to-back hold. Ms. Sorensen also suggests – in another footnote – that you prance on the *front* half of your feet or even flat-footed; she warns that dancing high on the toes can strain the Achilles tendon, the one that stretches from the calf to the heel. One is tempted to prance on the toes because most teachers ask students to lift their knees a bit as they jog, dance or run to increase their effort and juice up its training effect.

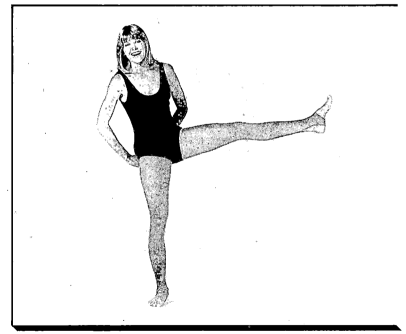

The right way—feet flat on the floor.

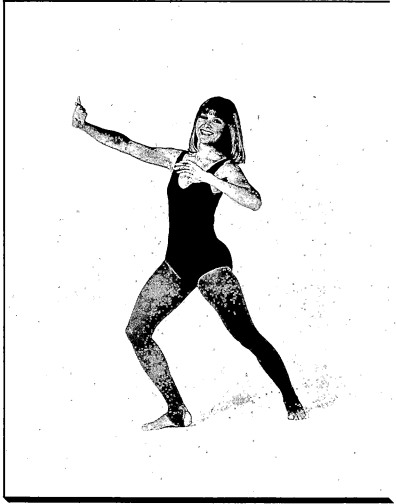

Weight can be on the ball of your foot.

Paying the Piper

You'll need music, obviously. Anything with a rapid disco or steady four-beat pace will do, and your own tastes can be your guide. If you can't keep up with your first choice, try something slower until you can. With dance music, of course, go dance steps, but we can't help you much there. We don't have the space to describe a whole routine, but most of the programs we saw combined the classic calisthenics everyone learned in junior high school with jogging and simple jazz and rock steps. The point is to keep moving,

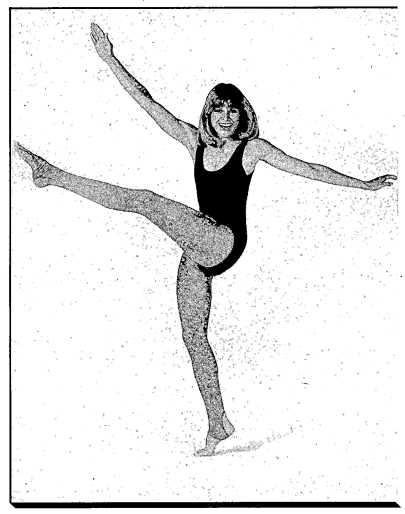

Don't dance on your toes.

and almost anything you do in time to the right music will get the job done. Some people we talked to took a few jazz dancing lessons to build up a fund of routines to do. One suggested that you buy a good dance instruction book for the same reason. She used *Jazz Dancing* (Vintage, 1978) by Robert Audy in her work. Professional aerobic dancers' books contain dance instructions and musical selections, and these firms will also gladly sell you records or tape cassettes with both music and narrated lessons. Here's the easiest solution we heard for the what-to-do dilemma: try the early 60s rock-and-roll records that teach a dance along with their lyrics. You know – "The Twist," "The Pony," "The Jerk," "The Frug," "The Mashed Potato," "The Stroll," "The Watusi." They're fast enough, and they combine music and steps in the same package. What you don't need in this regard is a special skill in dancing. The object in aerobic dance is health, *not* artistry. Ballet dancers are supposed to look good – and untaxed – as they float through the air, but you aren't. Your heart will never know that you looked dumb while helping it out.

The Heart of the Matter

One last piece of special knowledge before we get to how all this stuff fits together. Before you can aerobic-dance properly, you must know how to take your pulse, and you will have to determine where your pulse rate should be at various points in your routine. For, if the CooperGoal for all aerobic exercise is to have the pulse hover somewhere around 150 beats per minute, you must know when yours gets there, and, more important, you must know how close or how far away from 150 it should be, given your age and general health.

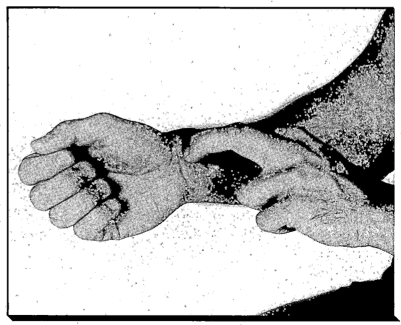

The pulse is commonly taken at the wrist.

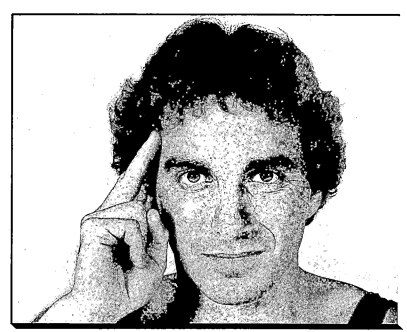

The correct method for taking the pulse at the temple.

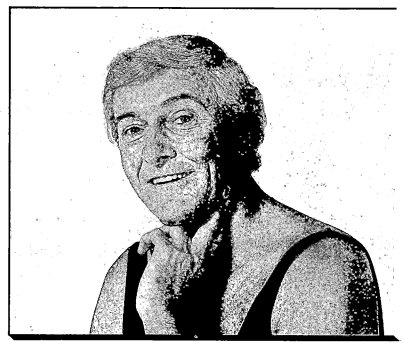

A strong pulse can be felt on the neck.

First things first: taking your pulse. Using your index and middle fingers, find your pulse's gentle throb (1) inside your wrist on the thumb side, (2) in the prominent vessel on the temple or (3) in the carotid artery on either side of the neck. The carotid artery is usually the easiest for beginners, but don't press hard, and do not put pressure on both sides of the neck at once. If you have trouble proving you're alive, try one of these shortcuts. On your wrist, find the central bone and move out until you feel the last band of connective tissue. Stop. Right there (or thereabouts) you should find a pulse with a light touch. On the temple, feel gently around the area just above the outside corner of your eye. And on the neck, touch gingerly alongside the windpipe until you feel a beat. Got it? All right. Count the beats for six seconds using a watch with a second hand to help you. Now multiply the total by ten – that is, add a

Working Heart Rate Range
Beats per Minute (BPM)

Resting Heart Rate*	30 and under	31-40	41-50	51-60
50-51	137-195	131-185	128-180	125-175
52-53	138-195	132-185	129-180	126-175
54-56	139-195	133-185	130-180	127-175
57-58	140-195	134-185	131-180	128-175
59-61	141-195	135-185	132-180	129-175
62-63	142-195	136-185	133-180	130-175
64-66	143-195	137-185	134-180	131-175
67-68	144-195	138-185	135-180	132-175
69-71	145-195	139-185	136-180	133-175
72-73	146-195	140-185	137-180	134-175
74-76	147-195	141-185	138-180	135-175
77-78	148-195	142-185	139-180	136-175
79-81	149-195	143-185	140-180	137-175
82-83	150-195	144-185	141-180	138-175
84-86	151-195	145-185	142-180	139-175
87-88	152-195	146-185	143-180	140-175
89-91	153-195	147-185	144-180	141-175

Do Not Exceed 140 BPM during First Two Weeks

*The ideal time to take your resting heart rate is before you get out of bed in the morning. Otherwise, make sure you sit quietly for at least 15 minutes.

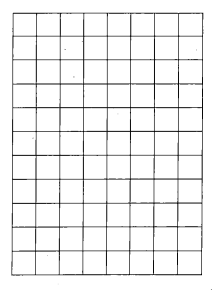

zero. Your answer will be a fairly accurate estimate of your pulse, and it's all you'll need for these purposes. In fact, this method is probably more accurate in inexperienced hands than trying to count a whole minute's worth of thumps.

If you were sitting still while you took your pulse just now (and had been inactive for a while before), what you've calculated is your *resting* pulse rate. Every aerobic dancing session should begin with such a pulse measurement. "Normal" for most women falls between 78 to 84 beats per minute. The average for men is 72 to 78. This resting rate will be used throughout the session as a comparison to the several *working* heart rate figures that are taken. They, of course, will be higher, because that's what's necessary for Dr. Cooper's training effect. But they shouldn't be too high. How high should they be? Well, most aerobic dancing books contain tables of working heart rates adjusted for all ages and stages of physical conditioning. We've included the one from the Aerobic Dancing, Inc., book.

To get a good idea of what your working heart rate should be, it is suggested that you take 220 – the maximum *safe* human heart rate – subtract your age and then subtract, say, 15 more. When using a book table and struggling under the burden of rotten conditioning, stick to the lower end of your pulse range at first. When doing your own estimates, keep your pulse under 150 to begin with – no matter what your calculations say.

To get a good idea of what your working heart rate should be, take 220–the maximum safe human heart rate–subtract your age and then subtract 15 more.

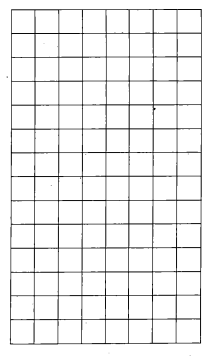

We Go Aerobic Dancing

Finally. You have everything you need but a routine, so it's time to go to class. The one we'd like to talk about was conducted by Sharon Holmes, an experienced dance teacher who has been certified to conduct aerobic dance sessions by several of the corporate dance companies. The class we attended was for beginners and met once a week for 90 minutes. This schedule – according to Dr. Cooper, most of the corporate teachers and even Ms. Holmes – is not the best idea. It is better to dance three times a week for 30 minutes a shot. That way, you have more energy throughout each session, can go harder and can stay in the training effect's grip longer. It's also true that the body is less stiff and sore after three short sessions spaced out over a week than after one long blitz.

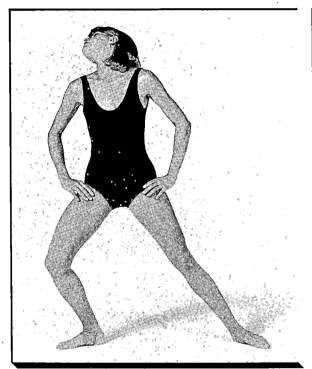

Rolling the head while dancing.

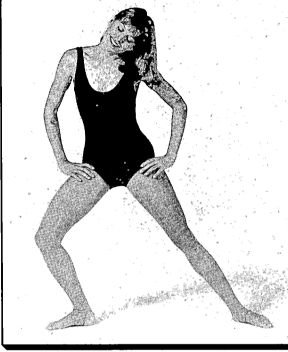

Keep muscles loose.

Ms. Holmes began her class by having us put mats down on the grade school gym floor where we met and by passing out 3 x 5 index cards to each of us. They would be used to record the many pulse readings we would take throughout the afternoon. Before we did anything else, she asked us to sit down, take a resting pulse and jot it down. It is important, she said, to have this point of reference later. A higher pulse now may mean a higher rate during the exercises and maybe trouble. Eating too soon before class, smoking or having something alcoholic all may mean an elevated resting rate and may lead to overtaxing. One embarrassed woman among us had munched a chocolate bar on the way in, and she constantly went over her target figure during the next hour and a half.

A Warm-up to the Warm-up
The class began at 3:30 P.M. At 3:40 we were into the first active phase, a group of stretches and flexes that were meant

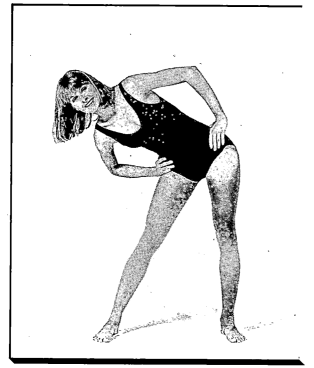

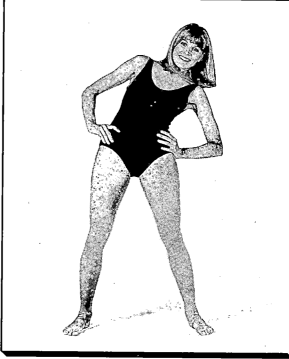

Rolling the trunk.

Bend from the waist.

to warm us up for the harder warm-up calisthenics to come. We rolled heads and necks, shoulders and trunks; touched our toes, stretched our arms (punching the air) – all sorts of mild things and all in time to a disco beat. The point was to take about ten minutes and move up and down the body, getting all of its parts awake and flowing. Since the body is an elaborate construction of bony levers and the muscles that move them, it's best to work on one set of muscles and levers at a time and then to move on to combinations of them – to let head rolls fade into shoulder rotations and on to torso twisters and so on.

After eight minutes of this, we took our pulses and were told to walk around the gym. Keep moving! Then we took our pulses again to see how well we had recovered from the activity, how quickly our pulses fell from their peaks. A recovery period that slowly gets shorter, say the experts, is a sign of improving condition, and a lowered resting pulse is a signal of being in shape.

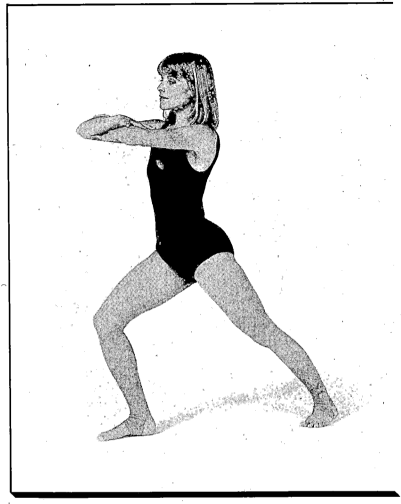

Stretching the feet and legs from a standing position.

The Warm-up

After that, we moved into the honest-to-goodness warm-up period, some old-fashioned calisthenics that grew harder and harder and more and more elaborate as their ten minutes wore on. On hands and knees, we did "hydrants"; we kicked our legs up and back; we rotated them; we bent them under us. Lying on our sides, we lifted one leg; we swirled it; we lifted both legs at once (groan). We pedaled

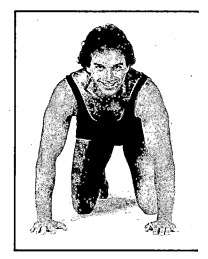
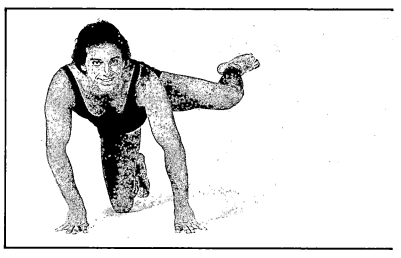
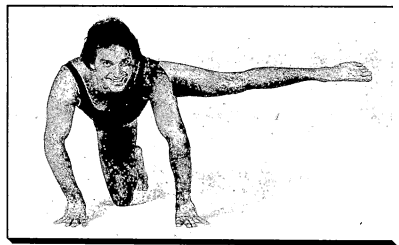

1. The fire hydrant exercise begins on all fours. 2. Lift one leg. 3. Extend the leg to the side.

bicycles on our backs. And every six to eight minutes we took our pulses again. This phase ended with some sit-ups done with legs bent at the knees (to prevent lower back strain) and went out in a blaze of effort, grunts and giggles. Everyone was pooped, and everyone was at his or her target heart rate. One nice touch, though, was Ms. Holmes's suggestion that we beat time to the music on the mat as we sat up. It was fun and made you forget about your stomach.

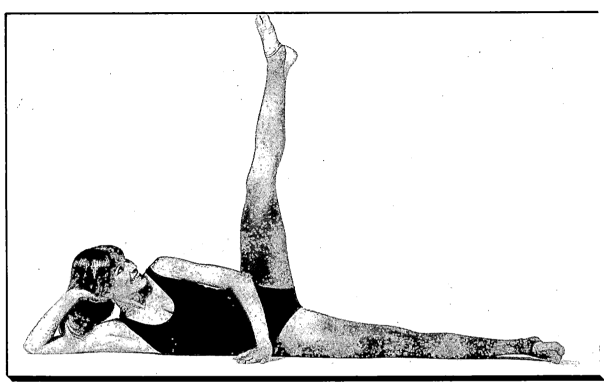

Side leg lift.

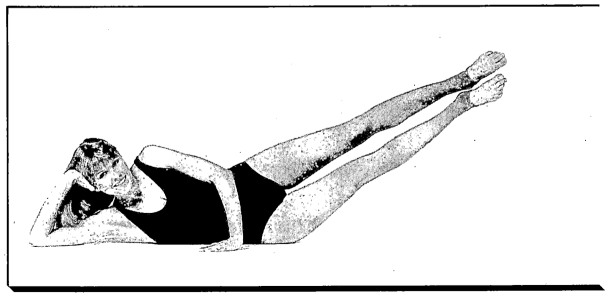

Side leg lift – raising both legs.

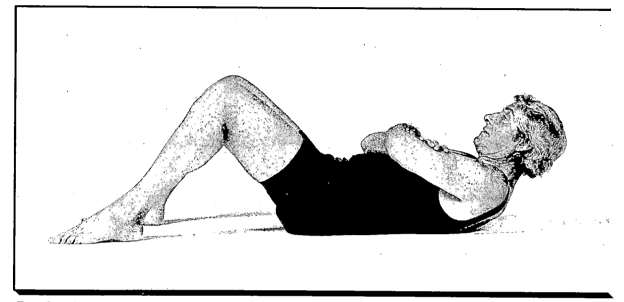

Bent-leg sit-up.

Some Jogging We Didn't Expect

After the sit-ups, we walked and jogged for 5 minutes around the gym to the blare of music from *Rocky.* More pulse counting. And then what passed for a "break." We were told we could get drinks from the water fountain, this after 45 minutes of class. In fact, Ms. Holmes made it clear that we could have water whenever we needed it. Contrary to old coachlore, when the body is losing water, there is no earthly reason not to replace it immediately.

Finally, the Dancing

Then back to work again, this time with 45 minutes of dancing. Each week Ms. Holmes teaches the class a routine or two of her own or of others' devising, and everyone goes through them all in turn. It's a good way of increasing the difficulty of the workouts as the conditioning of the class members improves. The better fit they become, the more routines they can get through – a maxim you should keep in mind when designing your own. We took off simply with "The Hustle" and then got down to business, which meant ending with a new Rockette number involving jump ropes and more skill than we visitors could manage. Still, it was evident that fitness, not disco expertise, was the object here, and there was no hooting at our clumsiness. Again, at regular intervals we took pulses, walked, recovered and pulsed again. And wrote it all down.

That's it, except for five minutes of cooling down at the end to a slow blues tune and another pulse. The cool-down routine was done in place and was filled with easy swoops and bends, a good suggestion for your routine. This has not been *all* that you need, of course, but with this outline and the books recommended, you should be able to get into aerobic dancing with comfort and style. And do try it. It's fun and terrific exercise. Our 3 x 5 pulse record said that we had had a stiff workout, but – wonder of wonders – we didn't feel it. We simply felt good and relaxed and satisfied with our afternoon.

BACK TROUBLES

I f it seems like just about everybody you talk to has a bad back, it's because just about everybody does. "Anyone who lives an average life span without suffering from backache belongs to a privileged minority," contends back expert Hamilton Hall, M.D., author of *The Back Doctor* (McGraw-Hill, 1980). Indeed, an estimated two-thirds of all adults suffer from back pain at some point during their lives. Like bunk beds, bad backs come in two layers, upper and lower. We'll talk about both here, but let's start with some general background information, then move on to lower back troubles, which seem to be more common, and finish up with – naturally – upper back problems. Along the way, of course, we'll have some remedies to suggest and some success stories to tell.

Some Background Material

Why are our backs so weak? Because we were a little hasty in getting up off all fours. About four million years ago, someone's brain said, "I think I could get more done if I didn't have to use my hands as feet." So that person stood up. And the rest of us followed. And our backs have been trying to catch up ever since.

Not that our backs are so archaic that we should be ashamed of them. The human spine is a wonderfully intricate structure (see illustrations). It's just that we are now asking it to function vertically when its basic design is still more suited for life on the horizontal. Indeed, virtually all common back problems are a result of downward pressure causing wear and tear on the bones of the spine (vertebrae) and the pads (discs) that separate them. Backache is a discouragingly "normal" development, Dr. Hall says.

So what do we do with these backs of ours that can lock up on us at the drop of a hat?

We learn to live with them, Dr. Hall says. We learn to sit, stand, bend, lift, sleep, brush our teeth, bowl, have sex, work and give piggyback rides with them. Because, in time, most back problems will cure themselves. Studies show, in fact, that backache is more of a middle-age than an old-age

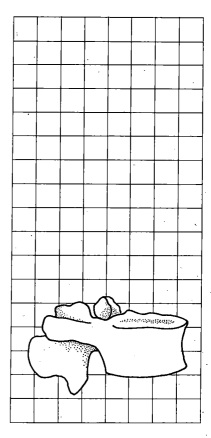

This is one of the lumbar vertebrae. Virtually all common back problems are from wear and tear on these bones of the spine and the pads (discs) between them.

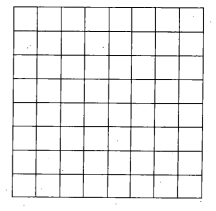

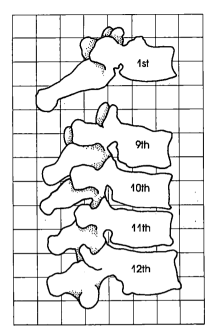

These are five of the thoracic vertebrae, the top part of your spine. As long as each part functions correctly, so does your back.

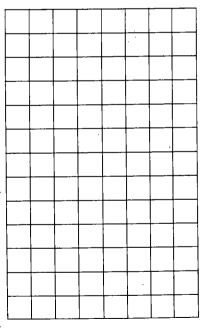

problem. By the time we turn 60 or so, our backs usually have made do with the imperfections that can cripple us in our thirties.

With that in mind, surgery, Dr. Hall says, should be avoided at all costs. "Fewer than 5 percent of all people with back pain are likely to benefit from surgery," he reports. "At least 19 out of 20, including serious cases, are better off with some combination of physiotherapy, medication, exercise and what we refer to as proper ADL–activities of daily living."

We'll explain those activities in a minute. But first we've got to determine what kind of back problem you have. Dr. Hall says all common backaches are due to either:

- A worn facet joint (which he calls Type One);
- A protruding disc (Type Two);
- A pinched nerve (Type Three); or, unfortunately,
- A combination of two of these, or even all three.

How can you tell which is you?

TYPE ONE back pain hurts most "when you arch your back, as you would when you lean back to look up at the ceiling," Dr. Hall says. The pain you feel is mainly at the top of your buttocks, and you find that bending slightly forward tends to relieve it. "Your trouble begins with a minor incident of routine exertion, such as picking up a garden hoe or retrieving a golf ball," according to Dr. Hall, and it usually subsides, if you rest it, within 4 to 14 days. If you're Type One, you probably experience such attacks two or three times a year.

TYPE TWO shares many of the symptoms of Type One, but it also has these distinguishing differences, Dr. Hall says: "A Type Two attack may begin with the same sort of incident as Type One, but the onset of pain is likely to be less sharp and immediate; more often it will build up slowly, over a couple of days, from mild discomfort to severe pain. The pain will recede noticeably in a week or two, but, unlike Type One pain, it won't disappear. Instead, it will linger on as a nagging backache or, in some cases, as an intense and constant pain." Unlike Type One, though, Type Two isn't aggravated more when you bend back; it's bending forward that intensifies the pain. "Like Type One, Type Two pain is felt mainly in the back, although it may radiate into the buttocks and legs," Dr. Hall explains, "just as Type One does."

TYPE THREE pain might be thought of as Type Two Plus, Dr. Hall says, because it involves a disc that has protruded to the point of pressing on a nerve. Hence, it has many of the symptoms of Type Two pain but also some of its own: pain can extend not just into the thighs but also lower, sometimes even to the feet and toes. Type Three pain usually comes on over a day or two, builds, and then stays for weeks. It is made distinctly worse by bending forward, and it is potentially the most serious of the three types because prolonged pressure can damage nerve function. It is also the least common, however, and it is responsible for only about 10 percent of all back woes.

What causes these three types of back pain?

In the case of Type One pain, it's usually a disc that has flattened to the point of allowing the bones of a facet joint to rub against one another. Discs can flatten because of a gradual drying-out process (a natural consequence of aging), and that process can be hastened by a life of hard physical labor and heavy lifting. It can also be aggravated by bad posture, pregnancy or a potbelly, because anything that causes you to arch your back causes facet joints (located at the rear of the spine) to press together.

Type Two back pain is the result of a disc doing more bulging than collapsing, because discs are not "dead" tissue. They contain nerve fibers, and they hurt when they get pushed out of shape.

Type Three back pain is the result of a disc bulging to the point of pressing on a spinal nerve – one of the few cases in which surgery may be required for repair.

Maybe now you can see why bed rest is so often recommended as the first order of business following a back attack. By lying down, you relieve pressure on discs, which in turn relieves pressure on spinal nerves, which should, in turn, erase the reason for the muscles of your back going into painful – but protective – spasm. Muscle spasms are your body's way of encouraging the very immobilization you need in order to heal. And not until those spasms relax is it time to think about doing some corrective exercises – exercises, as strange as it may sound, that concentrate not on the back but rather the stomach.

Why the stomach?

Because strong stomach muscles can provide a weak back with the additional support it needs. When stomach muscles are weak, greater pressure gets passed on to the discs, which are so important to spare.

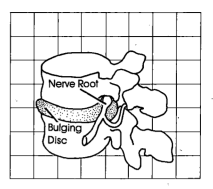

A backache caused by a bulging disc builds up slowly, over a couple of days, from mild discomfort to severe pain.

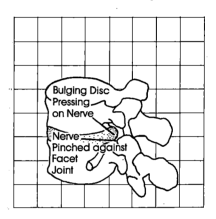

When a bulging disc presses on a spinal nerve, excruciating pain can result.

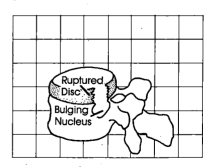

A ruptured disc is a serious injury and may require surgery to correct.

Abdominal exercises, however, are not the entire answer to getting along with a bad back. As we mentioned earlier, there are those all-important activities of daily living – ADLs, as Dr. Hall calls them. The idea is to make life as easy on your back as possible in as many situations as possible.

How to Sleep If you sleep on your back, roll a couple of pillows into a bolster to raise up your knees. Or, if you prefer sleeping on your stomach, "try sleeping with a pillow under the front of your pelvis to reduce the sag in your low back," Dr. Hall says. Side-sleepers should curl into a ball and place a pillow between their knees. The purpose of all these positions is to reduce pressure on spinal discs.

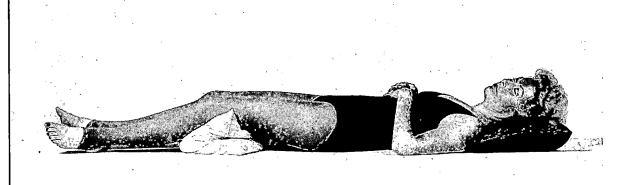

When sleeping on your back, a pillow under your knees takes strain off your lower back.

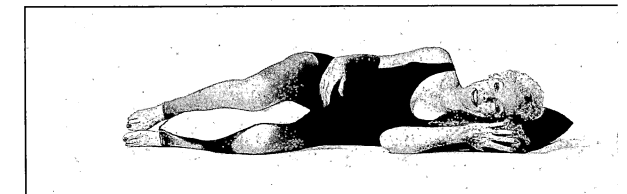

A comfortable way to sleep on your side is with a pillow between your knees.

How to Sit The first rule of thumb is not to sit for very long. Sitting can create a greater load on spinal discs than standing. You can reduce that load by making sure to support yourself with your elbows if you must lean forward to work at your desk. In other, more recreational sitting situations, try to keep your feet raised – on either a step stool or a stack of books – and place a small pillow between the back of your chair and the area just above your buttocks.

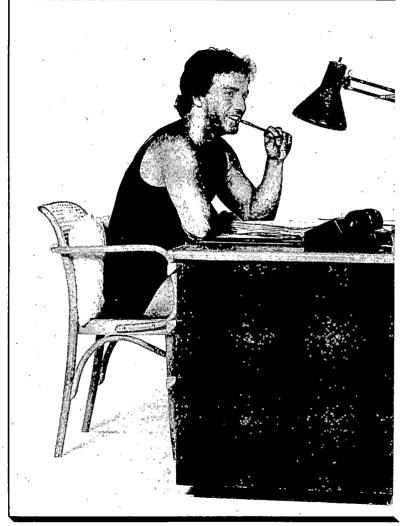

A well-placed pillow can ease back strain.

How to Stand "Never stand flat-footed if you can put one foot up on a stool or a low shelf – the posture drinkers assume at a stand-up bar. Saloonkeepers discovered the comfort of this position long before doctors developed the theory behind it," Dr. Hall says.

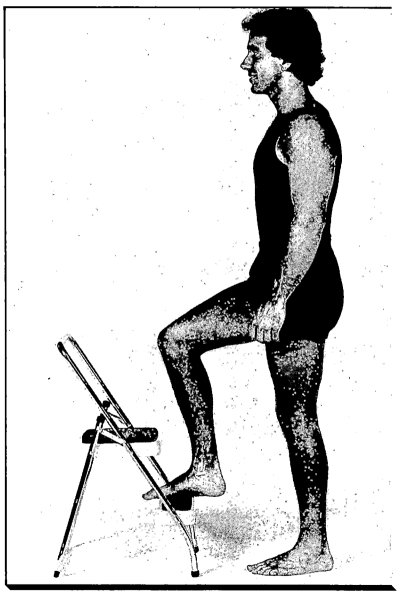

Putting one foot up takes stress off the back.

How to Lift Lift with the back as straight as possible. Squat, in other words, but don't bend over. The more work you can pass on to the legs, the better. "The most hazardous lifts are the ones for which you are unprepared," Dr. Hall says. And the most difficult, even when you are prepared, are the ones where you must hoist something over a barrier at arm's length – for example, a 40-pound nephew out of a high-sided crib. Make it a habit to think before you attempt a lift. If even the thought of it hurts, chances are that it will.

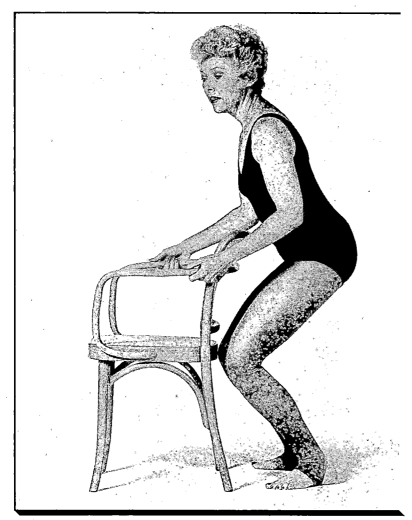

The correct way to lift an object – knees bent, back straight.

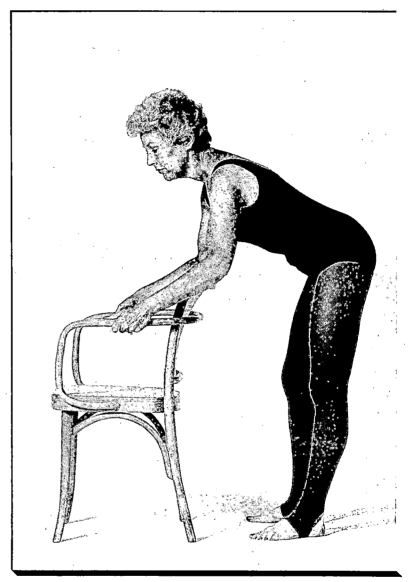

Never lift something without bending your knees!

How to Have Sex There are a number of painfree ways: face-to-face, with both partners on their sides; or face-to-back, in what is sometimes called the "spoon" position, with the female nestled against the male's lap. There are, of course, many other possible positions, and the key to avoiding strain "is to make sure you do not arch your back or your neck" in all of them, says Dr. Hall.

How to Keep Fit All sports involve some wear and tear on the spine. But that's no reason to sit on the sidelines, Dr. Hall says. "Apart from the trauma of an accident – which, after all, can happen anywhere to anybody – even the most vigorous sports activities won't harm your back; they may simply make it hurt for a few days." But "hurt is not the same as harm," Dr. Hall assures us, "and the trade-off may be worth it to you, in immediate pleasure and in feeling like a normal person instead of a semi-invalid."

Three forms of strain may be imposed upon your spine by your fitness efforts, according to Dr. Hall: "weight-loading, rotation and arching." Weight-loading, which happens during weightlifting and jogging, tends to compress discs and causes facet joints to settle even more tightly together. Rotation, a common maneuver in squash, racquetball, tennis and golf, can strain discs by tugging at the fibers of their outer shells. And arching, a common occurrence during hockey, basketball, baseball, rowing, canoeing, skiing, archery and certain forms of swimming, especially the breaststroke, tends – like weight-loading sports – to create friction between facet joints.

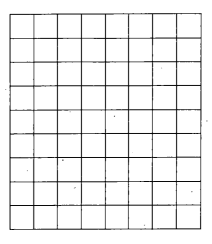

You shouldn't bend forward to pick up anything unless there's something there to support your weight.

Whatever you do for exercise, though, don't feel bad for learning to "cheat" in ways that minimize your discomfort. Hurt may not be harm. But it's not much fun, either.

Most of the things we've just ticked off might be considered first aid for backs, and their use – their successful use – implies that a back problem isn't too serious or too far along. Some of these first aids, however, deserve a second and closer look. Lots of bum backs come from poor lifting habits, and some attention to better practices in this common area could prevent some uncommon pain later on.

Some Uplifting Advice

One place to learn how to lift things without lowering your spirits is a book by a physics professor at Tufts University in Massachusetts. Physics is, among other things, the study of the movement of bodies in space, and so there is no better person to tell you how to lift the miscellaneous weights of your life than a physics teacher. Jack R. Tessman, Ph.D., in his practical and very likable volume *My Back Doesn't Hurt Anymore* (Quick Fox, 1980), strips the he-man show-off and the "Don't worry; I can do it myself" from most lifting jobs and treats them like the mechanical problems he teaches his students. What's the best, most efficient way to get this job done, he asks in each case.

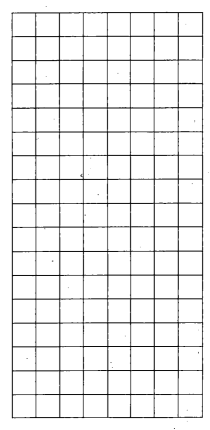

In brief, Dr. Tessman's advice is that you shouldn't bend forward to pick up anything unless there's something there to support your weight.

The physics behind this advice is simple and straightforward. Imagine that you and a friend want to ride on a seesaw at the neighborhood playground. Your friend weighs 100 pounds and sits down five feet away from the pivot point at the center of the plank. You sit down on the other side of the plank but only a foot away from the pivot point. To balance your friend, you would have to weigh 500 pounds.

Now imagine your body as a seesaw. Your arms, reaching down and forward, are like your friend's half of the plank. Your hips are like the pivot point. Now your lower back muscles strain to lift that load. But since they are close to your hips, they have no leverage. It has been estimated that, in an activity such as shoveling, the back muscles must pull with a force 15 times the weight of the object lifted.

The solution to this problem is simply to lift and carry things beside or behind you, making the load work with your back muscles instead of against them.

Specific examples, illustrated and explained, are the best part of *My Back Doesn't Hurt Anymore*. In the past, you may have received vague advice about not lifting heavy objects. But Dr. Tessman shows how to prevent back pain while dealing with the inevitable burdens that present themselves every day.

A Day's Worth of Lifting

Imagine, for a moment, a normal day:

The alarm clock is ringing; it's 6 A.M. Getting out of bed is your back's first test of the day. Push yourself up and forward with your hands, and swing your feet around.

Next stop is the bathroom. When shaving or washing your face, take a load off your back by flexing at the knees or supporting your weight with a free hand. Then, while you're dressing, bring your foot up instead of bending forward to slip on socks or stockings.

Outside, on the welcome mat, lies the morning newspaper. Instead of bending over, flex at the knees and keep your back as straight as possible.

At breakfast, even little exertions such as reaching into the refrigerator for a gallon jug of milk or reaching across

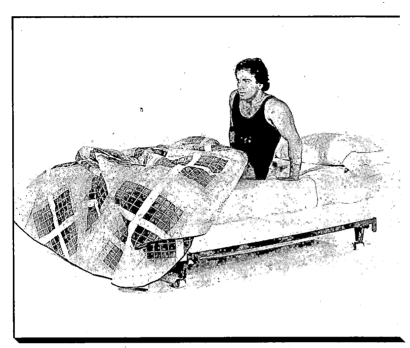

To get out of bed, first sit up.

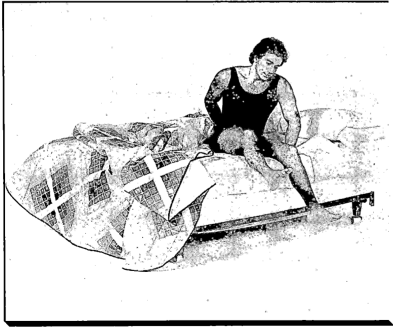

Then swing your legs over the side of the bed.

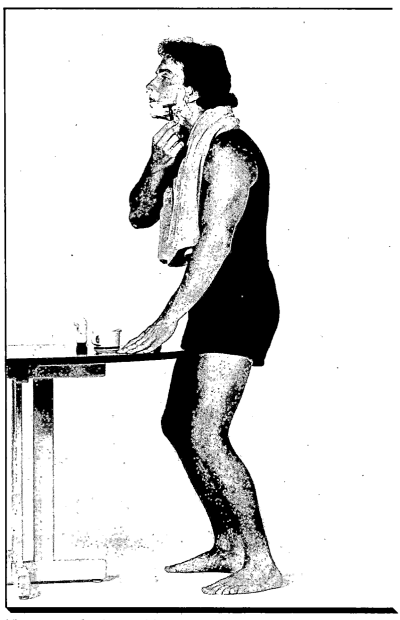

The correct shaving position.

the table for a platter of eggs could aggravate an existing back problem. Later, before you go out for the day, you might want to give your child or grandchild a bear hug. Avoid reaching over a crib railing or a safety gate to pick

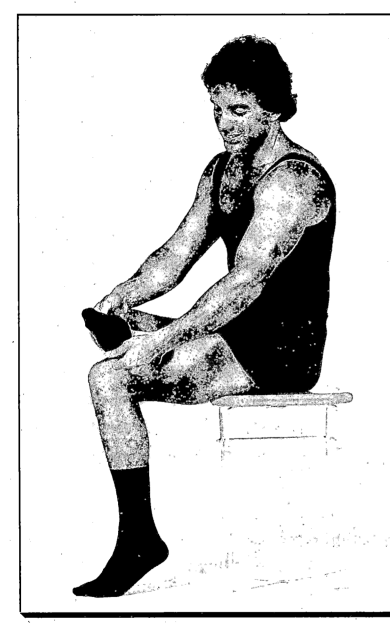

When putting on socks, bring your foot up. Don't bend over.

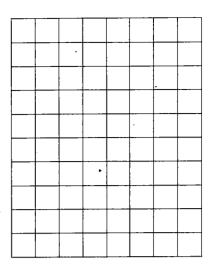

Someone with strong back muscles is more likely to pick up a load that's too heavy for the discs.

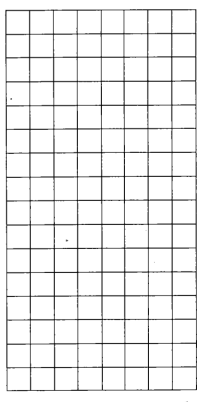

him up. Instead, lower the railing or open the gate, and flex your knees rather than bending over.

Assuming that you have been to work and are now ready to come home (there's no room here to cover the

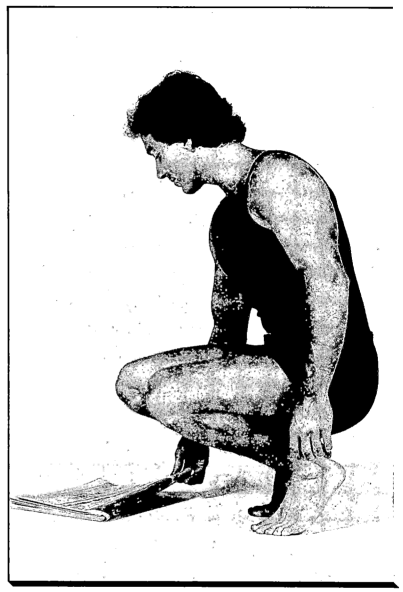

The right way to pick up a newspaper.

multitude of hazards on the job), you might stop to buy groceries. Supermarkets can pose a real dilemma for someone with a bad back. Heavy-duty paper bags are loaded too heavily, and deep-well shopping carts create awkward lifting situations.

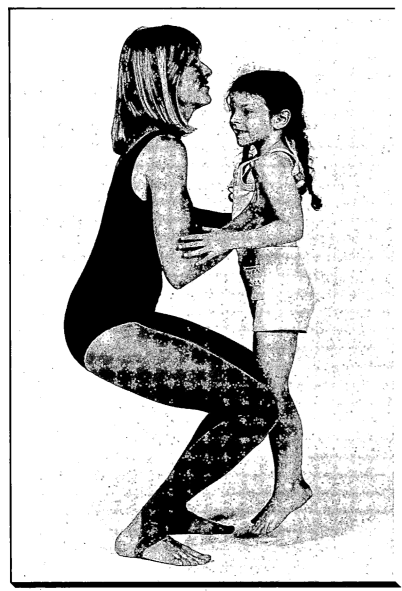

The proper way to lift a child.

Instead of one big sack, try carrying two smaller ones, one under each arm. If you can, use the new carts with waist-level bottoms. When loading bags into the car, don't put them on the floor. Put them on a seat, or on the rear deck if you have a station wagon.

In spring and summer, you may want to knock around the garden after work. If you're spading compost or soil, keep the payload end of the spade at your side or behind you. Dr. Tessman even suggests digging behind yourself, as if you were paddling a canoe. If you're putting in seeds, kneel rather than lean over and, if you kneel, use your forearm to prop up your weight.

Changing tires is another chore that can be a disaster for your back. To avoid the crunch, squat or sit on a stool when you pull off the tire and wheel. When loosening the lug nuts, always push down with the wrench.

Back inside the house, it might be time to open a window that's hard to budge.

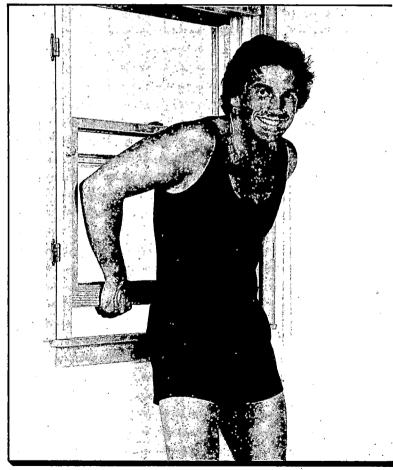

Opening a window behind you won't hurt your back.

If you face the window and pull up on the handles or grips, your back will think you're trying to lift the house. Instinct may tell you to do it that way, but it's far better to put your back to the window and raise it behind you.

The same principle applies to carrying a trunk, a sofa or an air conditioner. Hold the end that you're carrying behind you.

The day is almost done. You might want to give your child or grandchild a ride on your shoulders before he or she gets swaddled up and sent to bed. If you let the child use a sofa or chair to climb on your shoulders, you won't hurt your back. (For women who want to take infants with them during the day, what's best for their backs is to carry

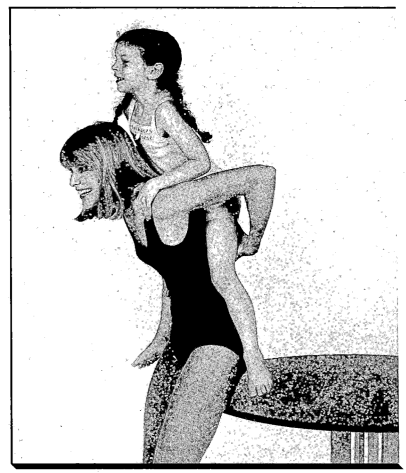

For piggyback rides, let the child first stand on a table or chair.

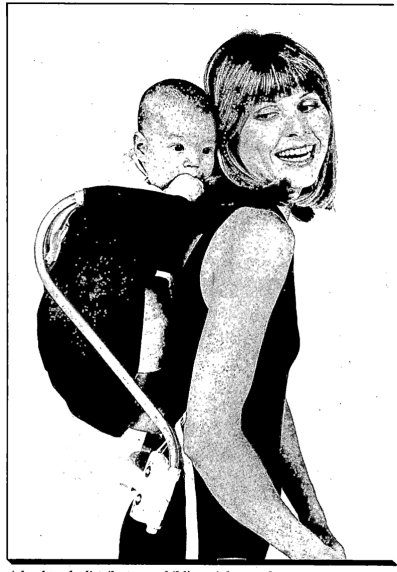

A backpack distributes a child's weight evenly.

the child on the back, in a knapsacklike affair.)

Your last chore of the evening involves that hallowed ritual: taking out the trash. If you try to carry a loaded trash can in front of you, by the handles, your back may never forgive you. Get your teenage son to take it down to the curb, or drag the can behind you, or best of all, put the can on a cart with wheels.

Myths Worth Puncturing

As well as giving advice, Dr. Tessman also punctures a few myths about the back. Strong arm and back muscles, he says, can't protect your discs. On the contrary, someone with strong back muscles is more likely to pick up a load that's too heavy for the discs.

Certain traditional exercises are also taboo. Dr. Tessman says that bending over to touch your toes and doing sit-ups place unnecessary strain on the discs. He prefers deep knee bends for strengthening the thigh muscles and deep breathing exercises for developing the abdominal muscles.

Doing the Pelvic Tilt

Another way to avoid back problems is by practicing the "pelvic tilt," a technique invented by Robert Lowe, M.D., an orthopedic surgeon and founder of the Low Back School at Cabell Hutington Hospital in West Virginia. Dr. Lowe explains that most of the forward and back bending of the spine takes place in the joint between the fifth (last) lumbar vertebra and the sacrum, which is the heavy bone forming the back of the pelvis. (It is really five vertebrae fused into one.) The sacrum is rather rigid compared to the fifth lumbar vertebra, and bending, lifting and even prolonged sitting put stress on the muscles, ligaments and disc which make up that joint. Ideally, strong stomach and buttock muscles will keep this part of the spine correctly aligned, but over time poor posture, sedentary habits and overweight can combine to accentuate the natural lumbar curve, producing a swayback, potbelly appearance. The stress from such a weakened condition falls most heavily on the joint between the fifth lumbar vertebra and the sacrum, and the pelvic tilt is an exercise designed to help reverse the curve temporarily, easing pressure on the discs and strengthening the supporting muscles. It is incredibly effective, considering its simplicity.

While lying on your back, bend your knees and place your feet flat on the floor near your buttocks. Raise your pelvis and "tuck" it under, concentrating on pushing your lower back gently to the floor. Your shoulders, legs, neck and upper back should be relaxed. As you gently push your lower back to the floor, three things begin to happen: your pelvis rotates forward (reversing the curve of your lower back), your buttock muscles tighten, and your stomach mus-

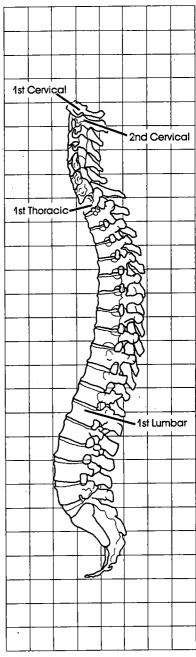

The vertebral column, your backbone, is normally an S shape. But its curves should not be too exaggerated, or structural problems will result.

cles are exercised. If it's easy, you're in pretty good shape and will be able to keep your back near to or on the floor without straining. If you find it difficult, your back needs work. For some people, the pelvic tilt becomes an automatic part of their posture with little training. For others, it requires a great deal of effort.

Inside your back, the benefits from this simple exercise are great: the pressure on the rear part of the lumbar discs is eased, the stretched muscles and ligaments are relaxed, and the supportive muscles of the stomach, buttocks and pelvis are toned and exercised.

You can, and should, perform the pelvic tilt while standing. Stand with your lower back against a wall and your feet six inches from the wall. Keep the lower back tight against the wall with your heels, buttocks and shoulders also touching the wall. Again, neck, shoulders and legs are relaxed, and stomach and buttock muscles are taut. In time, you should be able to assume the pelvic tilt posture without a supporting wall.

Can such a simple exercise really help? If faithfully practiced, the answer is yes. The benefits of the pelvic tilt have been documented by precise measurements of the pressure inside the spine. When you sit upright, 300 pounds of pressure per square inch is bearing on your lumbar discs (if you are of average weight); when standing, 200 pounds, and when lying flat on your back, 100 pounds is brought to bear on the area. But lying in the pelvic tilt position reduces the force to 60 pounds per square inch!

Now, the Upper Berth

So we've seen the good, the bad, and the achy in troublesome backs, and we're done, right? Wrong! We're only half done, in fact. Up until now we've talked mainly about muscular and skeletal distortions of the spinal column and those of just the lower back to boot. We must still talk about pains in the upper back and, of course, in the neck. Fortunately, much of that task is accomplished by merely saying, "Ditto." Most of the things that go wrong with the lower back can also go wrong with the upper back, and they're avoided and treated in the same way. One problem that's very common in the upper reaches of the spine (and not so common down below) is the tightness and pain that's caused by the stress, miscellaneous distress and fatigue of

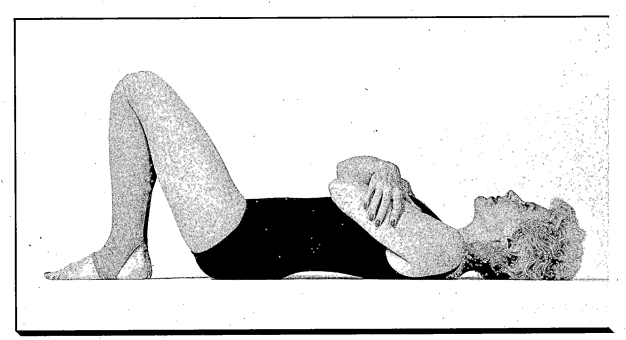

Here the lower back is in its normal position.

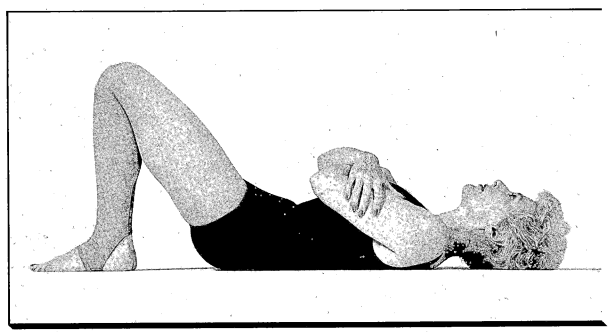

The pelvic tilt presses the lower back into the ground and straightens the spine.

getting through even normal days. *That* we must talk about.

Pain in the upper back and shoulders afflicts almost as many people as low back pain, which is the most common back problem. As in so many other illnesses, our backs are the victims of the city life, the sitting-down way of life.

The way we live and work in our modern society puts too much of the wrong kind of stress on this part of the body. For most of our daily activities, we sit over a desk, bench, typewriter, sewing machine or steering wheel. Washing dishes, cooking, typing, driving – our arms are always in pretty much the same position, straight out in front of us. If we lived a more rural life, our daily chores would guarantee plenty of twisting and very little sitting in the same tensed position.

Poor posture of this type causes a gradual buildup of tension, which affects the many nerve pathways in this area that control the hands, arms, head, heart, lungs and upper abdomen. Hour after hour of this tension builds up to a point where the tightness follows us to bed. We wake up with numb arms, a painful back or a headache.

You Are Your Back's Worst Enemy

Keep in mind that many of our daily routines are potential troublemakers and that taking early steps in strengthening the upper back will prevent attacks of severe stiffness and pain in the future.

Ask yourself if your working and playing hours put a lot of strain on this area. If you spend hours sitting in a stooped position over a desk or bench or steering wheel, you're probably giving little or no motion to the upper spine – motion it needs to stay healthy and loose. Of course, we occasionally have the natural protective reaction to this poor posture in the form of restlessness or the desire to get up and stretch. Giving in to that urge is sometimes all that's needed. But it's important to do it frequently enough to make sure the effects of poor posture don't climb into bed with you. If you don't get rid of them by bedtime, you may wake up with aching shoulders and a stiff, painful upper back.

There is nothing so helpful as regularly moving these tense areas, which is what nature tries to tell us with the "restlessness reflex." Truck drivers, for instance, can make a habit of turning their heads to look over their shoulders once every mile and to stop every two hours for a good five-minute stretch and a short walk. And this advice is

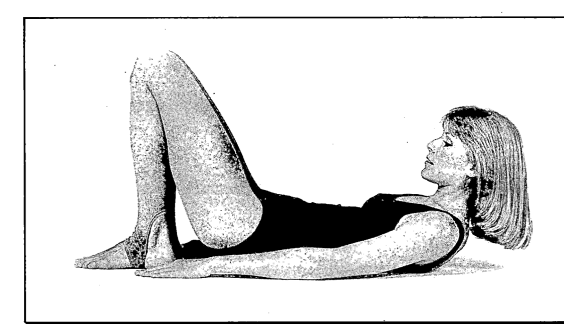

The curl-up is a good way to strengthen your stomach muscles and relax your back. Slowly lift your back off the ground, taking only three vertebrae off of the floor. Then slowly let yourself down.

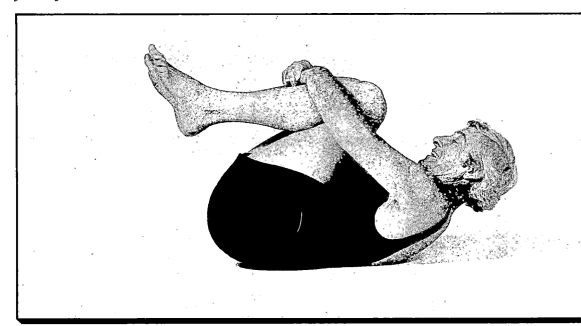

Rocking on the ground in this manner is a good back relief measure.

good for anyone who must be at the wheel for long periods at a time. Modern cars are made so low that the seats are more conducive to sleeping than to paying attention to the road. To overcome this, the driver has to thrust his or her head forward and concentrate, with little or no motion given to the upper back. This builds up tension. How often have you heard people say that they must rest up after a long driving trip? You won't need that rest at the end of your trip if you follow these suggestions for stretching and relaxing during the trip.

Treating Injury

In a manner of speaking, you could call this chronic, unrelieved stress to the shoulders an injury. But the usual, sudden type of injury or sprain can also lead to lingering pain and stiffness. Usually, the shoulder joint injury causes pain and swelling immediately. But a minor strain that might be caused by a sudden twist or jerk may go unnoticed for a day or more until pain, swelling and stiffness leave you virtually disabled.

First aid for an injury of this type – or for any sudden strain, sprain or bruise – is to apply cold in the form of ice or cold water packs for the first 12 to 24 hours. Applications of cold should keep the swelling to a minimum. Heat should be applied after a day or so, when you are getting the injured area back in operation.

The most important thing to remember in treating a sprain or injury to the upper back is to get those joints moving again as soon as possible. If motion isn't restored within a few days, tension and stiffness will build up as nerve reflexes reduce circulation to these parts. This condition can get even more debilitating if the pads of fatty tissue that surround the joints or the ligaments which connect bones to other bones become inflamed. It may then be called a "frozen shoulder," and it can take a long course of therapy to "break the ice."

Pain and stiffness across the back and shoulders can also be caused by an upper respiratory infection such as cold or flu. This is possible because the tissues in the nose, throat and chest are supplied by nerves centered in the spinal cord which come around from the upper back and neck. Messages sent over these nerve pathways go both ways, so we have the inflammation of the nose and throat tissues sending messages of trouble back to the spinal cord.

Some of these messages result in pain reflexes in the tissues around the spine, while others help heal the inflammation. But the messages to the upper back unfortunately result in aches, pains and stiffness, some of nature's warning signs.

Most likely, however, it's really posture that is giving your upper back a bad time. Check your posture for round shoulders or a stooped position. Does one shoulder tilt downward or more forward than the other? Do the head and neck assume an erect, straight position? Do you spend much of your time at a bench or desk? If so, your upper back pain is probably the result of poor posture. And the sooner you establish a routine that will prevent back and shoulder problems, the better your health will be.

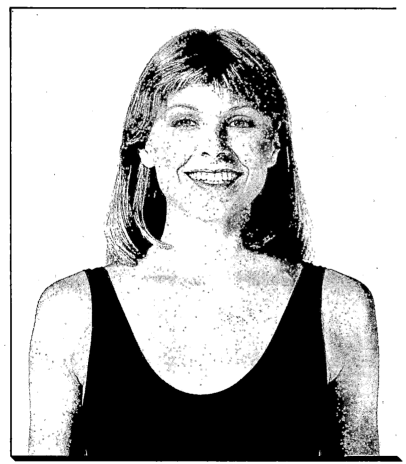

A straight neck feels good.

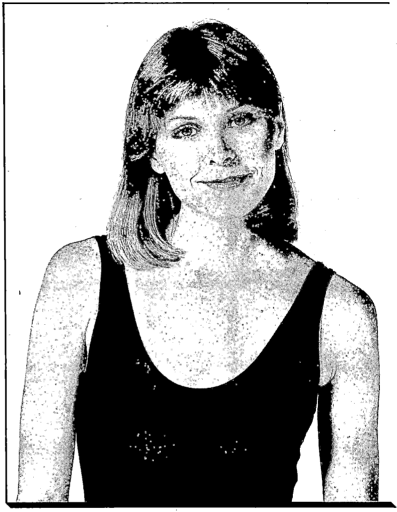

A curled neck stresses the body.

Preventive Exercises

Presented on the next several pages are some simple routines that everyone can do, that everyone should do to prevent the problems we have been discussing.

First of all, almost any exercise will do some good, by stimulating circulation and generally increasing motion in this area. Swimming, golf, tennis and walking all have this beneficial effect. But concentrating on the specific area can reduce the amount of time required to relieve or prevent shoulder aches.

For instance, if there is stiffness and soreness in the large shoulder joint, try bending forward and supporting yourself with the good arm and hand on a chair. Allow the afflicted arm to drop downward. Then swing this arm back and forth, side to side, and finally in circles both clockwise and counterclockwise. This gives the joint a gentle stretching motion without the added weight of the arm when you are standing erect. Bending over this way is more effective because it stretches the ligaments, where the swelling is.

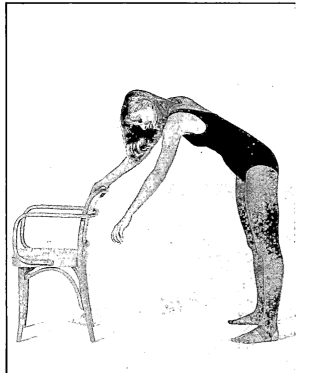 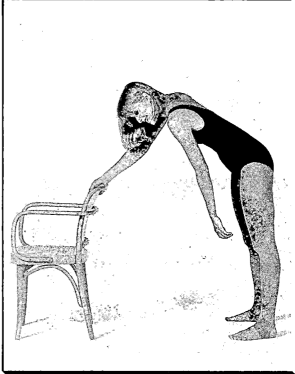

1. Lean on a chair to stretch your shoulder. 2. Gently let your arm swing.

Another gentle stretching exercise for a stiff shoulder joint is to lie down on your back with knees raised and arms out at your sides. Gently roll away from the stiff shoulder side until it feels ready to rise off the floor. Now gently rock back and forth. The weight of your arm is enough to stretch the tense ligaments of the shoulder. But in this case you are not really using the muscles around that joint, which might cause more harm than good.

(continued on page 82)   **BACK TROUBLES**   ·79

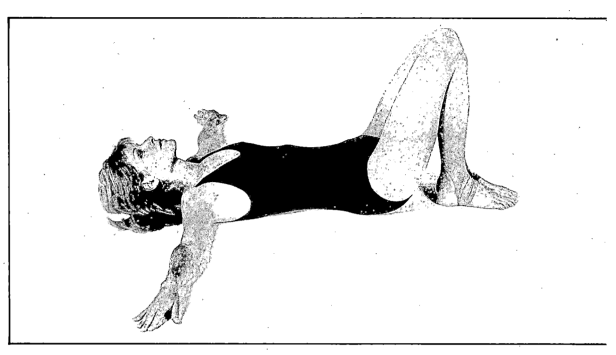

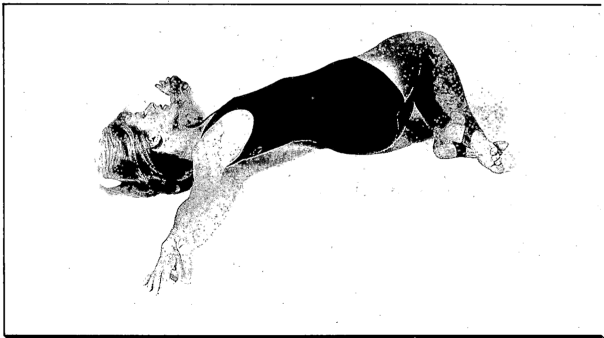

1. The shoulder stretch starts with your arms out straight. 2. Then roll to the side.

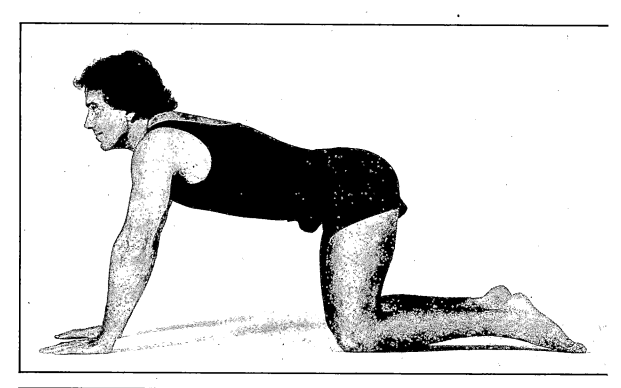

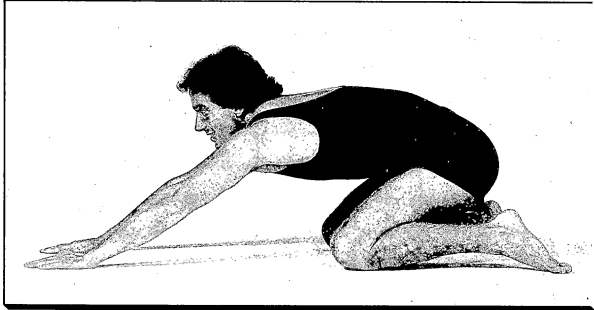

1. The cat stretch starts on all fours. 2. Then you come down and back.

One of the most effective primary stretching motions for all upper spinal tension as well as stiff shoulder joints is called the "cat stretch." Get down on your hands and knees, but with your hands forward. Keep your elbows stiff as you bend your knees and come down and back on your legs. This motion stretches the shoulders and upper back. While you're doing this, be careful not to hold your breath; just breathe easily. If you add a slight bouncing motion at the point when you begin to feel the stress, you will help release tight tissues.

The Peanut Roll

While you're down in this position, you can also try the "peanut roll." First, bring your hands back until both arms and upper legs are perpendicular to the floor. Now, from this neutral position, allow your elbows and knees to bend in order to bring your chin or nose close to the floor near

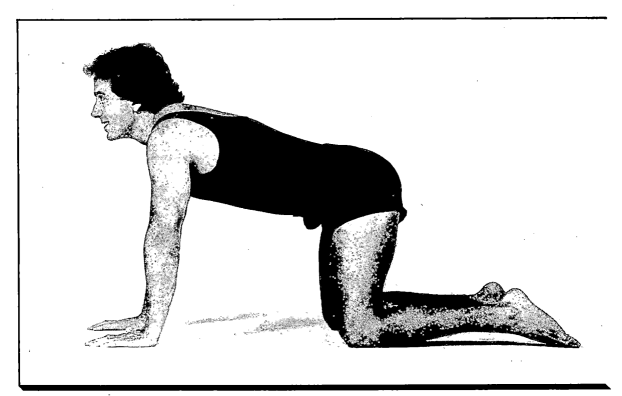

1. The peanut roll starts on all fours.

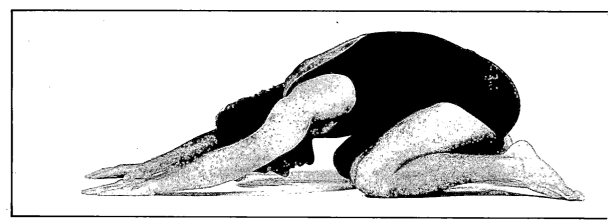

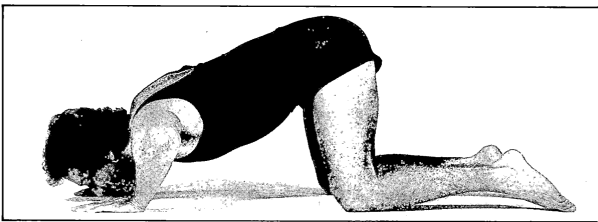

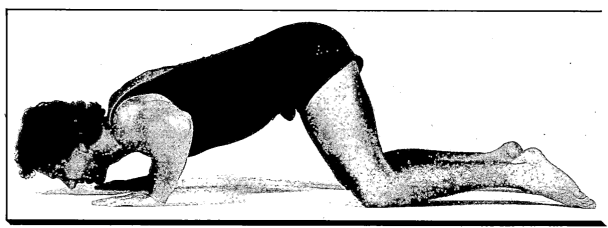

2. Bring your chin to the floor. 3. Have your chin forward as though rolling a nut on the floor. 4. Then raise your chin.

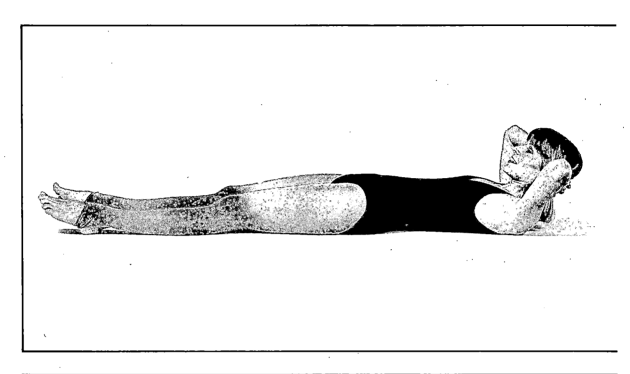

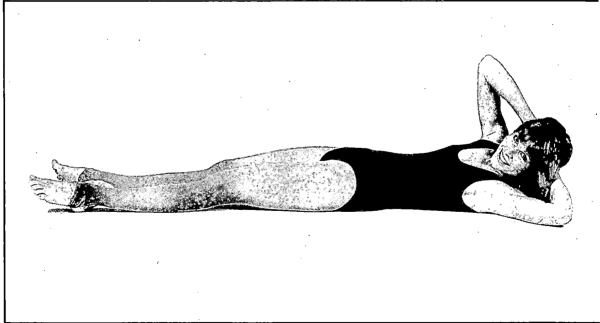

1. Start this shoulder roll on your back. 2. Then touch your elbow to the floor.

your knees. Now move your chin forward to your fingers, as if you were rolling a peanut forward on the floor. Then come up to the neutral position. Reverse the stretch by first getting down with your nose or chin near your fingers and then "rolling the peanut" back toward your knees, ending in the neutral position. The entire exercise should take only three to five seconds. Repeat it three or four times, and don't hold your breath.

If these exercises are going quite easily, you can add a different stretch by turning the head at the starting neutral position and rolling the peanut with one ear both forward and backward, then repeating with the opposite ear.

Another good stretching position is the "shoulder roll." Frequently a sudden release of tension is felt during this stretch as more motion is given to the upper spinal vertebrae. Lie flat on your back, with legs a little apart and hands clasped in back of the neck. Keep the elbows forward while you pull your head off the floor a few inches. From this neutral position, twist the head and shoulders to the right so that the elbow touches the floor. Then twist to the opposite direction, and touch the floor with the other elbow. As you go from side to side, rolling across the upper back from six to eight times will stretch and tone the upper spinal tissues. Again, let's emphasize that the ideal motion involves relaxed breathing and taking just one or two seconds to go from left to right.

Even if you don't have any pain or stiffness in the shoulders or upper back, these exercises can still benefit your health. Of course, they are not meant as substitutes for exercise such as running, cycling, walking, swimming and other sports. The healthy person who will best weather the effects of aging and stress is the person who gets as much motion as possible into his or her life.

BICYCLING

Just about every day at lunch a 52-year-old sheriff in the Los Angeles area rides his bicycle. He rides for pleasure, he rides to train for races, and he rides to save his heart. "It's amazing to me," Rudy Berteaux marvels. "About 15 years ago they discovered I had high blood pressure and problems with my heart cardiogram – it showed irregularities. In fact, I'd had a heart attack but we didn't realize it. I weighed 200 and some pounds. I had lots of trouble breathing, and I could barely mow the lawn, so they told me to exercise."

During the next five years he began jogging, improved his eating habits, and reduced to 185. Because his knees eventually hurt him, he had to give up running, but fortunately he had begun cycling for pleasure. He started enjoying the scenery and riding with a bike club. So he stepped up the cycling and began competing four years ago.

The man who formerly had to stay in bed just to keep his blood pressure down was soon winning medals. In the California Police Olympics two years ago, he took two silver medals in the over-40 category. Last year, just to see how he'd fare, he entered open competition and won a gold in the sprints, "which was a super surprise." He also copped two silver medals in the 10-mile criterium and the 30-mile road race. "So I've been getting better."

That is an understatement indeed. With the California team he entered the International Police Olympics, "and we had guys from all over the country and from Europe. I got a third place in the open in the 25-mile. The guys who beat me were 25 . . ." He's twice their age.

His training is regular and monitored by his doctor with twice-yearly stress tests. "He keeps telling me, 'Go at it! It's the best thing you can do.'" Mr. Berteaux smiles. Averaging about 150 miles a week, he rides back and forth to work 20 miles each way in summer. In winter he gets up early and bikes 10 or 15 miles on good mornings and an hour at lunchtime.

He is enthusiastic about the change in himself. "I look good, I feel trim. And it's nice to have a cardiologist tell you, 'You're in great shape. Go out there and ride that

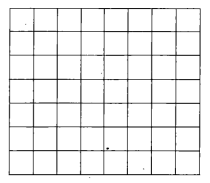

30-miler." I just can't get over the fact that people don't realize what they can do if they want to. If they get out there every day and jog, they'll get better; if they get out there on that bike, they can ride to work."

Bikers with Bad Hearts

It's exciting to know Mr. Berteaux and what he's done. It's equally pleasing to know that he is not alone. He told us, in fact, about the Rancho Los Amigos Hospital cycling club, comprised entirely of riders who bike for rehabilitation as well as sport. Organized in 1974 by Randy Ice, a therapist at the hospital, the club accepts cyclists only after their coronary disease shows some degree of stability. Most have participated in a training program conducted at the hospital; there they have been monitored while exercising on a bicycle ergometer or treadmill, and they monitor themselves at home. They get started on a proper diet and give up cigarettes if they smoke. Eventually they phase into the Saturday club.

Bike riding is pleasurable, and it's also a great source of aerobic fitness. You can get into the bike scene gradually and build up your endurance and ability as you slowly increase your fitness.

"The camaraderie in the group is just unbelievable," reports Mr. Ice. "The big thing for most patients when they have heart diseases is that they are very depressed and uncertain about what they can and cannot do. When they get into a group of people like this who are making incredible improvements – some rapidly and some slowly, but improving – it gives them the chance to talk to other guys about their problem."

Mr. Ice told us about one member, a 73-year-old, who recently completed his third "century," a 100-mile trip. "We rode from Fullerton to San Diego in one day; he found it was easy for him. He'd had a cancer operation in 1951 and about 2½ years ago had an aortic aneurysm as well as bypass surgery. He'd never cycled before. When he came to me, he was 69 years old and wasn't really doing anything. Now he's so interested in cycling, he knows more about the technical aspects of bicycles and components than I do. He rides about 500 to 600 miles a month."

It isn't easy to get started, but the supervision helps. Knowing how to pace yourself and how far to ride in the beginning are important. One plus-50 cyclist who began without such guidance describes how difficult it was for her at first. "I am a 'bikey' now," writes the woman, whose cycling is therapy for a cardiomyopathy – "a charley horse of the heart muscle," as she calls it.

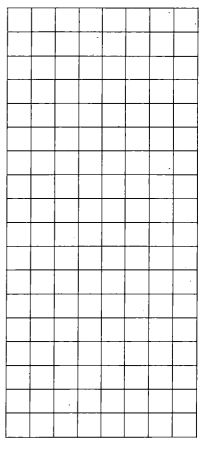

"Three years ago I just went in and bought a ten-speed, and with no technical knowledge purchased what I thought was suitable. I then attempted to participate in various club rides. This I did, always unsure as to the difficulty of the ride and my capabilities. I suffered them out, many times finding myself alone, trying to read the map. Sometimes I would cry right in the middle of a ride, wondering what I was doing to myself. Eventually I would find my way back, coming home tired and feeling so good about myself I knew I wanted to try again."

One afternoon on a ride she met a man who looked like Colonel Sanders on a bicycle. "He led rides independently and actually taught me how to use those gears – slow and easy. He had not taken up bicycling until his sixties and had experienced a previous heart attack. His rides were geared to his riders, the terrain, traffic and wind factor, if possible. This experience started me on my way, and I was now convinced I could be a bikey.

"Since that time I rode with another man, a loving friend who was a cyclist all his life. I was introduced to rides and outings on which mature bikeys take the time to look around and enjoy. We experienced bicycle rides that made a one-day outing seem like a whole vacation.

"Today, 2½ years later, my health problem seems to be gone. I no longer take any medication, and it is like I have a whole new body."

Rolling to Fitness

The main advantage of biking is that it is relaxing, fun and less straining on your joints and ligaments than many other forms of exercise. You're on wheels, rolling along rather than bouncing your legs off the pavement or asphalt. Bicycling opens up the fitness arena to many people who would be unable to do an activity like running.

And, while biking is pleasurable, it's still a great source of aerobic fitness. You can get into the bike scene gradually and build up your endurance and ability as you slowly increase your fitness.

When you finally decide that you're ready to start biking, the first question you'll probably ask is: what kind of bike do I get?

Different types of bicycles are best suited for different uses. For riding around town or short commutes, the three-speed bike, which requires little maintenance, is the most practical. But for recreational riding, hilly terrain or long distances, the mechanical advantages of the ten-speed make it the best choice. A ten-speed is far better if you seek to use your bicycle for exercise.

Finding a bike that's the right size for you is easy. While wearing flat-soled shoes, straddle the top tube of a men's bicycle frame. There should be about an inch clearance between your crotch and the top tube. (If you wish to purchase a women's frame, first make this test on a men's frame and then find a women's frame on which the seat tube is the same length as the proper-sized men's frame.) You'll find a too-small frame uncomfortable to ride, while a too-large frame is both uncomfortable and dangerous. You'll probably want to extend the seatpost a few inches when you have a frame that's right for you. And since not everyone's arms are the same size, you may need a longer or shorter handlebar stem than the one that comes with the bicycle.

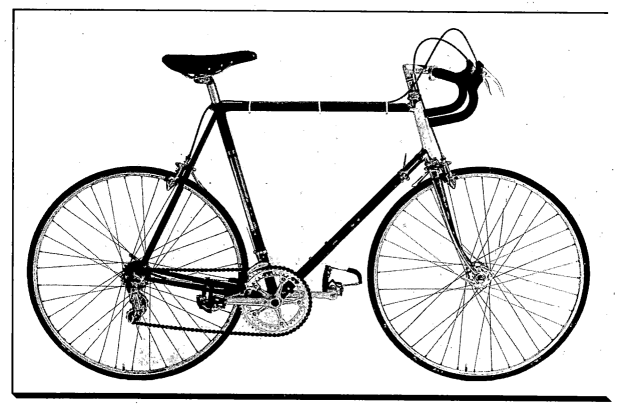

A ten-speed bicycle makes hills easier and trips less tiring.

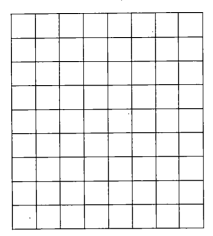

Bicycling is an excellent exercise. And you don't need fancy equipment to do it.

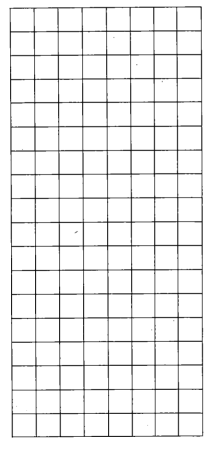

You Don't Have to Ride Tall in the Saddle

For the most beneficial exercise, for long rides and for hill climbing, you'll want to have the dropped (racing style) handlebars seen on ten-speed bicycles. Dropped bars look uncomfortable, and they are for your first few rides, but most cyclists grow to prefer them. They rearrange your body to provide many biomechanical advantages. But if your back can't get used to dropped bars or if you don't anticipate long rides, you may want to join the many people who stick with upright handlebars.

The kind of saddle that you use depends on the kind of handlebars you have. A wide saddle works well with upright handlebars. If you have dropped handlebars, you'll find the wide saddle uncomfortable. Racing-style saddles, like racing-style handlebars, are quite functional and more comfortable than they look. Women, who have wider pelvic bones than men, generally need a slightly wider version of the racing-style saddle.

Toe clips, those little gizmos that clamp your feet to the bicycle pedals, are handy for keeping your feet where they belong.

You'll probably want to start out without toe clips and get used to your bicycle first. But once you're used to your bike, you'll want clips. They increase your pedaling efficiency by holding your feet in the optimum position on the pedals. With clips, pedaling becomes a smooth 360-degree motion instead of a jerking push-push. They help you get more exercise out of your bicycle, and they help you enjoy an afternoon ride without getting tired.

Whatever you do, don't think that you have to get fancy when it comes to equipment. One disadvantage bicycling has in comparison to an exercise like running is the cost of a bike. If you want to run, all you need is a pair of running shoes and a pair of shorts. A bicycle, on the other hand, can be a substantial investment.

Be Safe, Not Sorry

When you ride your bike on the road, you should be sure to obey all the safety regulations. If you don't, you're asking for trouble. In a collision with an automobile, you and your bike will be at an extreme disadvantage.

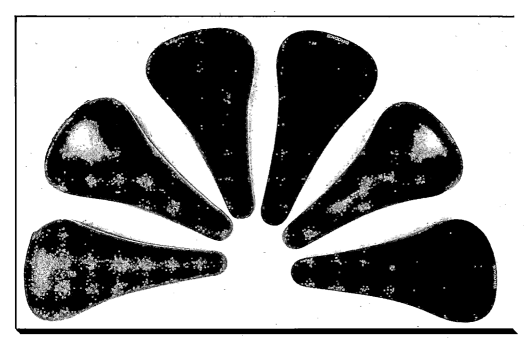

Bicycle seats, like people, come in all shapes and sizes.

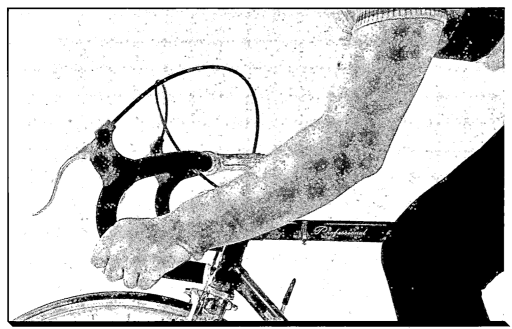

Dropped handlebars like these are usually the best choice for serious cyclists.

In general, the safety rules you should obey are the same as those that govern automobile driving. You should ride on the right side of the street and follow the directions of all traffic signs and signals. For details on the safety rules that bike riders should follow, contact your local police department. Most departments have traffic safety books especially geared for cyclists.

In addition to obeying traffic rules, bikers should also wear helmets for safety. Your head is the most vulnerable and most valuable body part that is endangered when you ride. Visit your neighborhood bike shop to find the helmet that best suits your needs.

Once you have all your safety measures taken care of, get out there and ride!

As Victor Hadlock, a born-again biker, puts it:

As I look back, I'm glad I didn't yield to that little demon voice that kept whispering, "You're too old for this foolishness; quit while you're ahead!" I shall be ever grateful to that doctor who said, "You ought to ride it every day." In return, when I looked at his ample paunch, I was tempted to say, "Why don't you try it, Doc?" But I kept my mouth shut.

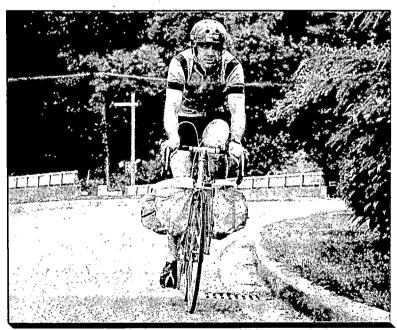

For safety's sake, wear a helmet when you bike.

BIOFEEDBACK

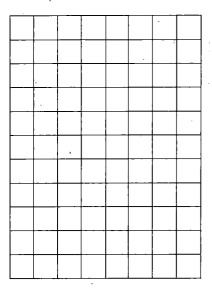

Biofeedback is an in-law of folk medicine. People use folk cures because they've worked for them before or they've been reported to work by reliable sources. But no one knows why or even how they work. The process is mysterious. And that's the way it is with biofeedback. It's a mysterious form of physical therapy, or perhaps learning, which has been used to treat all sorts of things with very reasonable success – things like tension headaches and migraine, cold hands and feet, anxiety and stress, irregular heartbeats, even the paralysis of cerebral palsy and the seizures of epilepsy. But it also has a dimension of hocus-pocus. No one knows whether biofeedback treats these ills directly or indirectly. Does biofeedback training allow a patient actually to control the inner mechanism that produces icicle hands, for instance? Or does it do something else entirely – something whose by-product is toasty fingers? As with most folk remedies, no one knows for sure. Fortunately, in this case, someone cares, and lots of researchers are trying to find out how and why biofeedback works. What we'll do in this chapter is look at some definitions of biofeedback and the explanations of how it works – or at least how it's supposed to work – that come with these definitions. And we'll make lists of the things it can do for you and those it can't do.

So what *is* biofeedback? Some would say that we don't know – now – what it is and that we can only describe how it's used and how it *appears* to work. So before we get to the definitions advanced by those who claim to know what biofeedback is, let's take a look at it in action.

Biofeedback increases your ability to control processes deep inside your body. It's been used to treat headaches, cold hands, anxiety, stress, and even cerebral palsy and the seizures of epilepsy.

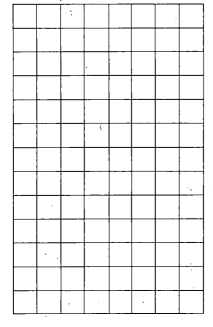

A Tension Headache

Fred suffers from tension headaches fairly often, maybe two or three times a week. *This* week the number went up considerably, because his daughter's orthodontia turned an expensive new corner and his seven-year-old car developed an oil leak that would require $139.50 to plug. So he went to his family doctor, who sent him to the headache clinic at a big university hospital nearby. The GP's reasoning was that Fred's drug dosage was already pretty high, and still the painkiller wasn't working. It was time to try something else. At the clinic, biofeedback was the "something else" decided upon. With feedback (we'll get to what *that* is in a second) from the muscles in his head and neck, Fred would be trained to relax the muscular bands that gripped him in times of tension and – it is supposed – produced his headaches.

First, the process was explained to him, and he agreed to try it. Then he was led into a small, soundproof, dimly lit room filled with blipping electronic hardware. He was introduced to the knobs, blinking lights and dials and was asked to lie down on a couch. Explaining carefully what was going on and working very gently with the spidery devices, a staff therapist taped three electrodes to Fred's forehead – one an inch above each eyebrow and one in the middle. These wires would pick up the electrical signals produced by the muscles spanning the forehead and take them back to a machine called an electromyograph (EMG), which would record and amplify (or strengthen) them. The theory was that if tension in Fred's muscles was producing his headaches, reducing that tension would reduce the headaches, too.

This theory became practice when the electrical charges from Fred's furrowed brow reached the electromyograph.

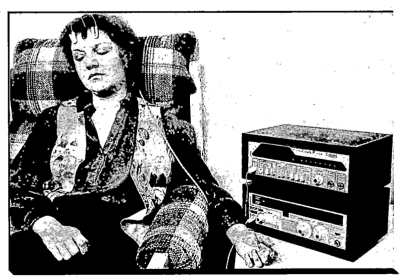

An at-home biofeedback machine can be used to induce relaxation.

The gizmo turned them into mechanical clicks, and they became feedback. The more tension in the muscles, the more pain Fred felt, and the stronger and harder came the clicks. The point, said the therapist, was for him to "see" and "hear" his discomfort in this indirect way – as electronic feedback – because soon he would be asked to slow the clicks and whittle away at the pain in an equally indirect way – *through* the feedback. While wired up and lying in the clinic, he would have to discover some way, any way, to relax the muscles, cut off their electrical activity and turn off the clicks. He was not given any hints on how to do it; he was just told to try. And he did it, over the next several days and weeks. Somehow, thinking of good times, of straight teeth and a new, leakless car, of lots of things, he managed to relax, to stifle the clicking machine and to end his pain.

The staff member working with Fred in the lab avoided talking to him about what he was doing to relax. He simply encouraged *whatever* it was, and he told Fred to concentrate on the telltale clicks. Of course, the real test of this or any biofeedback therapy will come in the weeks and months ahead, in seeing how well Fred can use his new shortcut to relaxation outside the clinic and away from the encouraging feedback. Biofeedback enthusiasts, of course, say that Fred's chances for success are good. Hardened disbelievers, naturally, say they are bad. But that's a story for later.

Getting Control of Yourself

The problem at hand is a definition of biofeedback to go with this demonstration of its inner workings. The definitions most widely circulated these days claim merely that it is any technique which *increases* the ability of a patient to *voluntarily* control *certain* physiological activities by providing him with information about them. We've used italics three times in that sentence to illustrate three important points. Biofeedback only *increases* your ability to control a process deep inside the body. It cannot provide you with a magic medical on-off switch or, for instance, absolute mastery over your blood pressure. It is also not a cure-all; as the rest of this section will show, only *certain* specific conditions respond to its blandishments.

And, finally, don't be fooled by the word *"voluntary."* The scientists, doctors and psychologists who use biofeedback have not yet agreed on what it means in this situation. They can't say whether the patient actually gains conscious

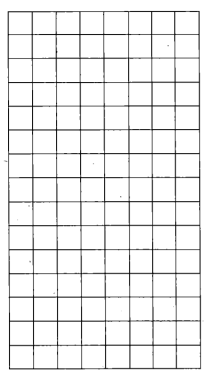

Biofeedback can free you from drugs and other invasive therapies.

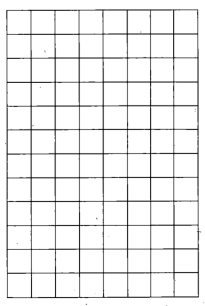

control over the temperature of his hands and feet – when suffering from Raynaud's disease – or if something else entirely happens, which only inadvertently produces a rise in these temperatures.

And there's a fourth thing we should highlight here. Biofeedback is a *cooperative* effort, both in the research that has created it and the medical practice that uses it. No one person should control your biofeedback therapy, because no one branch of medicine is responsible for its shaping. Medical doctors describe the symptoms of disease and the way in which feedback therapy modifies them. MDs often get the treatment process started with a diagnosis and a "prescription" for biofeedback. The machine used by whomever administers your therapy will have been designed by a biomedical engineer, and his role is crucial. The better the information you receive about your condition, the better your use of it is apt to be. The sooner you get it, the sooner you'll be able to react – and recover. And the more precise that information is, the more precise and steady your reaction and recovery will be.

A psychiatrist may also be called in to consult on your biofeedback treatment. Psychiatrists study the emotional aspects of disease states, and many conditions which respond to biofeedback have been labeled "psychosomatic"; they are physical conditions which have mental causes. Finally, a psychologist is often made part of a biofeedback team for his or her knowledge of the learning process. Biofeedback is, of course, a kind of learning, and psychologists frequently advise treatment groups on the organization of their therapies.

Biofeedback and Behavioral Medicine

What all that means is that the use of biofeedback has become a branch of behavioral medicine, which is one of the reasons it interests us. Behavioral medicine deals with illnesses in which a patient's behavior contributes to both declining and ascending health. Many forms of asthma, for example, are directly connected to emotional problems, and high blood pressure can come from a high-pressure life. But the part of behavioral medicine that intrigues us is its demand that the patient participate actively *in his recovery*. After all, the therapist can tell the patient how to use the equipment and its information, but only the patient can master the technique and produce the desired results. Of course, there's a catch here. If the patient must learn how to help himself or herself, he or she must also keep at the process long enough to get the job done – and then continue to practice it to keep the condition at bay. So biofeedback as a form of behavioral medicine has advantages and disadvantages. It frees the patient from drugs and other therapies that invade the body, strewing side effects in their tracks. But it also makes the patient dependent upon his or her own sense of self-discipline and self-control – a pretty good trade, we think.

The Uses of Feedback

There is a fairly lengthy list of conditions that have been treated by biofeedback, but one point should be kept in mind before being bowled over by it. Many of them are commonly associated with stress – tension and migraine headaches, ulcers and asthma are frequent targets – and biofeedback is used to attack the bodily consequences of that stress rather than the stress itself. Of course, biofeedback is also used in cases of serious injury and paralysis, such as stroke, accidental nerve damage, cerebral palsy and many other causes of physical impairment. But here, too, it is the symptoms of the disease or condition that are being attacked, not the problem itself. The assumption made by most biofeedback therapists is that the kind of self-control they teach can reduce the misery of illness no matter what the organic source of that misery. They do not say that their techniques restore the body parts knocked out of commission by disease or accident; they say, instead, that as long as there is some function in the affected system, biofeedback can help the patient use it to his greatest advantage. Biofeedback in most of its applications – whether it is for chronic lower back pain or Parkinson's disease or simple tooth grinding or jaw clenching – seeks to make the most of whatever resources the patient has.

A Sampler of Feedback Machines

No matter what your problem is, if feedback can help it, that help will get started with some type of monitoring equipment. Heart problems are worked on by a mechanical pulse-taker that continually monitors the contractions of the heart muscle. It is no more than an EKG (or electrocardiograph) machine like the one used to check your heart during your last physical, and it picks up its information through electrodes attached to the patient's chest. Similarly, blood pressure data used for biofeedback therapy comes from a specially modified blood pressure cuff which, though not unlike the standard item, is different, because it can *continually* measure both blood pressures (that is, the pressures with the heart pumping and at rest) without collapsing the vessels.

Another type of feedback comes from the EEG (electroencephalograph) machine, which records the electrical activity of firing nerve cells. It is used to monitor brain activity and reproduces signals that are commonly called "brain waves," pictures of particular kinds of brain goings-on. All EEG treatments allow patients to "watch" their brains at work and seek to train them to produce (on demand) certain wave patterns deemed desirable for one reason or another. Much excitement was generated several years ago when a special kind of brain wave, dubbed the "Alpha," was discovered. The Alpha pattern, some folks have decided, is very desirable, because they associate it with a very relaxed yet alert and creative state of mind. EEG electrodes are attached to the forehead and scalp of the patient.

Still another type of feedback comes from the EMG (or electromyograph) machine. This device picks up the electrical signals given off by moving muscles, and its information is used to retrain damaged limbs. It can help partially paralyzed or handicapped patients to find new ways of moving, and it has been used to reactivate nerve pathways in the stump of an amputated limb when the patient is fitted with a sophisticated artificial replacement. The sensors of an EMG device are taped to the skin over the muscle being investigated. Body temperature is recorded for feedback purposes as the amount of blood flowing through a particular area of the skin. A large and rapid flow indicates a high temperature to electrodes attached to the skin surface, and a low, slow flow suggests a heat loss.

Finally, we have one more machine to talk about. The GSR (galvanic skin resistance) is a measure of the electrical conductivity of the skin, and it is used as a sign of emotional arousal, of excitement and nervousness. When the skin's ability to conduct electricity goes up, our hackles, our guards, go down, indicating increased relaxation. The GSR is one of the things a lie detector measures. It has been used in biofeedback operations, both directly and indirectly – to record a patient's anxiety directly in stress-related illnesses and to determine in an indirect way when a patient is learning a feedback-controlled skill and when he is not.

What Biofeedback Looks (and Sounds) Like

No matter where your feedback comes from, in therapeutic situations it will appear to you in one of just a few forms – that is, it will become either visible or audible in one mechanical way or another. A light may go on or a tone may start sounding when some desired effect is achieved; or, the tone may alternately go up or down in pitch and lights of other colors may take over as the effect goes either up or down in intensity. For instance, if a patient is trying to raise the temperature of his or her hands, the biofeedback machine may change its tone (or color) only once at a predetermined point, say, after the temperature has risen to a level deemed acceptable by the prescribing doctor. Or the tone might continuously go up in pitch (or the lights march through a rainbow of colors) as the temperature gradually climbs.

How does the patient process this "space patrol" information? Let's pretend that our patient is being asked to slow the heart rate, a common demand in the lab, though not in the clinic. The patient is hooked up to an EKG machine with a control panel that features a red light, a green light and a yellow light. When his or her heart rate reaches the target figure, the yellow light will come on. Until then, the green and red ones work; when the red is on, the patient must try to raise his pulse, and when the green bulb flashes, he or she must lower it. Okay, the lesson starts. The yellow light is either go or no go. If it's no go, the patient looks at the other two for instructions and decides what must be done, either up or down, and tries to comply, checking the changing relationship of the three lights in order to monitor progress and to make whatever adjustments are necessary. How the patient does what he or she does, as we've said a number of times, isn't known. But *something* the patient does causes the heart to slow to the desired speed. This something is often called "feedforward." In some mysterious way, the patient processes the information provided by the feedback, and the brain turns it into messages that are fed forward to his or her heart muscle as instructions to cool it.

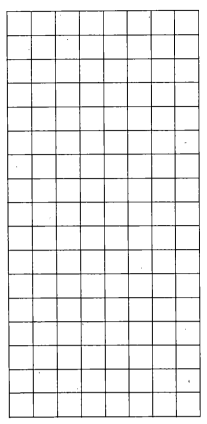

Migraine patients are taught to raise the temperature of their hands. Not much is known about why this hand warming works, but it somehow reduces the headache.

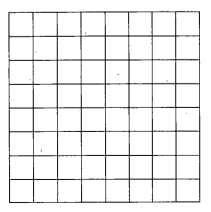

How Long Does Feedback Training Take?

When speaking generally, it's difficult to say how long clinical biofeedback sessions are; each learner and each treatment situation differs. One thing that's sure, however, is that sessions will be separated by periods at home without training, gaps sometimes called "rest" periods. Biofeedback therapy requires intense effort and demands these breaks. The intensity of the work also means that the sessions in the clinic may be short, especially at first. The patient's ability to concentrate will ultimately determine the best session length, but if his or her performance falls after 15 minutes, then there is no point going beyond this natural limit. Of course, after the patient gets used to the work, the sessions may grow longer. And it is true that many feedback therapists ask their patients to practice further at home on simple, portable and easy-to-use equipment. These efforts not only increase the patient's trial time but, more importantly, acquaint him or her with new control techniques in familiar and more normal surroundings.

Another part of most feedback training is a weaning process. The goal of this therapy, like any other, is to provide the patient with something that can be used without effort to achieve a more comfortable life. This means gradually severing the patient's connection with the feedback machine, such as alternating sessions with feedback and those without. It means teaching the patient the difference between a performance, which is rewarded by ringing bells and flashing lights, and genuine learning, which is rewarded by health and good feeling. And it means that the patient must develop some internal system for assessing the success of his or her efforts. Internal, personal feedback must be substituted for the external blips of the machine. As the therapy continues, the number of feedback-free sessions will increase until the machine is permanently unplugged.

Biofeedback therapy generally ends when the patient and the therapist agree there's no longer a need for it. That could come after only one session or after months of sessions – it all depends on the aptitude of the patient and the severity of the problem. The end can most often be seen, though, when the clinic appointments become further and further apart and when there is more and more home practice. Finally, the appointments are used simply to check the success of the home practice. This progression is also accompanied by an increase in the frequency of the feedback-less meetings. Once the formal get-togethers between professional and patient have ceased completely, most practitioners do insist on a series of follow-up contacts. These could be full-blown appointments or simple phone calls, but the goal is to check on the presence or absence of symptoms and the success or failure of the learned techniques.

Headache Treatment with Biofeedback

The two most common types of headaches are usually characterized by their symptoms and their suspected causes; they are both frequently treated with biofeedback. Migraine headaches are thought to be caused by the contraction or dilation of the blood vessels in the head, while tension headaches are supposed to come from tightly clenched muscles in the forehead and neck. Migraines produce severe and throbbing pain and can be accompanied by nausea, vomiting and sensitivity to light. Tension headaches tend to bring pain that is dull, persistent and undulating in nature; sufferers claim these attacks feel like bands pulled snugly around the head.

The biofeedback treatment of migraine headaches normally enters the scene through what is decidedly a back door; migraine patients are taught to raise the temperature of their hands. Not much is known about why this hand warming works, but it is almost always accompanied by some kind of relaxation exercise, and it is guessed that the technique is successful because it somehow reduces nervous system overload and, with it, headache. Most authorities do not believe, as they once did, that this biofeedback ploy reduces the flow of blood to the head and in doing so reduces the likelihood of these "vascular" pains in the head. How successful is this strange method? One large study that followed patients for a year after their feedback training ended discovered that *all* the patients had maintained the gains they had made during treatment – even the ones who did not continue to practice their hand-warming trick. This trial also compared the results of patients treated with feedback *and* relaxation techniques with those treated with relaxation alone. There was no difference in their successes, implying, we guess, that biofeedback is an elaborate way to beat stress.

Biofeedback training for tension headaches was pioneered by a group of doctors at the University of Colorado

Medical Center in Denver, but their methods are widely used elsewhere these days. They involve systematic relaxation and biofeedback reports on muscle activity in the forehead and throughout the neck and head. The word from Colorado suggests that feedback in this case, too, is a helpmate for relaxation, that it is not the main attraction. As with migraine headaches, studies of the success of feedback assaults on tension headaches generally say that machine-assisted relaxation or relaxation alone works, but only a few researchers have found that the machines work by themselves.

Raynaud's Disease

Cold hands have never killed anybody, but Raynaud's disease, which produces icy fingers and toes, can be very uncomfortable. The problem is brought on by exposure to cold or emotional stress and may occur frequently during chilly months. Simply warming the affected areas doesn't help much, because the blood that rushes in to meet the heat causes throbbing pain, swelling and unpleasant redness. Instructions to avoid cold, to use drugs or to try surgery (to cut off nerve messages to the hands) have been tried against Raynaud's disease without much luck; surgery, for instance, works in only half of all cases. Biofeedback treatments, however, have done considerably better. Using reports of the skin's temperature on one finger as a guideline, Raynaud sufferers are usually told to imagine that their hands are growing heavy and warm while practicing some form of relaxation therapy. Unfortunately, scientific checks on the effectiveness of biofeedback therapy for this complaint have not been very rigorous, and it's impossible to say how well it works. Many practitioners feel, here again, that relaxation or the feedback/relaxation combo may be the thing doing the corrective work.

Anxiety Attacked

This frequent pairing may have led researchers to try feedback on the psychological disorder often called, for want of a better term, stress or anxiety. It has also been used to treat insomnia, addictions of various kinds and phobias, those unnatural or unwarranted fears of relatively safe things that affect many people. In the case of some emotional disorders, feedback is used, more often than not, as a way into more conventional psychotherapy. Its ability to show people their own nervousness and tension in a graphic way sometimes convinces them that they need the counseling they have been resisting.

One phobia method we read about treats severe fears of flying with feedback from the muscles of the forehead, which technicians consider a good sign of tension. Five sessions, each 20 minutes long, are used to teach the patient to relax. The tightness of the patient's muscles is revealed to him or her by a steady, machine-made tone. First, the patient is taught to become calm (and turn off the tone) on the simple command of "Relax!" Then he or she is asked to obey the same command while reading about flying or seeing a film about it. Finally, the patient is instructed to take a commercial plane to give the technique the acid test. And it usually works.

Stressful Illnesses and Feedback

Two illnesses that have been associated with mental stress and are also frequently treated with biofeedback are asthma and stomach ulcers. Asthma has long been known to have an emotional or even a psychosomatic aspect. In some people it's more a mental disorder than a physical one. As a result, two biofeedback approaches have been taken to the disease. One attacks it indirectly, and one goes the direct route. The indirect treatment gives the patient information about the stress affecting him through readouts from the muscles in his or her head and neck. With this aid, the patient is taught to relax in the face of crisis and so to fight asthma attacks. The more direct gambit gives the patient information about the constriction, or pinching off, of the lungs' bronchial passages and, in a complicated process, teaches him or her to open them and to ease labored breathing. Both methods have produced what medical writers call "clinically significant" results; that is, they *really* reduce the number of asthmatic attacks suffered by trainees and improve their breathing. The bugaboo here is that most patients are also taking medication to do these same things while they're using biofeedback. Still, most trials claim that once the technique is mastered, medication can be reduced.

The treatment of stomach ulcers with biofeedback has been successful, too, but it's decidedly more uncomfortable for the patient than most other uses of these techniques. The pain and havoc caused by ulcers come from too much stomach acid. That's not news. It figures, then, that cutting down on the stomach's supply of acid will lessen the devastation; that's not news, either. In a number of recent studies, patients *have* been able to control the release of acid into the stomach using feedback readings of its contents; that's news, and good news to boot. What's also news, bad news, is that these readings come from instruments that must be *swallowed* (one unpleasant way or another) before they can send back their flashes from the interior. What's also discouraging about this therapy is that it's new. We don't know if patients can stop the acid flow completely enough to end their ulcer problems. We'll have to wait and see, but even if the tidings are very good, the instrument swallowing may always prevent biofeedback from becoming a staple of ulcer control.

The other conditions that are treated with biofeedback often enough to be mentioned here may be roughly grouped together as kinds of abnormal muscle activity. Some of them, like various types of paralysis, begin and end with the muscles. Others, like epilepsy, start in the head. Let's look at epilepsy first.

The ill effects of the disease, which range from nearly undetectable muscle quirks to brief blackouts to violent and frightening grand mal seizures, stem from the abnormal activity of certain brain cells. This activity, of course, can be seen (or heard) on an EEG record, and when this record is turned into feedback, it can be used to train a patient to suppress the destructive brain waves and encourage the normal ones. Control of these brain waves is, as you might imagine, one of the most difficult things for biofeedback users to learn. Training sessions can take more than an hour – *each* – and may have to be scheduled several times a week – for several months – before there is *any* change in a patient's pattern of seizures. These sessions *have* been successful, however. The number and frequency of seizures have been reduced for people who have not been able to control their illness in other ways. Still, active biofeedback practice may have to be continued indefinitely to preserve these gains, and it is still unclear whether biofeedback can replace drug therapy in epilepsy cases.

Feedback and Muscle Therapy

The other kinds of abnormal muscle activity tended to with feedback come from injury, stroke or debilitating illnesses such as cerebral palsy or Parkinson's disease. These applications are, without question, the most widely accepted uses of feedback, but even they are often termed no more than valuable additions to more traditional sorts of drug and physical therapy. The muscle disorders treated with biofeedback fall into three broad categories: muscles which contract when they should not, either continuously or sporadically and unpredictably; muscles which do *not* contract when they should; and muscles whose contractions are not well coordinated with those of others in the body. Using the information provided by an EMG machine of the electrical activity inside these balky muscles, the patient in each case is slowly taught to bring them in line. First the patient is trained to relax the target muscle group and perhaps his or her whole body. Then, he or she may be helped to loosen the chronically clenched muscle or to contract the permanently weakened one. Since muscle groups work in pairs – one, for instance, extends the arm, and another pulls it back – these procedures often require feedback from two locations at once. Finally, the patient is taught to produce coordinated movements with feedback from several areas in a long and very complex process. Many authorities claim that the visual feedback provided by joint movement is the most crucial factor in this type of rehabilitation. When it comes to assessing the overall success of biofeedback therapy in muscle reeducation, however, these same authorities are divided. Some say it is merely an experimental ploy, while others feel it is a proven addition to the physical therapist's tools. The procedure's greatest acceptance seems to be in cases of stroke-induced paralysis.

Should You Give It a Try?

Given all those possible uses for biofeedback – and all the reservations about them (not the least of which is that nobody really knows how they work) – should you try biofeedback? A report prepared for the U.S. Department of

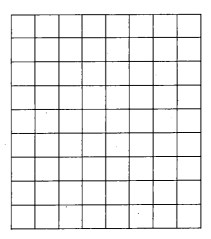

Biofeedback has reduced the number and frequency of seizures for some epileptics who have not been able to control their illness in other ways.

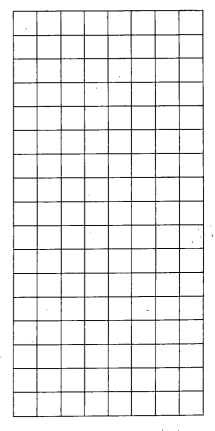

Health and Human Services, which was critical of biofeedback, steps back from its suspicions and says that the case for the clinical effectiveness of biofeedback is still open. Careful scrutiny has failed to substantiate the extreme early claims for its therapeutic potency. However, biofeedback has uncovered new possibilities – if not of complete control, then at least of some influence – over maladies and mechanisms which Western societies had traditionally considered immune to conscious manipulation. Even the strongest critics of research on the therapeutic effectiveness of biofeedback do not want to see the technique abandoned. They just want it demystified. In other words, this government body wants more information on what exactly biofeedback can and cannot do. So do we. But, we would add, if there is a possibility that feedback therapy might help you, it's worth a try, the *first* try, perhaps. Biofeedback treatment is cheaper than many medical and most surgical remedies; it's easier on the patient's mind *and* body; it has no known side effects; and it puts the patient in charge of his or her own destiny. All things which are worth encouraging, we think.

BIORHYTHMS

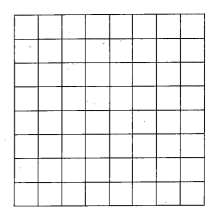

We got a little confused the other day while reading the Good Book, the chapter called Ecclesiastes to be exact. On one hand, we read: "Vanity of vanities, saith the Preacher, vanity of vanities; all *is* vanity. . . . One generation passeth away, and another generation cometh: but earth abideth for ever."

We read that, and we got depressed. Nothing changes, and nothing is worth doing as a result. But then we read more and cheered up. The Book continued: "To every *thing there is* a season, and a time to every purpose under the heaven. . . . A time to rend, and a time to sew; a time to keep silence, and a time to speak."

Everything changes, we decided now, but that replaced our depression with confusion. Everything changes, but everything remains the same. What did this apparent contradiction mean? We couldn't clear that obviously unclearable question up, but it did remind us of something else useful – biorhythms, or, more properly, the currently hot theory of biological rhythms.

All people, plants and animals change rhythmically along the time course of seconds, minutes, days, months and years. We're different at different times of the day, and so there are good and bad times to do all things.

The Science of Chronobiology

Even more properly, the *science* of chronobiology. The bright idea behind this sometimes heavy going is an old one. At least since the time of the Bible writers in Ecclesiastes, we have believed that things have seasons, that they go through cyclic changes during the course of their existences. As Lawrence E. Scheving, Ph.D., once told the International Society of Chronobiology, not just the earth but "all biological systems [animals, people and plants to you] change rhythmically along the time course of seconds, minutes, days, months and years." Change, he said, is "a fundamental property of life." Because this is true, an "organism is a different biochemical entity at different time points during the day." What that means is that there are seasons in the daily lives of all of us, just like the biblical scribe contended. And *that* means, to return to Dr. Scheving again, that the body "reacts differently when identical stimuli are applied

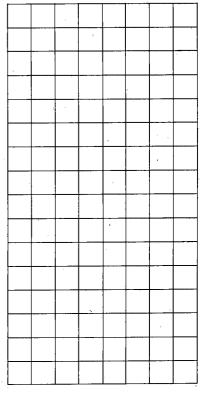

at different times." And there's good news in that dry pronouncement. If we're fundamentally different at different times of the day, there must be good and bad times to do *all* things. Like eating or sleeping or studying or working or falling in love. *Any*thing. As the biblical author said, "To every *thing there is* a season, and a time to every purpose under the heaven."

A Schedule for Health

That set us to thinking. Couldn't this information be used to set up a calendar for doing things *right*, even a daily schedule for taking the best care of ourselves? Yes, but someday, not quite now, say the chronobiologists. For now, our best bet would be to stop thinking so often about *what* we do for our health, or *how much* of it we do, and start thinking about *when* we do things.

A good example of that kind of thinking was in an article we read in a medical journal. It suggested that *when* you eat dinner might very well play a large role in determining whether those proverbial 14 angels guarding you while you sleep can spend their time humming Gregorian chants or must get their wings all aflutter giving you cardiopulmonary resuscitation. Or, perhaps, be forced to turn your case over to their Boss.

Paul B. Roen, M.D., recently retired as senior director of the Clinic for the Study of Arteriosclerosis at the Hollywood Presbyterian Medical Center in Los Angeles, draws attention to the fact that many people eat a very large meal shortly before going to bed. That style of eating, he says (and our own experience backs him up), is often characteristic of the high-powered executive or "the apparently healthy man past 45 who has a voracious appetite." And that style of eating may have unsuspected health implications, he suggests in the *Journal of the American Geriatrics Society* (June, 1978).

The absorption of food into the system is at its peak, Dr. Roen explains, about seven hours after eating. And dinner is typically not only the largest meal of the day but also the one that contains the highest amount of fat. While you're sound asleep, then, and the circulation of your blood is quite minimal, "this material, full of saturated fats, moves slowly through the arteries," creating a situation which "is ideal for clot formation, possibly resulting in a stroke, a heart attack or sudden death."

And, quite possibly, that high-powered executive or older person with a voracious appetite is unusually vulnerable to a heart attack to begin with. His arteries may already be occluded by fat deposits and covered with calcified plaques, inviting a clot. And that sudden infusion of saturated fats is custom-made to do the job.

Dr. Roen offers his analysis as a theory, but it does seem to make sense. We once knew of a grandfather-aged man, apparently in vigorous health, who ate almost an entire pie before going to bed one Thanksgiving evening and died of a stroke during his sleep. We could never understand why that happened; we thought that the pie might give him a stomachache . . . but a stroke? Dr. Roen's theory offers an explanation for that event as well as a possible explanation for the reason that a surprisingly high number of heart attacks occur during sleep, rather than during strenuous activity.

Eat Earlier, Lighter, Oftener

When *is* the best time to eat, we asked Roen. "Based on 30 years of work in the area of arteriosclerosis," he told us, "I advocate a number of small meals (five or six) a day rather than one or more large meals. This has been shown to cut down mortality due to atherosclerosis by 25 percent."

Besides that, he adds, "there is no question but that we feel better, sleep better and *are* better with a light meal in the evening. Personally, it is our experience that as long as your last meal is light, it doesn't matter how late it is. Around 6 o'clock is best, though."

But what about Spanish people and people in other cultures, we asked, who traditionally eat their big meal very late at night?

"It is a misconception that the Spanish eat their large meals late at night," Dr. Roen explains. "Only the upper class do that. Average people have their large meal at noon, then siesta, then return to work for several hours. Their last meal is not as heavy as their noon meal."

As for his own evening meal, Dr. Roen says he favors a small portion of cold, lean meat, a homemade soup, a raw salad and whole wheat bread. As part of his health program, he avoids white flour products, sugar, cakes and cookies. In addition, he always takes a walk in the evening, usually after supper.

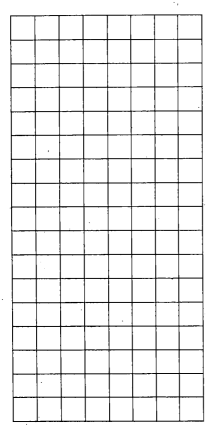

Research suggests that people who stay up very late at night studying or reading are doing themselves an intellectual injustice.

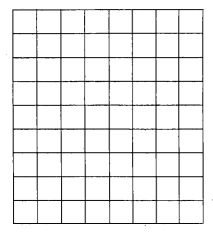

Dr. Roen's remark about always taking a walk after dinner made us think about the timing of exercise, as well as that of meals. One doctor who believes that walking after dinner is an excellent health practice is Vlado Simko, M.D., a specialist in digestive diseases in the department of internal medicine at the University of Cincinnati College of Medicine. Exercising after a meal, Dr. Simko believes, increases the flow of bile and improves the efficiency of digestion, specifically improving the intestinal absorption of fat.

To the extent that you may be prone to develop gallstones, exercise after dinner is an especially good idea, Dr. Simko suggests, because "exercise performed when no food is entering the body probably improves the cholesterol solubility in bile and helps in preventing formation of cholesterol crystals, perhaps the starting point for cholesterol gallstones." Going for a walk shortly before retiring, he believes, would probably help to "recirculate the bile and decrease the time span when bile is likely to form stones."

Like Dr. Roen, Dr. Simko feels that eating one big meal a day is wrong. "If you overload the gastrointestinal system with fats at any one time, it promotes diabetes and obesity as well as other diseases."

Eating a big meal late at night is also calculated to do nothing good for your sex life. A review in *Postgraduate Medicine* (July, 1975) mentions that practice as one possible cause of "secondary impotence," along with fatigue, overindulgence in alcohol and the use of drugs. But the real danger here is not simply the isolated instance of male sexual failure. It's possible that if a man habitually eats a heavy meal before retiring and also finds it very difficult if not impossible to make love, he may interpret that to mean that he is suffering from some kind of hormone deficiency or other underlying physical or emotional problem. That, in turn, can lead to fear, the expectation of failure, and the *guarantee* of failure.

The moral of all this? Eating and drinking by candlelight late in the evening may seem romantic, but it's not recommended if the romance is to continue after the table's been cleared.

Time and Alcohol

As most men know only too well, alcohol in amounts greater than one or two drinks might make your eyes sparkle but other parts of you sputter. But regardless of *what* your plans are, *when* you drink shapes your reaction to alcohol just as how much you drink.

John D. Palmer, Ph.D., of the University of Massachusetts at Amherst, in his book *An Introduction to Biological Rhythms* (Academic Press, 1976), points out that the length of time alcohol remains circulating in your blood varies throughout the day. And, naturally, the more time the alcohol spends in your·blood, the more time it has to act on your brain cells. The most vulnerable hours are between 2 A.M. and noon, while the most "tolerant" hours are from late afternoon to early evening. The alcohol you drink at dinnertime will likely be burned away 25 percent faster than the Bloody Mary at breakfast time. Not that you drink at breakfast, but if you *did* . . .

Writing in *BioScience* (February, 1977), Palmer adds, "It might also be worth mentioning that the last drink of a party – 'the one for the road' after the bewitching hour – is metabolized relatively more slowly than the preceding ones and will produce a more lasting rise in blood alcohol – a feature that could prove embarrassing and even expensive should one be challenged by a traffic policeman."

Or a bridge abutment.

Is it beginning to seem that doing things late at night often·gets us into trouble? When we began researching this section, we didn't have any conclusion in mind, but as the research progressed, that theme seemed to emerge again and again.

At this point, we are reminded of Ben Franklin's saying, "Early to bed and early to rise makes a man healthy, wealthy and wise." Is there really something to that, perhaps more than we think? Well, so far, we've seen that "doing it earlier" might make us healthier, perhaps somewhat sexier, and some of us, at least, a bit more sober. But wiser?

The Worst Time to Learn

Could be. Some very interesting new research suggests that people who stay up very late at night studying or reading are doing themselves an intellectual injustice. Researchers at the University of Sussex in England showed a training film to two groups of nurses. Both groups were accustomed to the usual day work pattern, but half of them were shown the film at 8:30 P.M. and the other half at 4 A.M. Immediately after the film was shown, the nurses were tested on its content. The 8:30 P.M. group answered 55 percent of the questions correctly, while, curiously, the 4 A.M. group scored an average of 59.2 percent correct answers. That difference, though, was not considered "statistically significant."

What *was* significant was the difference between the two groups when they were retested on the same material a month later. The nurses who had done their learning at 4 A.M. had forgotten more than twice as much, scoring only 15.5 percent correct answers vs. 39.5 percent for the 8:30 P.M. group.

As an interesting sidelight, further tests and analyses revealed that the time at which the nurses were tested on the material was much less important than the time the material was learned (*Nature,* May 25, 1978).

Quite possibly, studying very late at night is just as good, maybe even slightly better, than studying at a more normal hour – if the purpose is merely to do well on a test the next morning. But since the real benefit of knowledge can only be exercised in the real world, late-night studying is only half as effective as earlier study. Maybe Ben Franklin really did know what he was talking about. And, since knowledge is often the road to wealth in these days of intensive education and professionalism, maybe Ben was right on all *three* counts.

Maximum Personal Efficiency

If studying at 4 A.M. is the pits, when's the *best* time to try to learn something? Dr. John Palmer, whom we mentioned before, cites some now-classic research done back in 1916 which shows that the peak times for learning are at about 10 A.M. and 3 P.M., with the earlier hour being the most efficient. Interestingly, the worst time, at least during the day (this study did not include evening hours), turned out to be about 1 P.M. Efficiency began to fall off at about 11:30 A.M. and plummeted until 1 P.M., when it began to rise again. At 2 P.M., efficiency was still relatively low, but by 3 P.M. it was at a very respectable level.

It's difficult to say how applicable these results obtained in 1916 are today, but they do suggest that the millions of people in the world who take a siesta after lunch aren't being self-indulgent but are actually designing their work schedule to obtain maximum personal efficiency.

One of the most curious things about this 1 P.M. slump is that it is not, apparently, simply the result of having eaten lunch. According to Palmer, "The depression occurs even if the noon meal is skipped." There is, in fact, "no good explanation" for this phenomenon in Palmer's opinion; it is just another example of fluctuations under the control of what is now known as the "bioclock," the clock that controls our internal change of seasons.

If being healthy, wealthy and wise isn't enough for you, how about being slender? Yes, it's true: eating earlier in the day can actually help you lose weight.

Franz Halberg, M.D., and associates at the Chronobiology Laboratory, University of Minnesota, discovered that fascinating fact in a series of experiments carried out a few years ago. In one test, they fed a group of people just one meal a day, consisting of 2,000 calories, either as breakfast or dinner. When they ate their only meal as breakfast, all seven subjects lost weight. But when the same people ate the same meal in the evening, they showed either a smaller weight loss or an actual gain. The difference between these two ways of eating, the researchers concluded, amounted to the equivalent of 2½ pounds a week.

Big Breakfast vs. Big Dinner

Using a different group of test subjects, they varied the conditions somewhat, approximating real life a little more closely. Rather than giving each person 2,000 calories in the form of preselected foods (some of which may not have been to their liking), the second group was simply told to eat anything they liked, and as much as they liked, except that they had to eat all of their daily ration either as breakfast or dinner. This time, it turned out that eating only breakfast caused the subjects to lose 1.4 pounds per week more than they did when they ate only dinner (*Chronobiologica,* vol. 3, no. 1, 1976).

These results may be as important as they are astonishing. Is it possible that gradually shifting more and more of your daily food intake toward breakfast (we wouldn't advise making any great sudden shift) would be a relatively painless way of reducing? Is it possible that so many people in the industrialized nations are overweight because they eat small breakfasts and huge dinners? Are peasant populations throughout the world generally much more slender than us because, lacking electricity to light their homes, they are forced to do their eating – and everything else – at an earlier hour?

Possibly the most important implication of all lies in just the opposite direction. As Dr. Halberg suggests, people whose food resources are meager might be able to enjoy greater health and well-being by eating *later* in the day than they normally do, thus enhancing the caloric value of their food.

We like the whole idea of shifting most of our activities to an earlier time of day because it's more *natural* than our present lifestyle. What could be more natural than going to bed shortly after sunset and getting up with the sunrise? What could be a more *unnatural* thing to be doing at 1 A.M. than sitting in front of the TV set watching "The Mummy That Ate Mommy"? Or to wake up in the morning with the feeling that an energy vampire had sucked you dry?

Perhaps what the new science of chronobiology is telling us about ourselves is simply another lesson in the wisdom of living more naturally.

Of course, there's a catch here. This science is a very young one, and it's not ready *yet* to prescribe patterns for the rest of our lives. Oh, there are lots of people, with lots of charts and funny machines, who *are* ready to tell us what to do with the rest of today (or the month, anyway), but most chronobiologists say that they've only just begun to learn about their subject. So, before we totally readjust our existences, we'll have to let them catch up a bit.

BODY THERAPIES

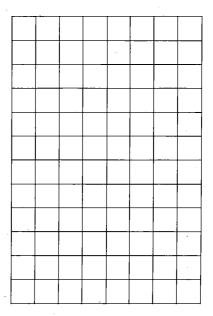

We have a problem here, a problem of definition. The two systems of physical rehabilitation and reeducation described here are called, for nothing more important than convenience' sake, "body therapies," but that's not a particularly meaningful term. *Any*body who does *any*thing to *any*body could be called a body therapist; the possibilities are limitless. So let's get a bit more specific.

What Are the Body Therapies?

There are many body therapies just now – with new ones developing practically each time a bad back gets worse or a trick knee starts to perform – but most of them have certain things in common. Whether they are the products of years of research and refinement or the property of three devotees in Toledo, most body therapies are firm in their belief in self-improvement – even self-perfection – for its own sake. Although all of the therapies we'll talk about have been used to treat physical disability due to injury, disease or birth defect, all of them were originally devised to treat the apparently whole and healthy body. Each of the treatment innovators we'll encounter was convinced that man did not automatically know (nor could he easily learn to know) how to use his body properly. They were – or are – sure that the combined effects of gravity, lifestyle, education and minor body imperfections work to throw this marvelous piece of machinery out of whack. Of the four time-proven, and fairly well-known systems we'll talk about here – the Alexander Technique of F. M. Alexander, Moshe Feldenkrais's Principles of Functional Integration, the fundamentals of Irmgard Bartenieff and the ideokinetic theories of Mabel Todd and Lulu Sweigard – all are concerned with how efficiently the upright human body deals with the downward pull of gravity. All contain definitions of "good" (or better, desirable) posture and explore whole-body means of achieving it which are decidedly *not* exercise programs. None of these therapies claims it will get you "in shape." They are not *at all* aerobic or muscle building. Rather, they each

Most body therapists believe that we don't know how to use our bodies properly. Gravity, lifestyle, education and imperfections throw us out of whack.

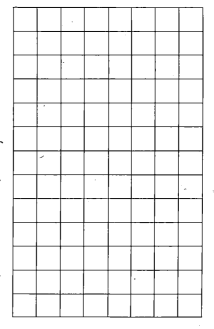

have an explanation for how the mind and the body interact which hopes to align the different muscle patterns that make up all human activity into a harmonious and stressless whole. The mind and body that work together, say these theories, will also play well together.

The F. M. Alexander Story

F. M. (Frederick Matthias) Alexander was an Australian actor who grew up in the bush country and made his living giving flamboyant readings of Shakespearean texts. He was a great success 'almost immediately and toured the nation constantly until, at age 19, he began to have trouble with his voice. This was in the days before electronic amplification in theaters, and Mr. Alexander was repeatedly plagued by shortness of breath, hoarseness and even loss of voice; if he couldn't be heard, he wouldn't be paid.

Mr. Alexander reasoned that something he was doing as he trod the boards was causing the problem, and he set out to discover what it was. He set up a series of mirrors in a large room at home and watched himself speak and recite. At first, he saw nothing. Then he noticed, as he boomed out *Hamlet* or *The Merchant of Venice,* that he was changing his posture and his whole manner of sound-making as he declaimed. He pulled his larynx *back* and gasped for breath. He lifted his chest and hollowed his back. And, most important, he changed the relationship of his head and neck, trying to lift his chin to an abnormally high position while counter-tilting his head "backward and down" (in his words).

What he was doing, it became clear, was squashing his speech-making apparatus, thus making making a living impossible. He tried to correct each of these bad habits separately but heard no improvement in voice and decided that he would have to change the use of his whole body to correct the situation. He added more mirrors to his system, watched himself from every conceivable angle and slowly developed what his disciples now call "Alexander's law"; "use," he decided, "determines functioning." How we use our bodies to achieve a particular end determines exactly how well we do it, how well we function.

With his mirrors, Mr. Alexander noted how parts of his body reacted to the process of speaking, picked out those things that added to his squashing tendency and tried to stop doing them. He tried for months, actually, but with no luck. His old bad habits, it seemed, were stronger than his good but new intentions. This lack of success led him to conclude that he would have to think consciously about *not* squashing his voice box *each* time he spoke, and to this end he designed a set of directions to send from his brain to the various muscle and bone structures involved, instructions to muscles in the neck to "release" instead of tensing (allowing his head to move "forward and up" rather than back and down), and to muscles in the back, allowing his spine to lengthen instead of arching into a question mark. When he gave himself these instructions (he called them "orders" when he wrote about the experience later), he found that he could override the bad habits and speak and recite without hoarseness and pain. He had "cured" himself by bringing an unconscious, involuntary process under conscious control. He had made an involuntary act voluntary and laid the cornerstone of his technique.

How the Alexander Technique Was Born

What happened next is unclear. How he got from his own remedy to a generalized plan of posture and body repair for everyone is not carefully documented in either Alexander's own writings or in those of his followers. Alexander's trouble was clearly centered on his head and neck, but so is his general body system. But why did he decide that all of man's mechanical problems could be solved by beginning with the head?

What seems to have happened is a story common to the development of all the body therapies and, indeed, to most kinds of physical therapy. Nearly everyone who deals with the use of the human body paints a picture of man oppressed by the forces of gravity, a glimpse of a frail little creature squished by an irresistible downward tug. The object of most of these systems, too, is to find a way of dissipating the effect of this force – to discover a way to use the equipment that man possesses to make the task as easy as possible, a way to bypass the pressure to the rigid bone structure, to the spongy, shock-absorbing discs between the vertebrae and to the fluid-filled joints between the limbs. The biggest obstacle to achieving this desirable end, Mr. Alexander (and many, many others) has decided, is the head, an eight- to ten-pound object that leads the body in most of its activities. If the head goes wrong, the body suffers. But if the

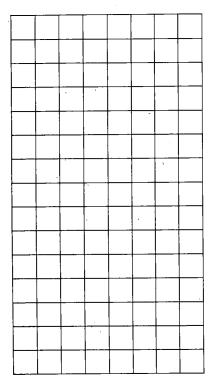

Alexanderians believe that many of the ailments we think come from specific sources— tennis elbow, for example— come from the general misuse we make of our bodies.

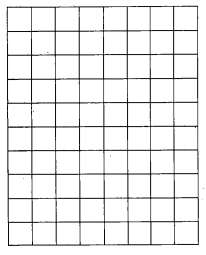

head is properly poised on the neck, and the neck is properly positioned on the spine, and so on down the body, most of the drag of gravity will be painlessly transferred from load-bearing structure to load-bearing structure.

Of course, the muscles will help in this transfer. They align the bones in such a way that the brunt of this burden can be passed efficiently from one to another. The posture sought by Alexander teachers is not the chest-out, spine-arched, arms-back pigeon-posture of the military academy but a stance that allows a straight line of force to be drawn from the back of the head through the neck, spine, pelvis, thighbones, shins and feet to the ground. So, if the head leads the body in running, walking and going around corners, it also shows the way standing still. If the body isn't carrying its brainy burden properly, it won't be able to do anything else well, either. This is the reason why Mr. Alexander felt all corrective work had to begin with a head-juggling act.

The Stupid Body

So far so good, but the next step in this saga (and in most body therapy stories) may be a little hard to swallow. According to one of Mr. Alexander's disciples, Wilfred Barlow, a British physician and teacher of the technique, the body is stupid, and it uses the remedial mechanisms at its disposal without a thought to the total health of its human inhabitor. Sometimes this tendency is harmless, as when some internal regulator senses a variation in the blood's chemistry and corrects it. But other times this process doesn't work quite so independently, and, unfortunately, muscular adjustments seem often to fall in this category. Faced with a particular physical task and being fully aware that it must work with an inherited muscular weakness in the right arm, for instance, or an old injury to the left knee, the stupid body may choose a simple but short-sighted means to its end. It may opt to do the task in a way that puts all the strain on one side – the strong side – of the frame. This may, if the task is frequently repeated, lead to a twisted posture and a weakness in the lower back – not to mention a hernia.

What's even worse is that the brain unconsciously aids the none-too-bright body with stupidities of its own. How we do certain things often has more to do with fashion and

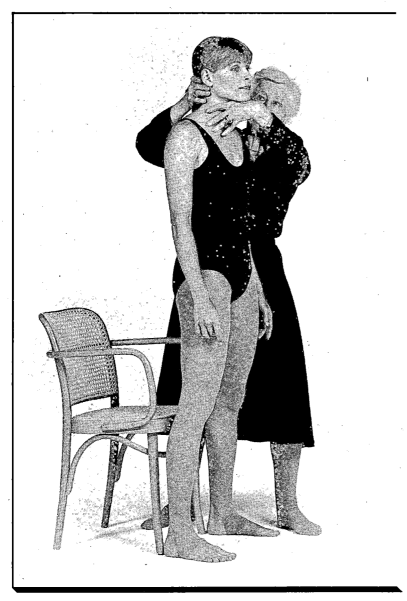

*The Countess Catherine Wielopolska shows a student how to
get in and out of a chair according to Alexander.*

imitation than it does with efficiency and comfort. We learn
to do things from our parents or from other people we
admire, and we seldom think to ask them if their back kills
them as they go through the task. The conclusion that convinced Alexanderians draw from this line of reasoning is

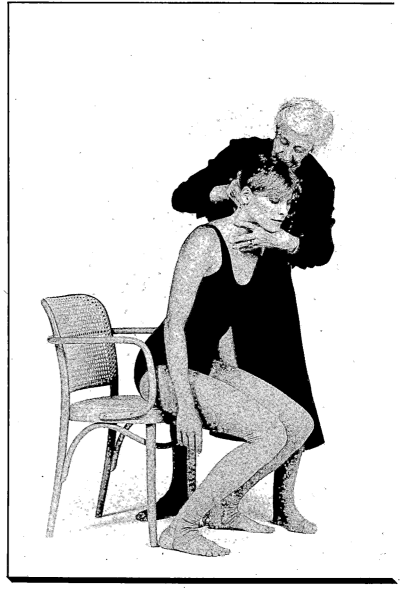

The direction of the head is all-important.

that many of the ailments we think come from specific sources – tennis elbow or football knee, for example – may be coming from the general misuse we make of our bodies while playing tennis or football. If use determines functioning, then misuse may determine almost all malfunctioning – or so say many true Alexander believers.

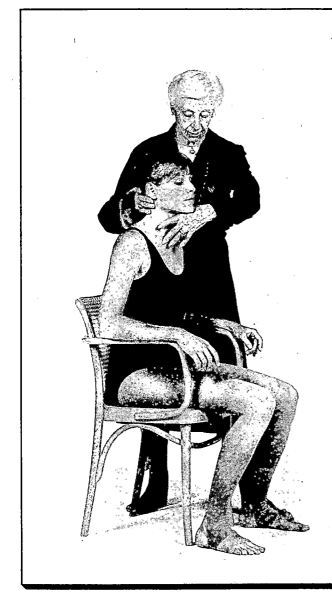

The student must slide all the way into the chair.

Alexander Students, Teachers and Student-Teachers

So, you're your own worst enemy, aided and abetted by your dumb-bunny body. Now what? You go to an Alexander teacher, who will take a practiced look at how you move and then seek to bring you to the point of self-discovery

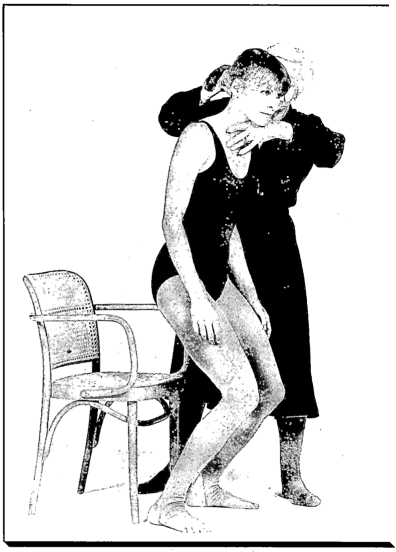

When rising, the head leads the way for the rest of the body.

that the Master himself achieved. This procedure begins with the head and neck and travels throughout the body, employing what has become known as the Alexander Technique. Partly, this is no more complex than "learning by doing," an element which attracted John Dewey, the American educational philosopher, to Mr. Alexander's work. But it is also not as simple as it sounds. In the words of Wilfred Barlow:

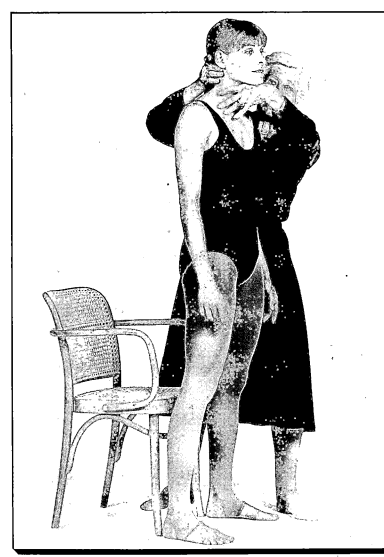

The correct Alexander style for standing after getting out of a chair.

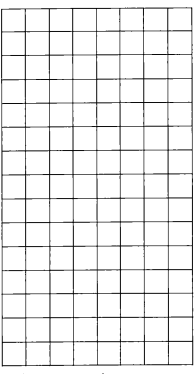

The Alexander technique shows people how they misuse their bodies and how they can prevent such misuse, during activity or at rest.

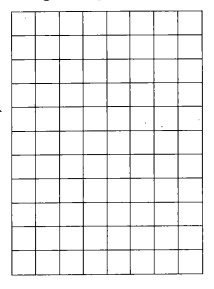

The Alexander technique is, briefly, a method of showing people how they are misusing their bodies and how they can prevent such misuse, whether it be at rest or during activity. This information about USE is conveyed by manual adjustment on the part of the teacher, and it involves learning of a new mental pattern in the form of a sequence of words which are taught to the patient or pupil, and which he

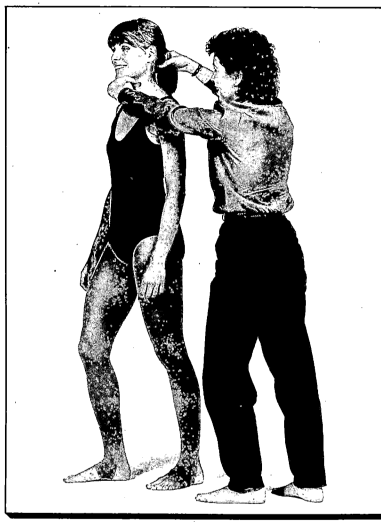

The head's direction also determines proper walking.

learns to associate with the new muscular use he is being taught by the manual adjustment. He learns to project this new pattern to himself not only while he is being taught but when he is on his own (*The Alexander Technique,* Alfred A. Knopf, 1973; reprinted with permission).

What this means is that Alexander teaching hopes to do two things at once: it wants to change the pupil's mental attitude about a movement at the same that it works on his

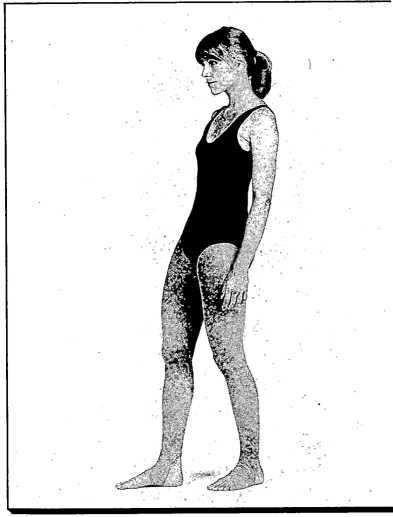

The wrong way to walk – leaning backward.

or her physical conditioning, or so-called "muscle-memory" of it. He or she is given verbal orders about how to stand up, for example, while the teacher gently guides his or her limbs through the act; the pupil both knows *and* feels what he or she must do to properly accomplish the motion. After many repetitions of this double-barreled process – so says the argument *and* a battery of scientific tests – the student takes over the role of teacher; the pupil gives himself the orders while correctly moving his or her limbs through the prescribed course of action.

Alexander's "Inhibition": How to Say "No" to Bad Habits

Now we've come to the moment of truth, quite literally, in this excursion through Alexander theory. F. M. Alexander and his brother, A. R., developed their method of bringing unconscious responses into conscious focus in order to give people an opportunity to choose between old behavior and new. Alexander teachers use their hands to let pupils experience in a quick, clear, "aha" way how both ways of doing something feel, how the new feels good and the old feels bad. When students can easily distinguish between the pleasure of one manner of acting and the near-pain of another, Alexander folks believe, they are in a position – the moment of truth – to stop taking the painful course and switch to the pleasurable one. This nay-saying is called "inhibition," and Alexander students, after many voluntary repetitions, are eventually able to return an act to its original unconscious, involuntary status with its changes intact. After deliberately choosing the good feeling, first under a teacher's guidance and then under their own power, pupils are finally able to do something the "right" way without thinking about it.

We Take Alexander to the Mat

This has all been pretty heady stuff, but now it's time to get down to the practical business of body work. We need to talk about what goes on in an Alexander lesson, and especially how it *feels*. To find *that* out, one of our authors subjected himself to the Body Therapy Workshop – which was led by practitioners of the four systems under discussion – of the American Dance Festival at Duke University in Durham, North Carolina. True to what we expected, most of the people in attendance were professional dancers or dance teachers. But, contrary to what we feared, the normal folks going through the week-long, ten-hour-a-day sessions were able to keep up with the (physically) abnormal folks without strain or exhaustion. The movements required by the Alexander Technique – and *all* the body therapies – contain much more enlightenment than sweat.

Our instructor was Deborah Caplan, M.A., R.P.T., from the American Center for the Alexander Technique in New

York City. She began by telling us many of the things we've just talked about. Then she told us that group lessons like ours – there were 75 people in the workshop – were frowned upon by most Alexanderians, because the technique's educational experience is necessarily an individual one. After that, she told us it would be better if we were lying on waist-high tables instead of the floor mats we had. The table position allows a teacher to see how a student's body reacts to the conditions of a lesson at the same time that it speeds communication between the instructor's sensitive hands and the pupil's muscles and muscle-memory – the chain of command that is the heart of any Alexander treatment. The teacher must be able to feel without straining what is right *and* wrong in the subject's actions, and the student must be comfortable enough to sense the subtle messages the tutor's fingertips are sending. How many times this quiet communication must occur to be effective is not a predetermined figure. Some teachers and pupils claim a feeling of improvement after the first lesson. But most students require at least 15 30- to 60-minute sessions to obtain the goals that brought them to Alexander. A few need many more, and one jaundiced reporter we read scoffed that the number of sessions prescribed often equals the number of years the client has lived. Of course, when the object of therapy is the reeducation of the whole body, even this exaggerated estimate seems conservative.

Finally, Ms. Caplan went through the crowd – along with an assistant, Jessica Wolf, another member of the New York Center's staff – and gave each of us a taste of individual Alexander attention. She and Ms. Wolf helped us to balance our heads properly and then to stand up and sit down without the usual burden on our neck and shoulder muscles. Here are the notes one of our authors made right after the experience:

The Alexander Technique: An Inside Story

Jessica (that's what she told me to call her) told me not to do anything. She told me to put myself in her hands – a pleasant prospect. Applying a powdery but unmistakably directive touch with her fingertips to the base of my skull, she lifted up, lengthening, it seemed, my neck and moving my head forward. My shoulders appeared to drop, and suddenly my head felt light; well, lighter. It almost bobbed on what

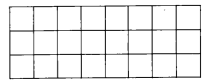

The Alexander Technique is used to help deal with many muscular and skeletal problems, for lower back pain, whiplash, postural imbalance, and misaligned feet and limbs.

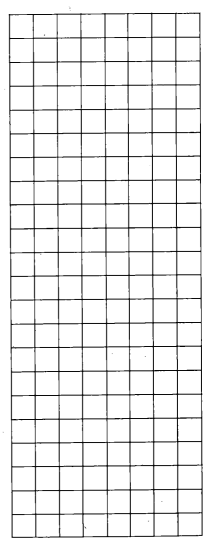

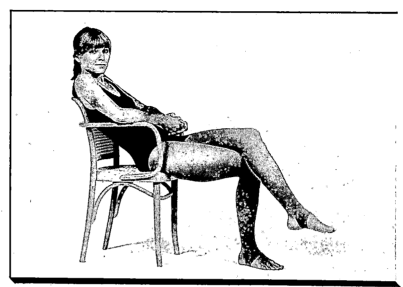

Sitting poorly stresses the whole body.

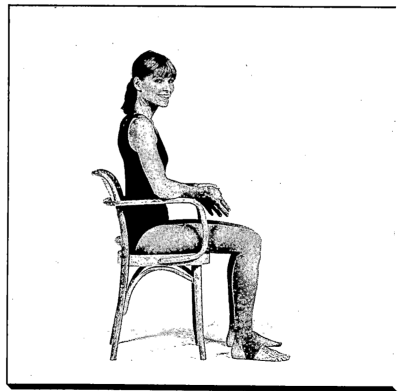

The proper way to sit.

may have been the point of my spine. I felt both good and like one of those dopey dogs in the back windows of certain cars. Then Jessica told me to stand up (I'd been sitting on a chair). As I did, she kept her fingerhold on my neck to remind me, she said, to "inhibit" any desire to change the position of my head. The first time up and down, it was tough. The unnatural situation I was in made me stand and sit in a pinwheel of angles, like a folding ruler falling down the stairs; I had to pitch my torso forward and throw my head back to get up enough steam to move. But I soon got used to having Jessica behind me, and I found her presence a help. I really did feel relieved of my head's weight and found I could glide up and down with a lot less effort than usual. I liked it. And I guess I'd been through an Alexander Experience. My first misadventures with getting up were attempts to move via my old habits. Ms. Wolf's hand pressure was an order to go at it in a new way, with my head properly held and balanced. And the pleasure with which I finally bounced up and down was the "aha" feeling that might eventually (if I kept at my Alexander lessons) teach me new habits. The whole experience was the difference between watching a parade with a child on your shoulders and watching it without the kiddo.

An Alexander Lesson You Can Try

All of which is fine, but one man's effusions cannot convince another that the Alexander Technique holds anything good for *him.* So here's a lesson you can try on yourself. It was designed as an introduction to the benefits of the system and printed in a textbook used by British students of the Master.

a. Find a place where you are not likely to be disturbed, and where, if necessary, you can lie down on the floor with a book under your head.

b. Lying down with a book under your head and with your knees pointing to the ceiling, decide consciously to keep quite still, and to inhibit reacting to stimuli; i.e., don't wriggle or scratch, and don't follow irrelevant patterns of thought. Give yourself the following verbal directions:

(i) "Neck release, head forward and up." As you give this sequence of thought, at first you will not "realize" what the direction means, but as you continue you will begin to associate it with an aware-

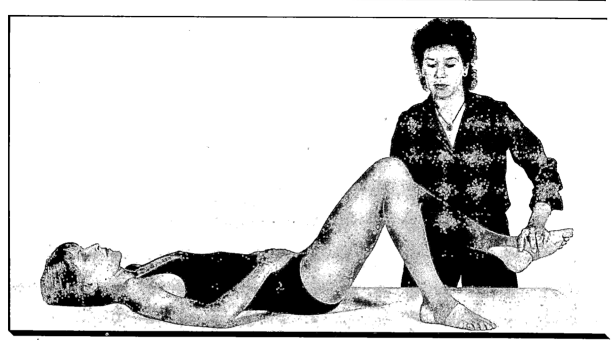

The Alexanderians like to use waist-high tables for body exams.

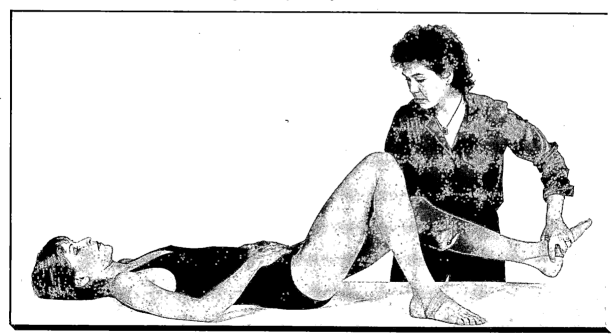

The therapist realigns the legs with the pelvis.

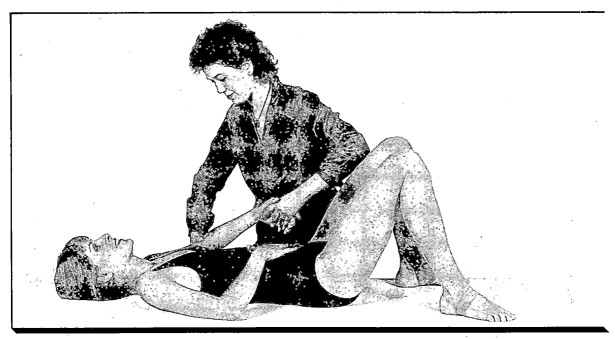

Releasing tense shoulder muscles frees the arms.

ness that you may previously have had either when working well on yourself or during a lesson. By "awareness" is meant what should be a normal sense of "being in yourself," as opposed to the state of mind-body split that is so often present in adults, if not in children.

(ii) While you are still preserving by direction this awareness of the head and neck – an awareness in which your verbal order will be part and parcel of the actual perception as the organizing component of it – add on the verbal direction "Lengthen and widen your back." Your lessons will already have made you familiar with the meaning of this phrase, and it is likely that fresh meaning and fresh simplification will accrue as you run over the sequence to yourself. For example, you may realize the whole of the back as lengthening in one unit instead of thinking of the upper back as separate from the lower back; or perhaps you may suddenly notice that widening the back includes releasing the shoulder blade and upper arm. At this point, your interest in the new realization may have caused you to "lose" the head direction, and it will be necessary to rein-

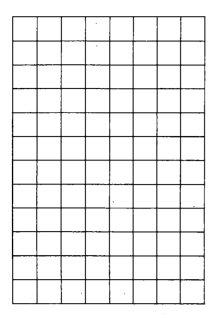

Certain respiratory illnesses, like asthma, can be helped by Alexander training, because its "release" of the chest and abdomen makes breathing easier.

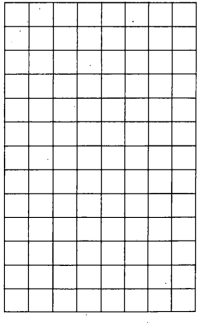

force it before returning to the lengthening and widening direction.

(iii) The process of adding together the direction to the head and the direction to the back may take several minutes or even longer: indeed, if it seems to take less time, you almost certainly have been making a muscular change by direct movement, instead of sticking to realizing the meaning of the orders. Remember that in this process we do not move our bodies in the same way as when we pick up an external object – a brush or a pen or a pail. To move our forearm is not the same as to move a spoon. Moving ourselves and bits of ourselves – as opposed to moving external objects – is always a question of allowing movement to take place, rather than of picking up and putting down somewhere else. Allowing the movement, say, of an arm will involve a total general awareness of the body; the active process involved in this particular movement is small compared with the active process of awareness that is going on in the whole of the body all of the time. Similarly, a movement of standing up after sitting down – a movement which involves mainly a leg adjustment – does not require only the leg activity, but primarily a maintenance of the awareness of the rest of the body while allowing the necessary leg movement to take place (*The Alexander Technique*, Alfred A. Knopf, 1973; reprinted with permission).

Going through these gyrations, of course, won't give you the sensation we had in North Carolina, but it will get you started on the Alexander jargon, and it will accustom you to concentrating on the tiny components of your body's movement while intriguing you with the possibility of interpreting them.

Some of the vocabulary here needs further explanation. The word "release" is used over and over again in the lesson. It does not mean "relax." It means that muscles and joints should be turned loose, should be free to assume their "natural" structural position, the position that best transfers the weight of the head from one bony element to another and then to the ground. The feeling of release around a joint or limb is actually the absence of muscle tension or contraction. As Ms. Caplan explained to us, there are four major areas of Alexander concern and four kinds of Alexander directions. They are:

1. The head – release the neck to let the head move

forward on the neck but up off the top of the spine. This is not a movement in space but a stable position of balance.

2. **The shoulders** – release the muscles of the shoulders so that they are free to go out to the side. The shoulder mechanism is actually a yoke – from which the arms hang – a yoke that must float on top of the torso at the spine just as the head floats on the neck.

3. **The torso** – release the muscles in the torso so that it may lengthen and widen and follow the head's direction, so that it may efficiently receive the head's weight. Remember that the head leads; the torso follows.

4. **The legs** – release the muscles in the hip joints until the knees (and legs) lengthen away from the pelvis. The pelvis is structurally part of the torso (in Alexander circles), and it should be allowed to act as a part of the torso. Proper torso-pelvic use frees the legs to act as independent load-bearing and bending joints.

The common factor in all of this is the goal of lengthening and lining up the body's parts. The most fundamental point in Alexander training is to change the balance of the head so that the muscles can align the bones and allow the body's weight to distribute properly. This, in turn, permits the body to move in its most efficient manner.

How the Alexander Technique Can Help You

So, what good does all this stuff do? To listen to a committed Alexanderian, nothing is beyond the ministry of the technique, not even organic disease or mental illness, the argument being that body misuse can cause weaknesses that reduce our resistance to bacteria or anxiety that becomes a chink in the psychological armor. Having seen a demonstration of the training, however, and having read its textbooks, we feel that the Alexander Technique is best considered a specialized form of physical therapy. That means that it can be used for the treatment of most muscular and skeletal problems, for lower back pain (for instance, lordosis and scoliosis, two kinds of spinal curvature), whiplash, all postural imbalance, misaligned feet and limbs, and the recovery from injury or broken bones. It is also commonly used to help "thaw" joints frozen by arthritis and rheumatism. Certain respiratory illnesses, like asthma, can be helped by Alexander training, because its "release" of the chest and

(continued on page 137)

BODY THERAPIES 133

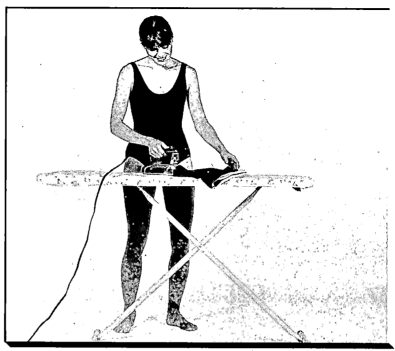

A good ironing stance.

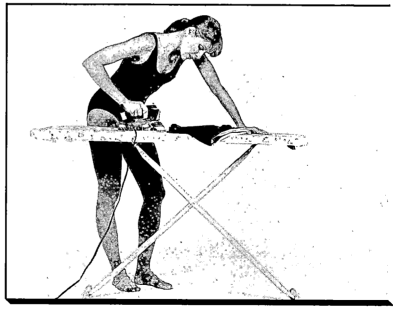

A stressful way to stand when ironing.

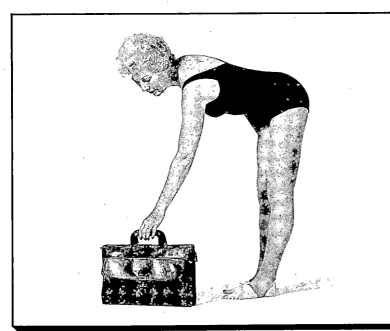

According to Alexander theory, this is the wrong way to pick up an object.

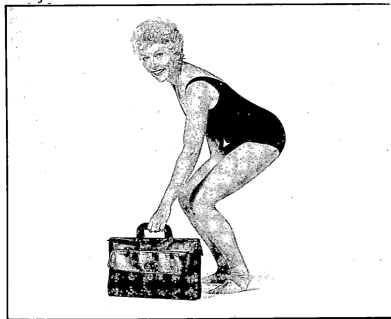

This stance agrees with the one favored by the Alexander Technique – knees are bent, back is fairly straight, feet are close.

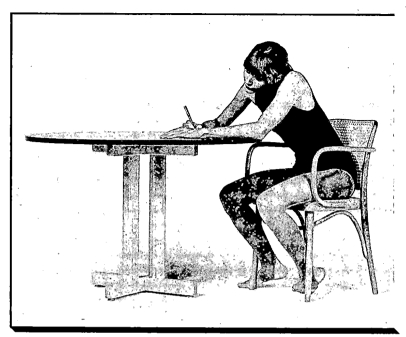

Don't slouch when working at a desk or table.

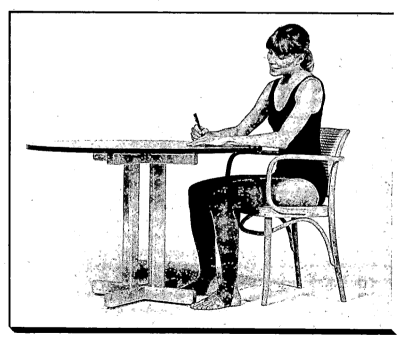

Sitting up straight is less stressful.

abdomen makes breathing easier. And, finally, there is some evidence that the freedom from muscular tension and fatigue that may accompany the mastery of the technique can help dissipate mental stress and depression.

Of course, what you need to get started in an Alexander way on whatever ails you is a teacher. You can find one of those by contacting the American Center for the Alexander Technique, 142 West End Avenue (at 66th Street), New York, NY 10023. The people there will give you the name and number of the qualified instructor nearest you.

The Moshe Feldenkrais Story

Moshe Feldenkrais is a fascinating man. He is so accomplished, so tenacious, so confident that will and intelligence can solve *any* problem man encounters, that one is almost inclined to believe in his Principles of Functional Integration *before* studying them. It's Dr. Feldenkrais, but his degree is a Ph.D. in physics, not medicine. Now in his seventies, Feldenkrais studied particle physics at the Sorbonne in France, attended lectures by Marie Curie, the discoverer of radium, and developed one of the machines that made experimental splitting of the atom possible. What's more, he is an innovator in judo, the holder of a black belt, and a doer of 007 derring-do for British Intelligence during the Second World War. He is clearly a developer of both mind *and* body.

Like Mr. Alexander, Dr. Feldenkrais's theories of physical therapy arose out of personal necessity. As a young man he was a skillful and maniacal soccer player. He chose to ignore the numerous injuries that went with the game, thinking they were no more than standard nuisances, but in 1940, at the age of 36, the accumulated damage of several years nearly crippled him. Doctors gave him a 50-50 chance of walking normally again after a new and risky surgical procedure, but the odds didn't appeal to him. So Dr. Feldenkrais – like Mr. Alexander again – decided to cure himself. He taught himself medicine, anatomy and physical therapy, then body mechanics, plain mechanical engineering and electrical engineering, even venturing into the then-virgin territory of learning theory. What came of this eclectic hodgepodge, this flurry of inspired pick-and-choose, was a school of thought which, in some ways, is the direct opposite of the Alexander Technique.

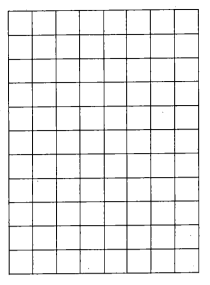

Feldenkrais believes that the solution to the body's troubles comes in an expansion of the brain's capacity to think its way through them. You reprogram the brain with new ways of sending messages to the rest of the body.

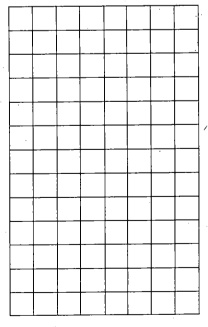

If the Alexander teacher seeks to put the student back in charge of his or her body's use, the Feldenkrais teacher wants to bypass certain of the student's conscious thought processes and *trick* his or her mind into new and more efficient control of the body. Although the Feldenkrais client is usually aware of what the instructor is doing, the teacher's goal may be to reprogram the movement centers in the patient's brain with *or* without his or her cooperation. You see, in Dr. Feldenkrais's system, tight, frozen, awkward – in some cases, even paralyzed – joints and muscle arrangements *do not exist.* According to the good doctor, these foul-ups actually occur in the brain, where some pattern of electrical relays, some bit of the soft computer's programming, has been destroyed, bungled or rearranged. To overcome movement problems, then, it is necessary to reprogram, to provide the brain with new options and new ways of sending messages to the affected bones and muscles. Physical training isn't what's required, because the problem isn't physical; it's mental. The solution to the body's troubles comes in an expansion of the brain's capacity to think its way through them. Stephen Appelbaum, Ph.D., a psychoanalyst who went into Feldenkrais therapy to say bad things about it, says (with considerable disbelief but clear admiration) about his experience:

> . . . we worked for some forty minutes on relaxing one shoulder so that it could meet the floor, but needed only a few minutes to do the same thing with the other shoulder. The brain had already learned the muscular arrangements that facilitated what seemed at first an impossible bodily position (*Out in Inner Space,* Anchor Press/Doubleday, 1979).

He didn't want to admit that Feldenkrais was on to something, but there it was.

Alexander and Feldenkrais

Reading Dr. Feldenkrais's most popular book, *Awareness Through Movement* (Harper and Row, 1977) – the one you should read if you'd like to introduce yourself to his techniques – can be a puzzling experience. In some ways, it sounds like a thank-you note to F. M. Alexander. Dr. Feldenkrais compares the efficient body to a well-oiled machine and claims that the goal of the exercises in his book is to eliminate all unnecessary effort and motion from human activity, to make man move in an ideal way. The book even argues that this ideal posture is one that transmits weight from bone to bone and allows the body to follow the lead of the head – just as Mr. Alexander did. According to Dr. Feldenkrais:

(continued on page 142)

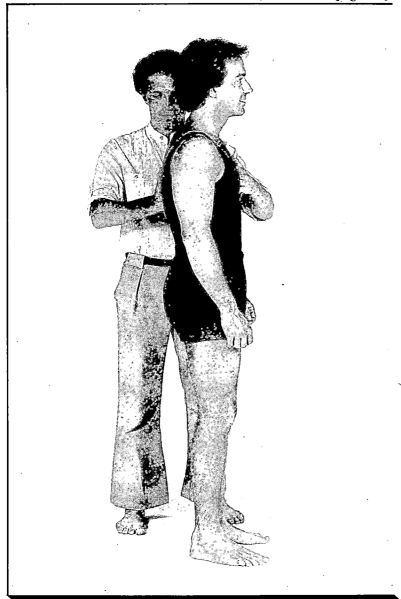

Russell Delman guides a patient through Feldenkrais movements.

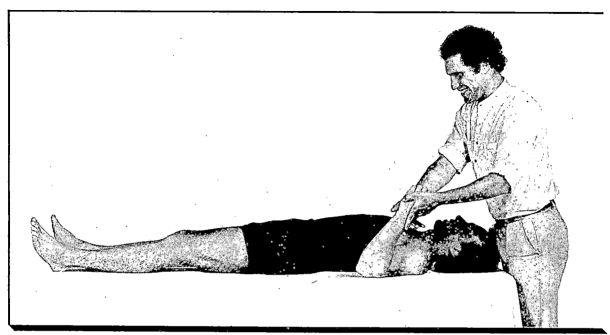

The therapist checks the function of each arm.

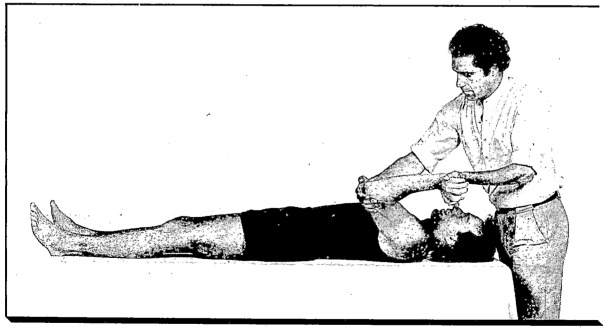

This gentle manipulation helps correct arm stiffness.

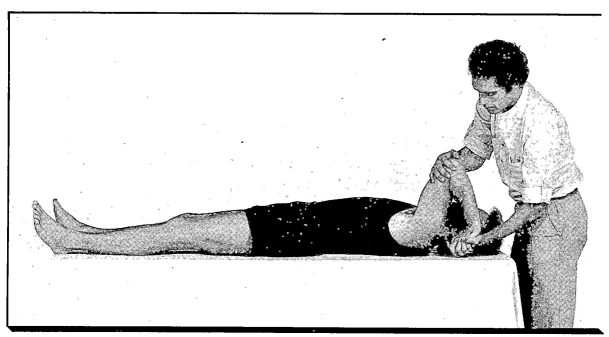

Rotating the arm teaches the brain new and more natural ways of controlling the limbs.

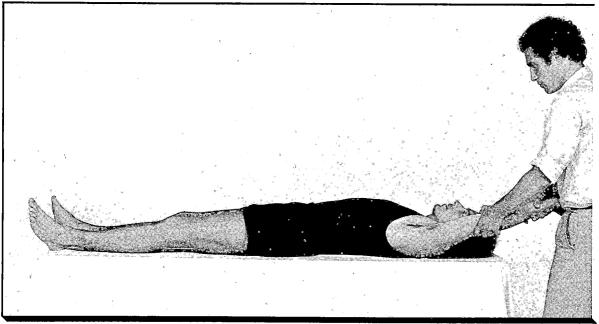

The therapist inspects the body's head-to-toe alignment.

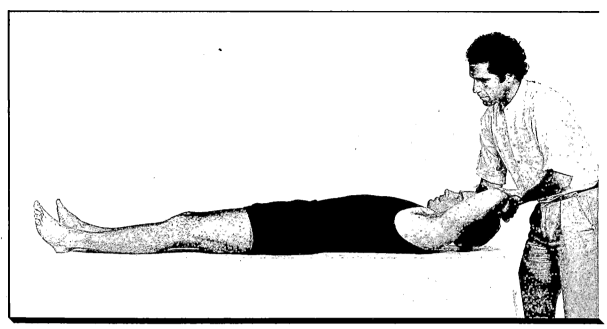

As the Feldenkrais therapist moves the arm, the rest of the body shifts, revealing muscular imbalances.

The ideal path of action for the skeleton as it moves from one position to another – say, from sitting to standing or from lying to sitting – is the path through which it would move if it had no muscles at all, if the bones were linked only by ligaments. In order to get up from the floor by the shortest and most efficient path, the body must be organized in such a way that the bones will follow the path indicated by a skeleton pulled up by its head (*Awareness Through Movement,* Harper and Row, 1977; reprinted with permission).

This means that most Feldenkrais treatments begin with attention to the head and neck, like Alexander treatment. On the other hand, Dr. Feldenkrais contradicts Mr. Alexander on important points. He feels that it is *not* possible to change bad physical habits by relying on "aha" sensations alone. Man becomes so used to the *feeling* of his habits, good or bad, that anything new will automatically seem abnormal and undesirable. As a result, Dr. Feldenkrais concentrates on brain changes rather than muscle changes. When "we refer to muscular movement," he writes in *Awareness Through Movement,* "we mean the impulses of the nervous system that activate the muscles, which cannot function without impulses to direct them. . . . Improvement in action and movement will appear only after a prior change in the brain and the nervous system has occurred."

Fooling the Body's Computer

Which leads, finally, back to trickery. In this example, which has been repeated with religious devotion by Feldenkrais converts, a writer who is taking the therapy for help with multiple sclerosis describes how the Master goes about convincing a reclining patient that she is standing up:

In his class the following day, coincidentally or not, he demonstrated the same thing with one of his students. "What am I doing?" he asked without pausing. "I know, I'm doing this damn silly thing with a breadboard. But what am I doing?" There were no answers.

"What's the function of a foot? To support a standing human. How does it function?" He got up and pretended to ski. "See? The ankle adjusts to keep the foot flat upon the ground and its owner from slipping. No matter what the angle. Now" – he went back to the girl's foot – "to make a perfect foot we must first relieve it of the weight of the body. One of Freud's most propitious discoveries was the couch. You see, I contend that all successful analysis is accompanied, and probably preceded, by a change in posture and muscular habits of the body and face. By laying his patients down and relieving the major extensor and flexor muscles of the habitual patterns of standing, a change could occur. Freud didn't know this, of course. He laid patients down because he didn't like looking them in the eye. Particularly when they were talking about sex.".

The old man looked pleased by the laughter and turned back to the girl. "So we lay her down and then, by touching her foot like so, convince her cerebral cortex that she is really standing. On a slope. Look!" He touched the outside edge of the sole with it as he spoke and the girl's foot turned to meet the board full face while she watched, as much a spectator as the rest of us. He took the board away and touched the inside edge, and the foot turned to flatten itself against the board again.

He teased the foot with his board. "We have made this an intelligent foot. Her brain is working it perfectly, because there is no possibility for the habitual mistakes this girl makes in standing."

When the student on whom he did the breadboard demonstration in class stood up, it was obvious that, through her foot, Feldenkrais had changed the organization of her entire neuromuscular system. Her left eye was visibly larger, the left side of her mouth more relaxed, her left shoulder several inches lower than her right (*Quest/78,* December, 1978-January, 1979).

The goal here is to teach the woman new ways of standing. By working with a breadboard while she lies before him, Dr. Feldenkrais can teach her brain how to say "Stand up" to her feet, and he can do it without tiring her (with struggles against gravity) or frustrating her (with difficult commands to follow or actions to imitate).

We Get Down on the Floor Again

Now it's time to go back to the Body Therapy Workshop at Duke. We've come about as far as we can with theory here, and it's time to get down on the floor again. The Feldenkrais instructor at the workshop was Norma Leistiko from San Francisco.

Ms. Leistiko began her presentation by laying some ground rules. Feldenkrais people do *not* frown upon group lessons, and the "Awareness Through Movement" program is designed specifically for them. But they do recommend individual treatment, called Functional Integration, for serious defects. There is no established number of sessions in a Feldenkrais "cure," and there is no age requirement for patients. Dr. Feldenkrais, we were told, has a large practice involving children, infants and people over 80 years old in Israel. Treatments for little ones tend to last about 15 minutes apiece, but the optimum length for an adult lesson seems to be somewhat under an hour; about 40 minutes is the average. The Master's teaching says that the patient's ability to perceive and absorb dwindles after that. Most Feldenkrais sessions begin with a very brief discussion of why the patients are seeking help and then move on to a series of exercises on the floor. At first, the teacher merely wants to see how the patients mold to the floor while lying on their backs or

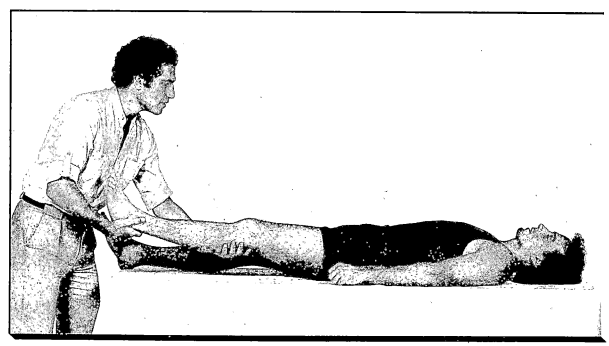

Stiffness reveals body areas that need work.

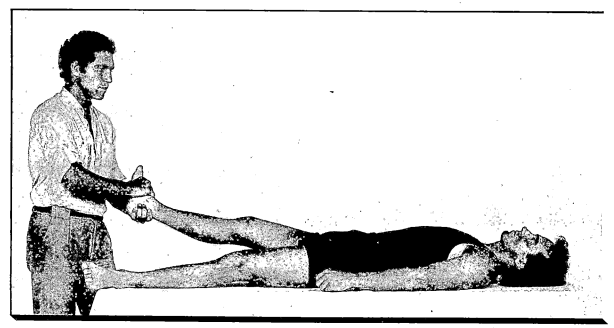

Improving how the foot works can relieve aches and pains in the rest of the body.

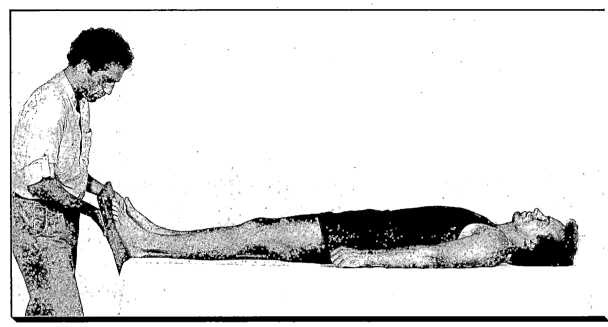

The therapist uses a breadboard to teach the foot a new way of standing.

sides and then while sitting. The teacher is looking for stiffness and imbalance, whether both sides behave in the same way, and whether one side is more or less supple and responsive.

Once this step is out of the way, some additional but equally simple exercises are asked of the patients, exercises that may or may not be guided by the instructor's hands. The purpose here is to watch how the major joints of the body slide in and out, open and close, to detect stiffness – if it's there – or to note ease – if *it's* there. All these manipulations, of course, are diagnostic as well as therapeutic and will help the teacher plan later sessions. Those sessions will contain more of the same kind of exercises, but they are chosen and ordered in ways that will show the student what the teacher has learned, ways that will eventually teach the brain new ways of commanding the body.

How a Feldenkrais Treatment Feels

The mood that descended upon us as Ms. Leistiko led us through these sequences was extremely pleasant, even luxurious and languorous. Her voice was soothing. The movements were small and easy to make. We got sleepy, despite the hard gym floor and the miserable summer day. But, strangely, we *did* feel what we were supposed to feel: that one hip (perhaps) moved through its range of motion more easily than the other, that one shoulder relaxed into the mat while the other could not. For this kind of Feldenkrais attention, obviously, one needs a trained instructor. To contact one of those, one needs the Feldenkrais Guild, Ms. Leistiko's organization, in California. A letter or call to the folks there will get you a "Directory of Guild Members" across the U.S., Canada, Europe and Israel. The address is 1776 Union Street, San Francisco, CA 94123. The directory is regularly updated.

Practicing Feldenkrais on Your Own

To practice Feldenkrais on your own, you need the book *Awareness Through Movement,* its sample of the Feldenkrais exercises published, and this warning: self-treatment is *not* as effective as guided treatment. Beyond those things, some simple basics should get you going. Dr. Feldenkrais feels that if you are putting yourself through his training, you should plan to run through the paces just before bedtime (at least an hour after eating) and turn in after finishing. His reasons are apparently twofold: he clearly hopes that the exercises will relieve some of the tension and fatigue of the day, and he also may feel that the mind is more receptive to his information at that time.

Students guiding themselves through the 12 stages of *Awareness Through Movement* are also told to wear as little as possible during their efforts. The goal is to eliminate all sensations but those provided by the movement of the body through the routines. Any confinement, most buttons and all zippers can produce messages of discomfort that may obscure the real subject of the program. For similar reasons, a large floor area is required. Dr. Feldenkrais wants to avoid information from bumped furniture, and, of course, he feels you should be exercising alone or with just a single helper to read his instructions. It's your body he wants you to hear. As you can see, Feldenkrais lessons take time, up to 45 minutes for a self-taught session, because he wants students to go through the sequences in short bursts, reading a portion of the directions, doing their bidding and

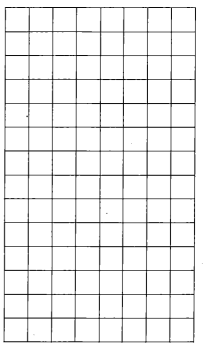

During Feldenkrais exercise, the goal is to eliminate all sensations but those provided by the movement of the body through the routines.

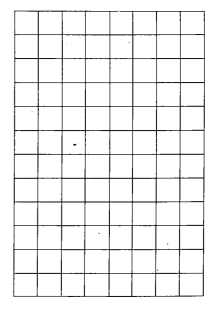

then moving on. But even that's too simple. He feels that his motions should be repeated a number of times – at first 10 times and then 25 – until they feel "normal" and natural. Only when all the strangeness and self-consciousness has gone out of the process will it begin to speak to the doer. This, however, will not be tiring, because Feldenkrais exercises are, by nature, easy. Their inventor believes that difficult maneuvers teach people about difficulty instead of about their bodies.

A Feldenkrais Lesson to Try

There you have it: Moshe Feldenkrais's Principles of Functional Integration. To understand more, you will have to try some of the doctor's movements, and so, to finish off this section, you may want to window-shop through this lesson entitled "Some Fundamental Properties of Movement":

In this lesson you will learn to recognize some of the fundamental properties of the control mechanisms of the voluntary muscles. You will find that about thirty slow, light, and short movements are sufficient to change the fundamental [tone] of the muscles, that is, the state of their contraction before their activation by the will. Once the change of [tone] is effected, it will spread to the entire half of the body containing the part originally worked on. An action becomes easy to perform and the movement becomes light when the huge muscles of the center of the body do the bulk of the work and the limbs only direct the bones to the destination of the effort.

Scan the state of your body
Lie down on your back. Place your legs a comfortable distance apart. Stretch your arms out above your head, slightly apart, so that the left arm will be approximately in a straight line with the right leg and the right arm in line with the left leg.

Close your eyes and try to check the areas of the body that are in contact with the floor. Pay attention to the manner in which the heels lie on the floor, whether the pressure upon them is equal, and whether the point of contact is at exactly the same points at both heels. In the same way examine the contact made with the floor by the calf muscles, the back of the knees, the hip joints, the floating ribs,

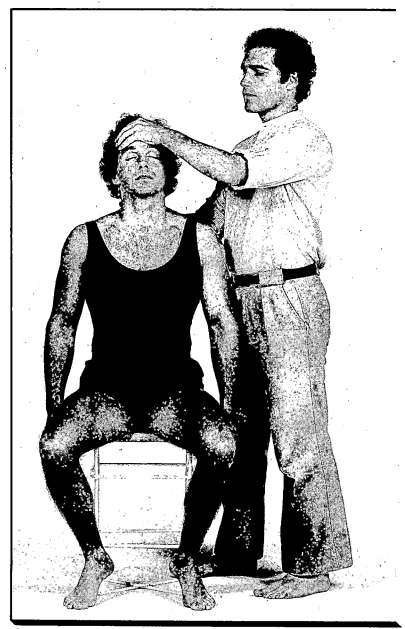

The therapist realigns the neck and upper back.

the upper ribs, and the shoulder blades. Pay attention to the respective distances between the shoulders, elbows, wrists and the floor.

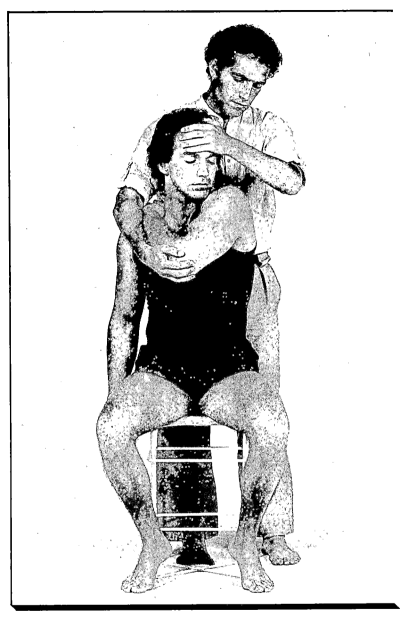

This unusual movement helps the upper body to function as a stress-free unit.

A few minutes of study will show that there is a considerable difference between the two sides of the body at the shoulders, elbows, ribs, and so forth.

Many people will find that in this position their elbows do not touch the floor at all but are suspended in space. The arms do not rest on the ground, and it becomes difficult to maintain them in this position until the examination is over.

We have a coccyx, five lumbar, twelve dorsal, and seven cervical vertebrae. On which vertebrae in the pelvic region is pressure heaviest? Do all the lumbar vertebrae (girdle) touch the floor? If not, what is raising them above the floor? On which of the dorsal or back vertebrae is pressure heaviest? At the beginning of this lesson most people will find that two or three of the vertebrae make clear contact with the floor while the others form arches between them. This is surprising, because our intention was to lie at rest on the floor, without making any effort or movement, so that in theory each of the vertebrae and ribs should sink to the floor and touch it at least at one point. A skeleton without muscles would indeed lie in this way. It seems, therefore, that the muscles raise the parts of the body to which they are attached without our being conscious of it.

It is impossible to stretch out the entire spine on the floor without a conscious strain upon several sections. As soon as this conscious effort is once more relaxed, the sections affected will again move up and away from the floor. In order to settle the whole of the spine on the floor we must stop the work the muscles are doing without our knowledge. How can we do this if deliberate and conscious effort is not successful? We shall have to try an indirect method (*Awareness Through Movement*, Harper and Row, 1977; reprinted with permission).

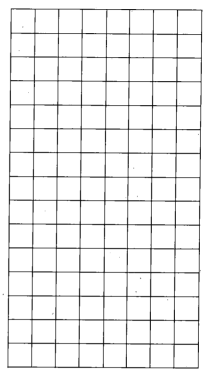

According to Feldenkrais, difficult exercises teach people about difficulty instead of about their bodies. So he makes his exercises easy.

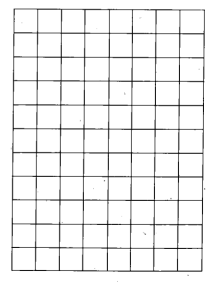

But let's stop here. We have only the first two of what become nine closely linked pages, but you get the idea. Dr. Feldenkrais is asking you to interpret answers provided by your own body, but he is asking the questions in such a way that it is difficult to miss the point.

And now we get to the minor leagues, not in quality, certainly, but in quantity. The methods of body therapy devised by Mabel Todd and Lulu Sweigard and the system developed by Irmgard Bartenieff have both supporters and success stories aplenty. They seem to have the product. What they *don't* have is distribution. It's very hard to have either of these things done to you outside of New York City.

Irmgard Bartenieff's Fundamentals

Bartenieff Fundamentals is the body therapy most closely associated with professional dancers, because Ms. Bartenieff is a student and disciple of Rudolf Laban, a refugee from Nazi Germany and a god in dance circles. Laban, who is also revered by physical therapists, invented Laban Movement Analysis, or Labananalysis. This system studies how well (or ill) people move by breaking their motion into component parts and records the effort involved. The hieroglyphics (called Labanotation; Rudolf liked word collisions) he developed to write down the things he observed in his patients is the most widely used method of recording dance steps and is still a valuable tool in the laboratory study of movement. Despite Laban's impressive pedigree, though, Ms. Bartenieff, now in her eighties, may be the more imposing figure, for she has turned Laban's concern for nearly weightless (and boneless) dancers into practical stuff that helps less-than-perfect bodies move and feel better. One has only to see her in action, as we did in North Carolina, to be bowled over. The hip joint is an important focus in the Bartenieff Fundamentals. During a lecture about the hip, she: (1) lifted the leg of a volunteer guinea pig at the joint and, with *one hand,* (2) practically removed it from the pelvic socket in order (3) to use the now-free limb as something like a pointer.

Of course, she also wanted the victim-volunteer to experience, as she said, "the ease and free range of movement *possible* with the joint by eliminating all superfluous muscle tension around it." Ms. Bartenieff is a wonder.

The idea that lights the bulb in these fundamentals says that if we are to get rid of the bad movement habits that parents, gym teachers and trick knees have given us, we'd better also re-create many of the situations that produced the learning in the first place. We'd better relearn the way we learned as a child. Children, of course, don't master twirling spaghetti around a fork on specific Tuesdays. First they acquire basic movement patterns – to scoop and then to grab, to lift their heads, turn over, creep, crawl, stand, and finally to walk. And then, as this piling-on process proceeds, other activities the child sees and tries to imitate serve to combine basic patterns into more complex behavior. Catching and throwing a ball inspires hand-eye coordination and lower-body cooperation. Tag, baseball, leap-frog, statue and so forth add other new and more compli-cated skills like running, twisting and falling in a painless heap. Learning goes on and on, until the child's whole complement of adult capabilities is available. The nice things about this process are that it takes place in small, non-threatening chunks and that it's fun. These are also the nice things about the Bartenieff Fundamentals. This relearning system asks a patient to dice his movement habits into tiny, tiny pieces that can be remastered without sweat or strain, and it often employs big, swooping, even dancelike motions which are fun to do.

The Principles of Bartenieff Therapy

Although Ms. Bartenieff and her colleagues at New York's Laban Institute break their training into four principal areas, those of us who attended her demonstrations at the Body Therapy Workshop got to see only one of them, one which

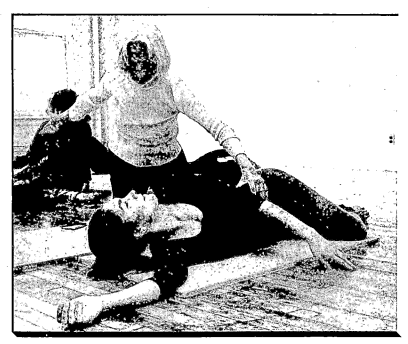

Irmgard Bartenieff instructing a pupil.

showed the techniques involved in shifting the body's weight from side to side and front to back. But before we get to that experience, let's talk briefly about the other three.

1. "Dynamic alignment" is what passes for posture build- ing with Bartenieff. It aims to create a stance in each patient which is literally *ready for anything*. It is *not* a stand-up/don't slouch! proposition but an arrange- ment of muscles, bones and brain messages that makes an individual flexible and able to react to anything his surroundings throw up, be it a dirty trick or a pleasant surprise.

2. "Body attitude" is an airy concept which seems to be the emotional counterpart of "dynamic alignment." It deals with the way our bodies reflect our feelings and produce a personal and fleshy signature: it's not for nothing, for instance, that we say a person is "up" or "down." We don't know about you, but we're more used to seeing personal signatures in professional danc- ers than in CPAs, but there *is* a point here. One's way of holding his or her body should not mask or stifle emotions. The more freely the emotions can escape or express themselves, the better one feels.

3. Lots of attention is given to the "initiation of move- ment" in the creation of exercise sequences in Fun- damentals training. This is true for a very simple reason. How well we do something – whether it's serving a tennis ball, running a 60-yard dash, leaping across the stage or getting up out of a sofa – depends on how well we get the whole business started. If the tennis player flubs the toss-up or the TV watcher his or her pitch forward to the edge of the couch, the rest of this person's action will be more tiring, less efficient and more embarrassing than it needs to be.

A Fundamental Experience

The segment of Ms. Bartenieff's therapy we encountered at Duke deals, as we said, with the transfer of weight in space and is probably the most playful of the four. While the other areas of Fundamental concern use the small, subtle movement of the other body therapies, the exercises designed to train students to move their bulk properly are large, fluid and fun in a swirling, dervish sort of way. We know what you're thinking. You have a desk job, and you don't shift weight that often, but – sure, you do. You transfer weight from position to position each time you swing a baseball bat or golf club; each time you go up or down the stairs; each time, in fact, you walk or stand up or sit down. So, the transfer of weight is crucial to most activities, and it's important, according to Bartenieff teachers, to do it smoothly, even flowingly, and with an evenness of effort and force. Once again, the efficiency with which the job is done is the telltale factor.

All of which sounds pretty dull – but isn't, really. The gyrations we were asked to go through in order to, first, test our own weight-transfer habits and, then, to oil them required pleasant cartwheels of action. We were asked to reach down to the floor with our right hand, bending at the knees and waist and stepping up with the right foot. And then to swoop back, with the right arm coming across the body and moving over the head, all the while stepping back with the right foot (again). This led to a quarter turn on that right foot and a whipping around of the left. Which led to . . . well, the idea was to put us in scrapes in which we *almost* lost our balance and *had to* shift our weight quickly – and however gracefully – to keep from flopping. This funny and silly series of predicaments made us look like clumsy discus throwers until Ms. Bartenieff began to tinker with our weight-shifting efforts; then, they smoothed out. There were no Nijinskys, but there was a good deal of comfortable, refreshing motion.

If this seems appealing – and it should – you might try finding a Bartenieff-trained teacher to help you into it. To do that, contact the Laban Institute of Movement Studies, 133 West 21st Street, New York, NY 10011. Ms. Bartenieff's book *Body Movement: Coping with the Environment* (written with Dori Lewis, 1980) can be obtained from Gordon and Breach Science Publishers, 1 Park Avenue, New York, NY 10016.

Mabel Todd and Lulu Sweigard

Let's be straight about this. When the letter came from the American Dance Festival about its Body Therapy Workshop, the Todd-Sweigard technique *sounded* crazy. The letter said we should bring along a floor mat, a pillow, a pair of knee pads and a rope or belt to bind our legs. Crazy, right? Not so crazy, it turned out.

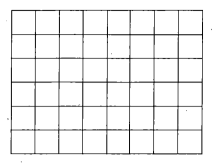

Irmgard Bartenieff teaches that to get rid of the bad movement habits we learned when we were young, we have to relearn them as if we were children again.

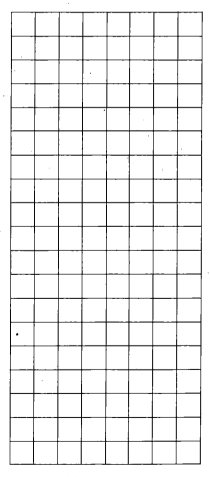

Todd-Sweigard therapy, or ideokinetic therapy, is even more closely associated with New York City than the Bartenieff Fundamentals. Mabel Todd taught physical therapy at Columbia Teachers College, and her movement theories were developed in classes there. Lulu Sweigard was Todd's student at Columbia, a teacher in New York University's physical education department, and later a PT teacher in the dance department of the Juilliard School of Music, where she helped Ms. Todd's ideas grow up. And the Todd-Sweigard collaborations are now being kept alive by André Bernard, who studied with both women, in his work at New York University's School of the Arts and School of Education.

How the Thinking Body Moves

The point of Ms. Todd and Ms. Sweigard's work is best expressed in the title of Ms. Todd's first book, *The Thinking Body: A Study of Balancing Forces of Dynamic Man* (Dance Horizon, 1968). The human being is a coupling of body and mind; it is a machine with the ability to think complicated thoughts, the tin woodsman in *The Wizard of Oz*. Which is also to say that between the desire to move in a particular way and the execution of that act comes a picture in the mind, of the hop or jump or whatever way we happen to move. This being true for Ms. Todd and Ms. Sweigard, they decided that the best way to change how people moved, or to teach them difficult new maneuvers, was to alter the mental picture – at least to go through it to the body's muscles, bones and joints. Like Dr. Feldenkrais, they guessed that to change movement one had first to change the brain impulses that triggered that movement. As a result of all this, we have "ideokinetic therapy," a word and a treatment philosophy that combine "ideo" (the idea, or stimulator of action) and "kinesis" (physical movement).

A major brainstorm which follows automatically from these decisions is that change in movement habits is *not* something that can best be accomplished by conscious effort; practice does not make perfect in this case. So Ms. Todd and later Ms. Sweigard, like Dr. Feldenkrais still later, set about creating unconscious, involuntary ways to do it, ways of *fooling* the body into change. They drew up games to be played with mental suggestions. But stop. To see this we have to leave the textbooks and go back to North Carolina. Todd-Sweigard seems goofy until you feel it with your own body.

A Crazy Experience That Made Good Sense

André Bernard asked us to team up with partners and pick one from each couple to lie down and be worked on. We did. We lay on our backs, put pillows under our heads, bent the legs at knees and tied them together – to avoid having to hold the legs up, Mr. Bernard said. Then he switched to an anchorman's voice and gently told the reclining member of each team to think of himself or herself as a suit of clothes. What? Yes, an *empty* suit of clothes suspended by the knees from a hanger dropped from the ceiling. What would it feel like, said he, to have the arms and legs – pardon, *sleeves* and legs – collapse against themselves? Relax. How does it feel? Pretty good, but . . . Yes, there are *wrinkles* in the suit, and they're uncomfortable. Let's smooth them out. He asked the kneeling partners, who were wearing knee pads, to reach under shoulders, backs and then legs to lightly smooth out coats and pants down the back. They did, and the strangest thing happened. Our wrinkles *moved* out with their hands, and with the wrinkles' exit came a feeling that the back's muscles were going out, too, relaxing, widening, moving into the floor. For that, Mr. Bernard explained later, was the goal of all this make-believe: to make backs that were tight with tension and bunched with stooping longer and wider, to put them in what Todd-Sweigard considers a more natural and efficient condition. And it worked. Oh, the feeling wasn't earth-shattering – it was more like water or suntan oil trickling, then flowing across the muscles – but it was there nonetheless. In fact, the feeling was there repeatedly for three hours as we continued to be imaginary suits of clothes, as we unrumpled pants, pulled shirt collars out of jackets and did countless other sartorial and postural refurbishments. Crazy it sounds, but it seems to work.

Anyway, if this sounds good to you, get in touch with André Bernard at New York University's School of the Arts, 40 East 7th Street, New York, NY 10003; he may have the name of a Todd-Sweigard therapist near you.

CALISTHENICS

Calisthenics – the sound of the word is enough to make grown men tremble. Grown women, too. Even the thought of these feared exercises has been known to set off loud groaning in children. But why all the negative vibes? Where have all the bad feelings about calisthenics come from? The answer is: drudgery and pain. That's what you associate with calisthenics.

Remember when you were in junior high, waiting in line to get into the auditorium to hear Mrs. White's ninth grade class whine through the overture to *Swan Lake* on their recorders, and Charlie Jones, the kid with the wart on his left ear, started misbehaving, having the audacity to poke and tease the pretty little red-haired girl after Mr. Catatonic, the guidance counselor, had just asked everyone to PLEEEEZE stop fidgeting and be quiet? And do you remember Charlie's punishment?

"Okay, Jones," bellowed Mr. Catatonic, his skinny little tie bobbing over his Adam's apple. "Twenty-five push-ups! Now!"

And poor Charlie, president of the Future Construction Workers of America and treasurer of the Russian Club, would be down on all fours pushing up and down on the dusty linoleum, trying to keep his nose out of the discarded bubble gum.

What did Mr. Catatonic have in mind? Charlie's physical fitness? His mental acuity? No way. What Mr. Catatonic was aiming for was *torture*.

But while Mr. Catatonic thought that he was punishing Charlie Jones, the truth is that he was probably doing him a favor.

"Some favor," you might snort. Yet, the fact is that calisthenics can be *good* for you. They don't have to hurt. And they aren't just for torturing classroom smart alecks.

Keeping Your Joints Limber

One of the most important things that calisthenics can do for you is help preserve the "range of motion" of your joints. That means the movements you perform during many calisthenics actually preserve your ability to perform that motion *any*time. Instead of your joints rusting up – instead of arthritis setting in, for instance – they remain flexible and painfree. "The one thing all your joints have in common is their need to be put through their full range of motion in order to function properly," says Rex Wiederanders, M.D., author of *Biotonics* (Funk and Wagnalls, 1977).

Dr. Wiederanders points out that babies' joints are "marvelously fluid and free from pain" because they "run their joints through the full range of motion almost instinctively." They flop and twist and stretch and bend like rubber mannequins.

With calisthenics, you can "baby" yourself at any age.

You can also increase your strength. Done properly, calisthenics are as effective as weightlifting – without the expense of buying weights. A push-up, for instance, can be the equivalent of lifts such as the military press or the bench press (described in the chapter on weight training).

Before you try a full-fledged push-up, however, try the modified variety. Kneel down and then lean forward, with your hands on the floor, your arms straight and your weight on your hands and knees.

Try to keep your back straight. Your hands should be directly under your shoulders. Bending your arms slowly, let your body down until it is just above the floor. Then straighten your arms to bring your body back up to the starting position. For starters, do five modified push-ups.

How did they feel? If they were difficult, but you could manage to do five of them without feeling like you were pushing yourself to the limit, then you've found a good level at which to start regularly performing the exercise. But if doing five of these modified push-ups was impossible, don't despair. All you need is a little work to get your neglected muscles back in shape. At the onset, however, you want to do only as many repetitions of a particular exercise as you can without feeling strained. (With time, you'll probably be able to do as many repetitions as we suggest.) Do more, and chances are you'll only succeed in hurting yourself. This advice, of course, goes for all the calisthenics in this chapter.

The modified push-up primarily develops the muscles of your chest and on the back of your arms. Your ability (or inability) to do it measures the strength you have in these areas.

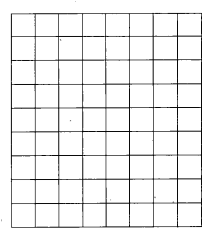

Calisthenics help keep your joints flexible and painfree instead of letting them rust up.

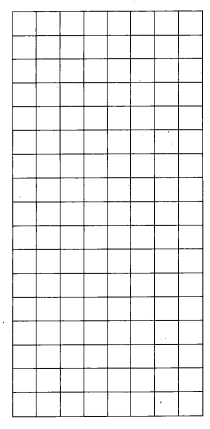

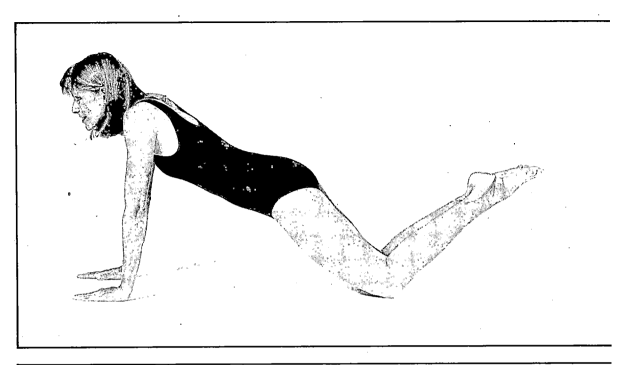

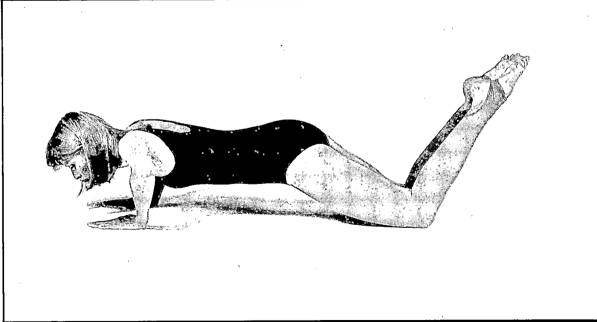

1. You begin the modified push-up on your hands and knees. 2. Lower your chest to the ground.

A Push in the Right Direction

When the modified push-up starts to feel easy, you're ready to advance to the regular push-up. But don't move on too soon. You should be able to do around 15 modified push-ups comfortably before you tackle the full push-up.

During the full push-up the upper half of your body is in the same position as during the modified: hands on the floor, arms straight. But this time, you keep your knees *off* the floor, supporting your lower half with your toes (see photo on next page).

Once in the position, slowly lower your body to within an inch or two of the floor by bending your arms, and then push your body back up into the starting position. Do not bend your knees or hips at any time.

How did that feel? A push-up not only gives your back and stomach muscles a workout but also develops the triceps, the muscle along your upper arm. You'll know you're well on your way to developing strength in those areas when you can do ten or more push-ups.

For Fast Progress, Go Slow

Before you move on to the other calisthenics, here are some rules you should follow when doing the exercises.

Don't work yourself into a state of sweaty exhaustion. Especially not the first few sessions. That's just asking for sore, tight muscles. Your body will adjust to tough physical workouts if given the chance, so give it the chance.

Some people still think of themselves physically as young kids with bodies that can take a lot of punishment and quickly rebound. When you're a little older, particularly if you've been relatively inactive, that kind of thinking can literally hurt you.

So take the advice of *The Official YMCA Physical Fitness Handbook* (Popular Library, 1975): "Avoid working without letup. Work, then rest, then resume work, and so on. The adult body can adapt to effort if a rest period permits it to accommodate to exercise before starting again."

Don't work one muscle or set of muscles to the exclusion of the others. You've got a whole body to strengthen and tone, not just arms or legs.

As a general rule, don't do more than two consecutive

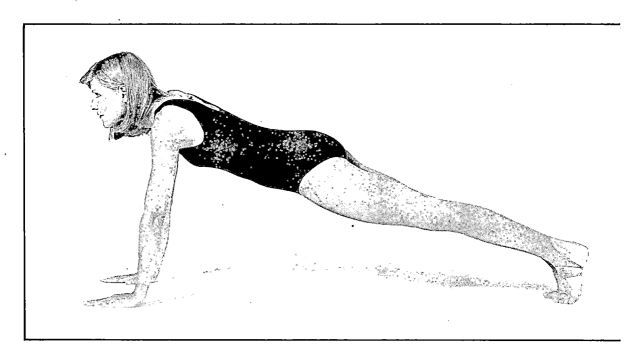

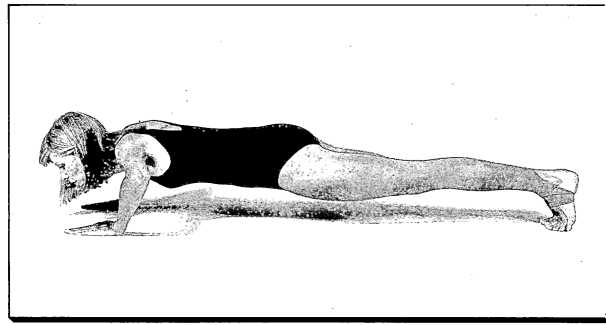

1. A regular push-up begins on your hands and toes. 2. Bend your elbows and almost touch your chest to the ground.

exercises that work on the same body area. Switch to a movement that uses a fresh set of muscles and then come back to that area if you feel it needs more work. For instance, if you do thigh tucks and then side leg raises (which we describe later), both of which develop – and put strain on – the leg muscles, you won't want to immediately follow them by another exercise that uses leg muscles. Instead, switch to sit-ups.

Don't bounce – push. If, for instance, an exercise calls for touching your toes with your knees straight and you can't quite make it down there, the worst thing you can do is bounce to get your fingers where you want them, because bouncing makes muscles *tighter.* You want to *tone* your muscles, not *tighten* them. Tight muscles put a strain on your joints, ligaments and tendons, leaving you prone to injury.

What's more, even a bounce on loose muscles is like a quick pull on a delicate piece of string; it's likely to snap! So if you can't make it into the position that an exercise calls for, *compromise.* If you can't touch those toes, bend your knees a little. That's not cheating. It's just a shortcut to help you get started. And even if your hands don't quite touch your toes with your knees bent, don't despair. Just reach down as far as you can without hurting yourself, and realize that sooner or later, if you persevere, those beautiful pink fingernails are going to meet their cousins down under. You gotta believe!

A Weekend Is Not Enough

What would happen if you took an ice-cold dish of food from the freezer and stuck it into a red-hot oven? You'd probably end up with a cracked dish. Well, as you start to exercise, it's important to remember that your muscles are like that dish (and for muscles that means tight, too). You have to warm them up *gradually.* If you move cold muscles fast, they're going to resist, and maybe even tear. So don't jump out of bed and start a set of jumping jacks. Warm up first!

A good way to start your warm-up is with the "neck roll." If your neck muscles are tight, many of the calisthenics we describe are hard to do, or even uncomfortable.

For the neck roll, stand with your hands at your sides, and gently lean your head forward. Then slowly rotate it

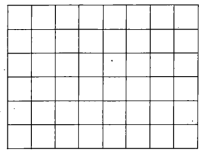

When you do exercises, don't bounce–push. Bouncing is like a quick pull on a delicate piece of string. It can make your muscles snap!

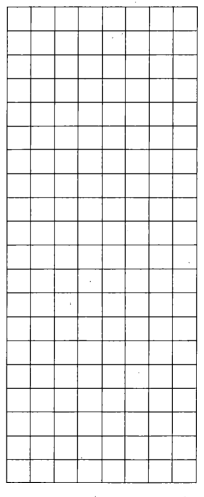

toward your right shoulder, your back, your left shoulder, finally bringing it back to your chest. (Some people find that they can relax more easily during this exercise if they close their eyes.) After one rotation, repeat the exercise in the opposite direction. Alternate rotations until your neck is completely relaxed.

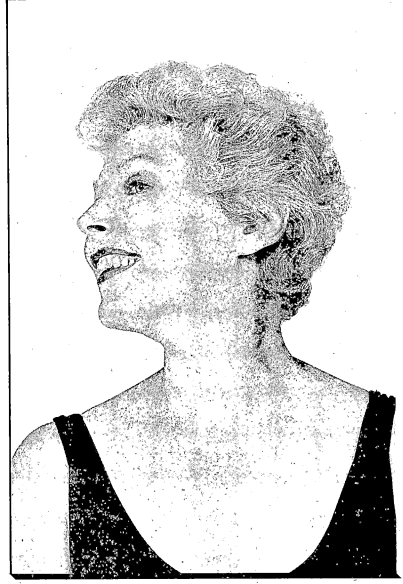

Roll your neck to loosen your muscles.

The next warm-up exercise is for your arms. With your arms extended to the sides, shake them up and down and back and forth in order to promote your circulation and to loosen the arm muscles. Think of it as if you were shaking yourself awake.

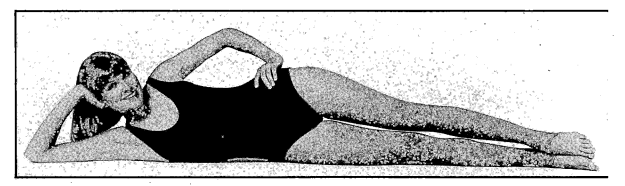

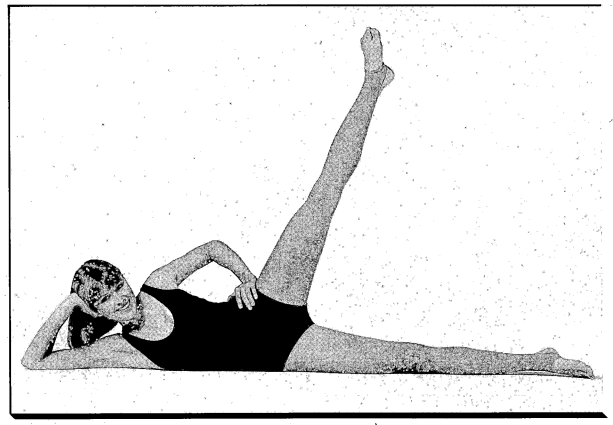

1. The side leg raise starts with legs together. 2. Lift the upper leg.

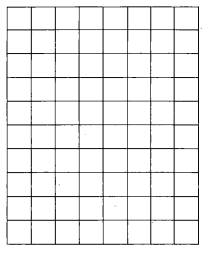

You should spend at least five to ten minutes warming up before you're ready for more strenuous exercise.

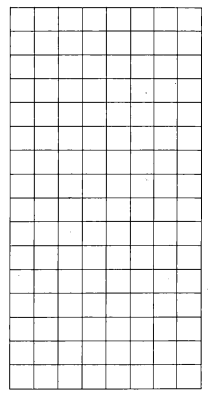

After you shake your arms, start circling them in front of the body in the same direction and in small but widening arcs. (You can, if you like, keep shaking them.) Reverse direction after every few swings and, when you start to feel a little warmed up, do make-believe golf swings and tennis backhand shots in order to add a little variety to the circling. But remember to keep the movements gentle. Don't go for a 400-yard hole in one!

To warm up your hips and legs, try a set of "side leg raises." Lie on your side with your back straight, supporting your head on your hand. Now, without straining, raise the top leg as far as it can comfortably go. Then lower it gently and slowly; don't just let it fall. Do ten of these on one side, and then flip over and do the other leg.

Continue your warm-up with the "thigh tuck and stretch." Lie on your back with your arms at your sides, and look toward your toes so that your neck is raised slightly (see photo). Now point your toes (this is called flexing your ankle), and, keeping your arms at your sides, slowly bring your left knee toward your chest. When you've brought it up as far as you can, reextend your leg so that the toes point toward the ceiling. Then lower your leg to the floor. Repeat the exercise five times with each leg, and keep every stage of the exercise slow, relaxed and controlled.

How Jack Got Nimble and Quick

Once you're warmed up – and don't spend any less than five to ten minutes on this important phase – you're ready for more strenuous exercises. A good one to start with is "jumping jacks."

Jumping jacks, for those of you who never took a high school gym class, consist of jumping up and down while bringing your hands over your head and back to your sides, landing with your feet together when the hands are at your sides and apart when they're over your head.

Start with your feet together and your hands at your sides. As you jump up, keep your arms straight and swing them out to either side and up over your head, clapping your hands together at the top of their arc. (Your arms can be slightly bent at that point.) At the same time as you bring your arms out, spread your feet so that they land about shoulder width apart. Your hands should clap at the same time your feet land.

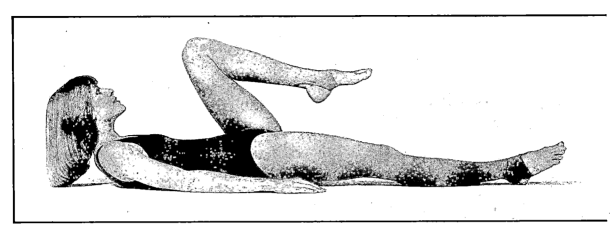

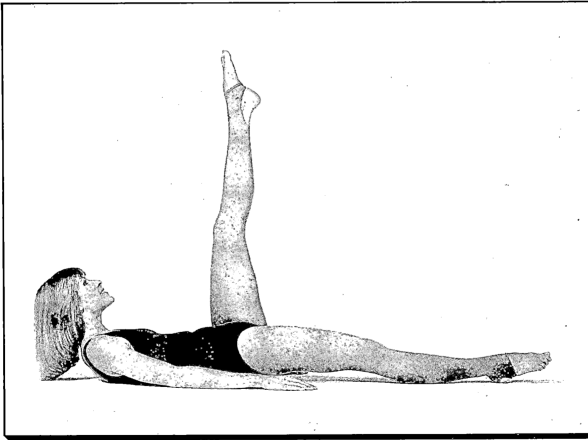

1. Raise your head and bring your knee up for this leg stretch. 2. Point your toe upward, leg straight.

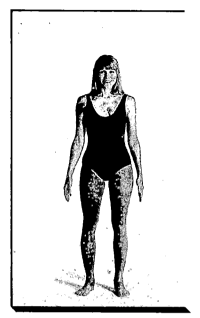 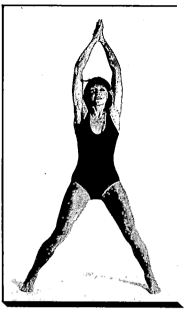 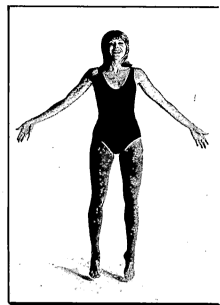

1. The jumping jack begins with your arms at your sides. 2. As you jump, spread your legs and clap your hands over your head. 3. The second half of the exercise is the reverse motion.

The next jump reverses the process. Jump up, bringing your arms back to your sides and your feet together (see photo).

If you are out of shape, do the jumping jacks slowly and carefully, trying for a total of about 25, but don't do more than you can do comfortably. If you are in reasonably good condition, you could aim for doing 500 in about eight minutes. But be careful. If jumping jacks haven't been a part of your fitness routine, 500 of them may leave your legs a little sore. So listen to your body and don't overdo.

Sit Up and Take Notice

After you finish your jumping jacks, you're ready to launch into "sit-ups," an important exercise. Stomach muscles help support the back, and sit-ups tone and strengthen those muscles. In fact, back pain often starts when stomach muscles weaken and droop. Sit-ups can help relieve back pain – or even prevent it.

Like push-ups, there are two kinds of sit-ups: modified and full. The modified variety is less strenuous, but it actu-

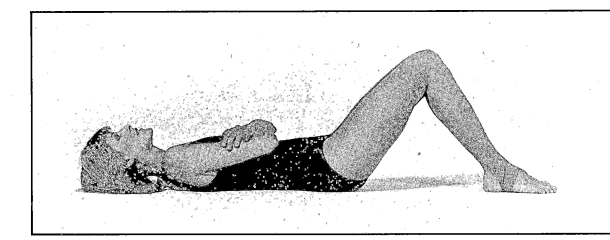

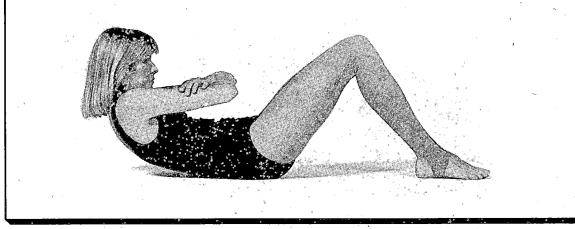

1. The modified sit-up starts with arms folded. 2. Then you come up to a 30-degree angle.

ally tones your stomach *more* than the full sit-up. That's because while the full sit-up is more work, a lot of that work is done by your back and legs.

Begin both sit-ups lying on your back with your feet flat on the floor and your knees bent (see photo). Cross your arms on your chest and sit up until your torso forms approximately a 30-degree angle with the floor. That's the modified sit-up. At the 30-degree mark your stomach muscles should feel very tight. From that position, slowly lower yourself back to the floor.

The full sit-up is basically the same motion, but this time sit *all* the way up, then twist your upper body and

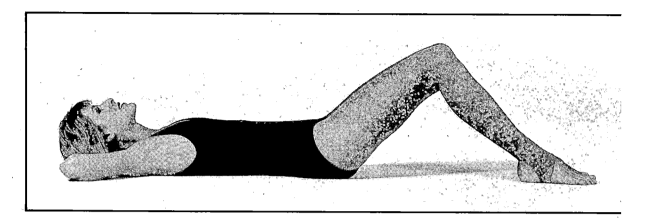

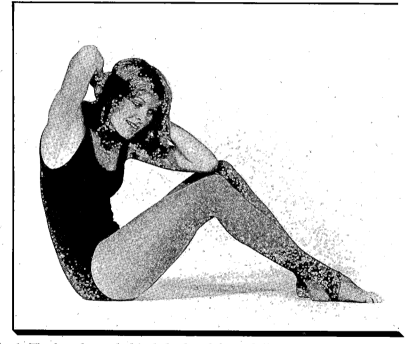

1. The hands are behind the head for a full sit-up. 2. Opposite elbow touches opposite knee.

touch an elbow to the opposite knee. Next, lower yourself to the floor. Alternate elbows with each sit-up.

If you can do 60 full sit-ups in three minutes, you're improving your aerobic capacity and burning about 12 calories.

Beginners, though, should definitely start with the modified sit-up. These give your stomach muscles a good workout and aren't so demanding on your back and legs.

At this point in your routine, you're probably feeling very "up," so to stay exhilarated, move to another up, the "push-up." Do these as we described earlier – the modified push-ups for beginners, the full push-ups for those who are already fit. Done in a minute, a set of 30 push-ups burns six to seven calories. Modified push-ups use up somewhat less.

The Squat Thrust

After the push-ups, try the "squat thrust." Starting in a standing position, you lower yourself to a squat, placing your hands on the floor. Next, thrust your feet backward so that you assume the push-up position. Then return to the squat position and stand up. If you're in good shape, you can do this exercise rapidly. If not, move slowly from pose to pose. If you want to add a little bit of extra difficulty to your squat thrusts, do a push-up (while you're in the push-up position).

Up, Up and Away

A "chin-up" – grabbing hold of a chinning bar and pulling up with your arms to get your chin tucked over the bar – is a good part of any calisthenic workout. If you're out of shape, you might not be able to do any chin-ups at first. But as your fitness program progresses, you should find them easier. It takes time to develop those arm muscles.

In order to strengthen your entire arm, alternate your hand position on the bar. During one set, keep your palms up, the backs of your hands facing away from you. The next set, reverse your grip, keeping the backs of your hands toward you, the palms away.

As you develop your calisthenic program, aim for a good, solid, 20-minute workout. But remember: that's your *goal.* As you progress toward it, keep in touch with your body, and don't rush into tough workouts that it's not prepared to handle. To pace yourself, stay constantly attuned to what your body is trying to tell you. Does a particular exercise make you sore? Does a particular part of your body feel weak? You should tailor your exercise routine to those messages.

And don't forget to take a few minutes to cool down at the end of your workout; use the warm-up exercises for

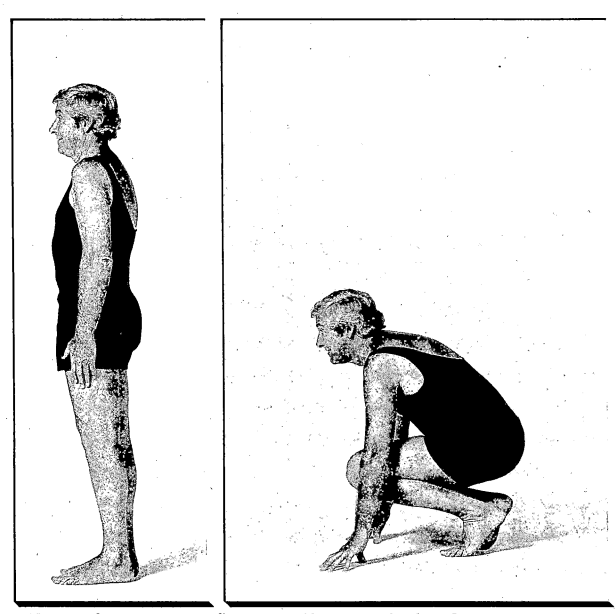

1. The squat thrust starts out standing, arms at sides. 2. Squat, hands on floor.

this purpose. Also, don't hesitate to include some stretching along with the calisthenics (refer to our chapter on stretching for some good exercises). Stretching at the end of your workout can help you avoid the soreness that the exercises might cause.

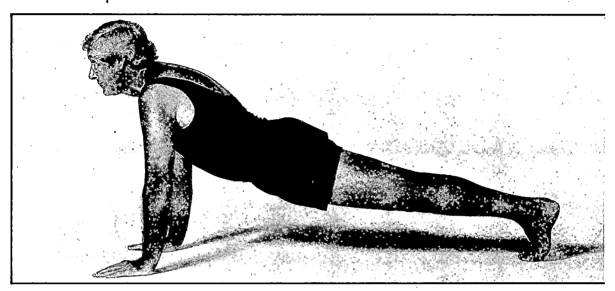

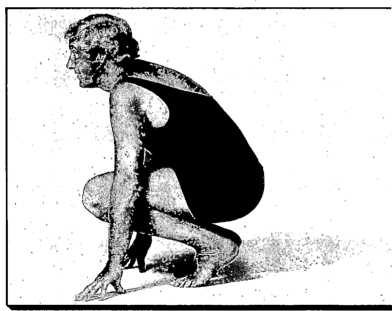

3. Thrust the feet back into the push-up position. 4. Then come back into a squat before rising.

Remember, if you can get through a strenuous, 20-minute calisthenic workout, you'll have performed the equivalent of a moderate run. And you'll develop muscles that jogging neglects. So put on your favorite record, take a deep breath and join Charlie Jones for some good, honest exertion!

CHIROPRACTIC

by Nathaniel Altman, author of *The Chiropractic Alternative: A Spine Owner's Guide* (J. P. Tarcher, 1981)

middle-aged executive nearly gave up his job because his migraine headaches were, as he said, "driving me up the wall." After six chiropractic adjustments, both the frequency and intensity of his headaches were sharply reduced.

A young woman had not had her period for three years. After four months of chiropractic care, she resumed her normal menstrual cycle.

A handyman sprained his back lifting machinery and could barely walk. Five minutes after a chiropractic adjustment, he was playfully lifting the chiropractor's child and tossing him into the air.

A 50-year-old man was told that he needed surgery to repair a herniated disc. After only two chiropractic adjustments, he returned to his amazed medical doctor, who canceled the operation.

If you walk into a chiropractor's office, the chances are good that patients will eagerly relate the "miracles" they attribute to chiropractic. "Chiropractic cured my back trouble." "It gave me sleep after years of insomnia and sleeping pills." "It lowered my blood pressure." "My arthritis is finally under control." "My child is no longer hyperkinetic and is doing well in school."

Although nearly everyone has heard about chiropractic and over ten million Americans chose the alternative of its ministrations at one time or other last year, many are unfamiliar with the theory behind it and are confused about what chiropractic can or can't do. Some feel that it is intended only for treating stiff necks and sore backs, while others believe that it can cure any disease known to humanity, including cancer. It has been variously seen as a form of massage, a process featuring acupressure and herbal remedies, a branch of medicine designed to stimulate nerves, or a painful and dangerous procedure of manipulation that cracks bones and loosens teeth. In the following pages we will explore what chiropractic is (and what it is not). We will also outline conditions that respond to chiropractic care and discuss the claim of many chiropractors that one can achieve an optimum level of positive wellness with their aid.

Chiropractic Roots

Chiropractic traces its modern roots to September 18, 1895, in the middle of a busy workweek in Davenport, Iowa. On the second story of an office building on Brady Street, a virtually deaf janitor related the story of how he became deaf to his employer. The employer was Daniel David Palmer, a magnetic healer singular for his knowledge of anatomy and his inquisitive mind. Seventeen years before, the janitor, Harvey Lillard, had bent under a stairwell to reach some cleaning supplies when he heard a loud "snap" in his back. Immediately he lost most of his hearing, which he was not able to regain.

Mr. Palmer examined the area where Mr. Lillard could remember feeling the "snap" at the time of the incident. He found a bump on the spinal column, which, according to his knowledge of anatomy, should not have been there. He associated the bump with the janitor's deafness, and he reasoned that if its appearance could *produce* deafness, its disappearance might *reduce* the affliction. With an action of the hands that would later become the basis of chiropractic manipulation, Mr. Palmer carefully pressed Mr. Lillard's back and, with a firm thrust, reduced the bump. For the first time in 17 years, Harvey Lillard said he could hear the sounds of the street below. This event led to the development of what Mr. Palmer later called "chiropractic."

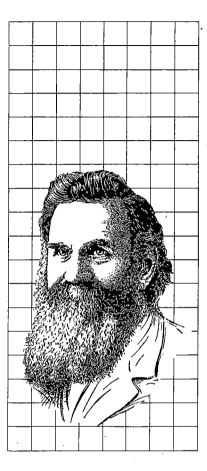

Daniel David Palmer, early pioneer of chiropractic treatment. Furnished by the Association for the History of Chiropractic.

The Meaning of "Chiropractic"

The word "chiropractic" was derived from the Greek terms *cheir* (hand) and *praktikos* (practical), which were combined by Mr. Palmer to mean "done by hand." He defined the body of belief that grew up around his practice as "that science which concerns itself with the relationship between structure (primarily the spine) and function (primarily the nervous system) of the human body." Chiropractic study was important to Mr. Palmer because he felt that the structure-function relationship might affect the restoration and preservation of health.

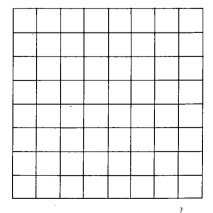

The basic philosophy of chiropractic, as first set forth by Mr. Palmer, says that we should look to the spinal column for the cause of disease – an idea, so chiropractors claim, first suggested by Hippocrates, the father of medicine. In Mr. Palmer's time it was already well known that the central nervous system – the brain, spinal cord and nerves – is the master control of the entire body. The brain serves as a generator of energy that is directed down the spinal cord in the form of electrical impulses or messages. These impulses leave the spinal cord at various points between the vertebrae and travel along nerve pathways to body organs and tissues to guide their every function. There is a return cycle as well. Every part of the body is constantly sending messages regarding its function and environment back to the brain. The brain processes this information in a fraction of a second and responds appropriately in order to protect and maintain that organ or tissue in good condition. For example, when the brain hears "hot" from the hand on a hot pot handle, it sends back an urgent request to "move!"

The Body's Ability to Heal Itself

Mr. Palmer turned this common knowledge into one theory of chiropractic treatment because he felt that we should pay special attention to the spinal column. It contains and protects the spinal cord through which these controlling nerve impulses flow. He maintained that misalignments, or *subluxations,* of the vertebrae could crowd the nerves that branch out from the spinal cord and reduce their ability to supply an organ or tissue with the correct amount of energy it needs to function properly. By extension, this theory says that most illnesses may be traced to vertebrae-cramped nerves. If an organ is not being properly supplied from the home office, it may malfunction or fall victim to disease. This statement, of course, does not sit well with most MDs. Mr. Palmer believed, as most chiropractors do today, that as long as the nervous system is free of interference, the body's innate intelligence will properly direct all body activities and maintain a harmonious order throughout the system. For that reason, the primary goal of the chiropractor is not to stimulate or inhibit the workings of the body, as they maintain other practitioners do. Rather, they want to remove the interference of vertebral subluxations so that the body's inborn wisdom can perform its task of keeping the body healthy.

The Causes of Subluxations

There are many ways in which the spine can get out of alignment and produce these subluxations, chiropractors claim. Accidents, both serious and minor, are probably the most common cause of subluxation. Improper lifting, slipping on ice, and various occupational hazards that involve subjecting the spine to unnatural stress (such as auto mechanics, plumbing, carpentry and homemaking) are all major causes of subluxation, they say. The psychological stress of our hectic society causes the muscles of the neck and back to become tense, and this also increases the risk of misalignment. Finally, some chiropractors argue that environment is another source of vertebral subluxations. Solid, liquid or gaseous toxins from food additives, tobacco, alcohol, exhaust fumes, other environmental pollution or drugs may cause nerves to react so violently that body muscles in the neck and back are affected enough to move a vertebra out of alignment. Lest we see life as a series of perils, chiropractic workers say that most minor subluxations are corrected naturally by the body (especially when we stretch), while others may require professional care. Of course, many medical doctors and lots of environmental chemists would dispute this claim. They might even retort that this is a circular argument. If subluxations usually cause pinched nerves, can it be said that irritated nerves sometimes cause subluxations?

The main task of the chiropractor is simple but exacting: to carefully locate and adjust the subluxated vertebra causing problems and to realign it once more, thus releasing pressure from the impinged nerve. The chiropractor first examines the spine in order to determine which bones are out of alignment, using his or her hands or a variety of specialized instruments. X-rays of the spine are often used as an aid in locating and analyzing the extent of the subluxation. When the chiropractor determines which vertebrae are out of whack, corrective adjustments are made to realign the bones and reduce pressure on spinal nerves. When the body's organs and tissues can receive an unobstructed nerve supply from the brain, chiropractors believe that the body will return to a state of health and will protect itself from illness.

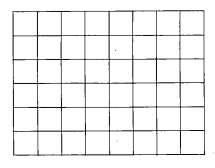

The main task of a chiropractor is to adjust the spine and realign it, releasing pressure from the spinal nerves.

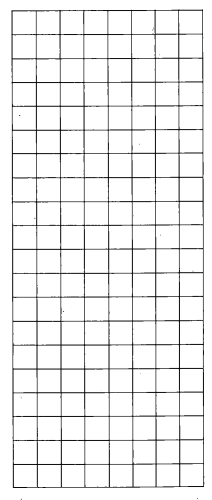

Adjustment vs. Manipulation

A chiropractic *adjustment* is different from a *manipulation*. An adjustment is a rapid, sudden and precise force (known in the profession as a "dynamic thrust") to a specific point on the vertebra, removing nerve interference. It is the body's healing reaction to the applied force that is important, chiropractors say. The realignment of structure is only a first step. A manipulation, on the other hand, is often a nonspecific, generalized procedure that resets bones, increases range of movement and realigns joint structure with the intent of stimulating or inhibiting body functions. For example, a practitioner who massages and then twists the neck and head in order to bring about a greater range of movement is performing a manipulation.

So far, we've talked about controversial matters, but the heat they generate is generally manageable. Now we must get into still hotter issues. A large number of chiropractors perform more than adjustments. While the more conservative members of the profession (known as "straights") concentrate on the detection, analysis and removal of subluxations, most chiropractors today (known as chiropractic physicians, full-service chiropractors or "mixers," depending on how you feel about them) utilize one or more adjunct therapies (including manipulation, acupressure, applied kinesiology, massage, water therapy, heat treatments, vitamin therapy and traction) to treat any number of painful or disease conditions. Many of the straights and most medical doctors contend that chiropractic training does not prepare the mixers to provide these services, and the fights begin.

Straights vs. Mixers

The positive aspects of the straight, or traditional, chiropractor include a respect for the innate wisdom of the body to heal itself. Because the straight believes that his or her "educated" intelligence has no right to determine what your body needs, the straight's goal is to remove nerve interference rather than to stimulate or inhibit body functions. Since his or her training is largely confined to chiropractic adjustment and technique, the straight often has a greater degree of expertise in this specialty than other chiropractors. Critics, however, charge that straights ignore additional therapeutic approaches that may be of benefit to the patient, and thus offer too limited a range of care. Straights reply that their specialty is the removal of subluxations and that they will often refer their patients to another specialist, such as a massage therapist or nutritional counselor, for that kind of treatment or advice.

A mind open to new health trends and a desire to integrate several natural therapeutic approaches into their work are the positive aspects of mixing chiropractors. The negative aspect of these chiropractors is not unlike that of some medical doctors: they are apt to say, "I can do anything." They provide many services which are not ordinarily available. In offering a wide variety of therapies to "fix up" the patient, the chiropractor takes on the role of magician with a bag of so-called "miracle" cures. Some mixers use adjunct therapies to justify a higher fee (a concern among critics), and the fact that chiropractors can legally perform certain adjunct procedures (like acupuncture and vitamin therapy in some states) does not necessarily mean that they are competent in these areas of treatment.

However, all chiropractors are licensed to perform chiropractic adjustments of the spine. If chiropractic interests you and you want care that specializes in the removal of nerve interference (or vertebral subluxations), you may need the services of a straight chiropractor. If you prefer more symptom-oriented health care that involves one or more natural therapies, you may want the services of a mixer.

There are no hard-and-fast rules that can help you differentiate a straight from a mixer, but a few key words in their advertisements often reveal their basic orientation. Mixers use terms like "holistic approach," adjunctive therapy, treatment (for specific things like back pain, headache, nervous tension, etc.), acupressure, massage, physiotherapy, "applied kinesiology" (simple forms of muscle testing), traction, nutritional therapy or counseling, vitamin therapy and "ACA (American Chiropractic Association) member" in their advertising.

Straights omit all the above terms but may include claims for the removal of nerve interference, "preventive" chiropractic care, restoration of nerve function, correction of vertebral subluxations or spinal misalignments, "straight chiropractor," "family chiropractor," "ICA (International Chiropractors Association) member" and "FSCO (Federation of Straight Chiropractic Organizations) member" in their ads.

The Scope of Chiropractic

One of the features of their system to which chiropractors point with pride is a health maintenance plan that helps the body remain free from nerve interference, rather than a "disease care" system designed primarily to remove symptoms. Indirectly, however, symptoms often disappear soon after chiropractic care begins because, as practitioners are equally quick to point out, the newly unobstructed nervous system has the ability to restore the body's functioning to normal. For this reason, they say chiropractic patients report being "cured" of a wide range of physical and emotional conditions (including cancer, diabetes, depression and hyperactivity) that did not respond to traditional medical treatment.

Most people think that chiropractors work with orthopedic (musculoskeletal) cases, such as backache, whiplash, disc pain and sciatica. Although this is true to a large extent, people also go to chiropractors for functional disorders that involve major body organs and processes. According to Chester A. Wilk, D.C., in his book *Chiropractic Speaks Out* (Wilk Publishing, 1976), the following ailments have responded favorably to chiropractic care:

- headache
- lower back strain or sprain
- other low back syndromes
- neck syndromes
- gastrointestinal disorders
- nervous disorders
- mid-back conditions
- cerebrospinal disorders
- heart trouble
- neurological disease
- bronchial asthma
- whiplash injuries
- extremity trauma (sprains)
- respiratory conditions
- sacroiliac strains
- high blood pressure
- torticollis (wryneck)
- emotional problems
- rheumatism
- spinal distortion
- sinusitis

- bursitis
- common cold
- strains
- neuritis
- arthritis
- sciatica
- migraine

Although millions of patients swear by chiropractic care for the removal of symptoms, practitioners like Dr. Wilk warn that chiropractic is not a miracle cure. They point out that symptoms are the final stage of disease and that most patients consult a chiropractor after traditional medicine has failed to help them. Many demand that chiropractic succeed where medical therapy did not. Although dramatic results have sometimes followed chiropractic adjustments, chiropractors maintain that such results are indirectly due to the restoration of normal nerve transmission. When the nervous system is free of interference, the body's inherent ability to heal itself is unimpeded and a state of health is more likely to exist. Of course, this argument also allows them to slip off the hook when their work does not lessen symptoms.

You as a Chiropractic Patient

The reality of a chiropractic visit is very different from most preconceived ideas. New patients soon discover that their visit is neither as painful nor as dangerous as they feared, and a good many, of course, find that chiropractic care can be a valuable experience. To them, the chiropractor is a highly trained specialist with a thorough knowledge of the spine and nervous system who is able to recognize conditions that are beyond his area of expertise and refer them to others. Let's explore the case of Kenneth Morrison (not his real name), who is typical of many chiropractic patients.

Ken's Stiff Neck

Ken, a 32-year-old house-painter, appeared to be in satisfactory health. He often complained of neck pain and occasional early morning headaches, however. One of his co-workers suggested that Dr. Roberts, a local chiropractor, might be able to help him. Ken set up an appointment for the following Thursday after work.

After receiving a welcome from the receptionist, he was given a case history to fill out. Although the form was similar to those used by medical doctors, it went into specifics about musculoskeletal complaints and asked him to make note of any fall, sprain or accident he could recall. Although Ken had a good safety record on the job, he remembered that at 17 he was involved in a minor car accident. His head bumped against the windshield, causing the glass to shatter. Although Ken suffered only a few scratches and a headache, his father took him to the hospital emergency room, where he was examined and sent home with a clean bill of health. Until he filled out the case history form, Ken hadn't given the accident a second thought.

By the time Ken completed the form, Dr. Roberts was ready to see him. The chiropractor's adjusting room looked more like a living room than a clinical office. It lacked the antiseptic odors, sterilizers and needles often found at a medical doctor's. A large adjusting table stood at the center of the room, and a model spine lay on the doctor's desk. Using the model spine as an example, Dr. Roberts showed how vertebrae become misaligned and impinged on spinal nerves. With the aid of a chart depicting the distribution of nerves throughout the body,-he-showed Ken how nerve interference in one part of the body can alter the function of an organ or tissue in another. "Even a childhood fall from a bicycle can cause a spinal misalignment that can impinge a nerve," he said. "You may not feel the effects for a long period of time, but I think your car accident 15 years ago may have been the beginning of your neck problem."

The doctor asked Ken to remove his shirt and lie face down on the adjusting table, which was heavily padded and fitted with a special notch to cradle his head. Dr. Roberts then proceeded to examine his back by hand, carefully palpating (examining by touch) each vertebra for tenderness or bumps. He asked Ken, "Does it hurt here?" when he found a tender area, and he recorded his findings.

Special attention was paid to the cervical (neck) region during the exam. The second cervical vertebra appeared to be out of alignment. The length of Ken's legs was compared – one leg was one-quarter inch shorter than the other – and his pelvis was found to be slightly askew.

Dr. Roberts then had Ken stand up and bend to the left, the right, forward and back. Using a plumb line to determine overall spinal alignment, he found that Ken's left shoulder was slightly lower than the right and that his head tilted a bit to the right.

After this postural analysis, Ken sat on the table while his skin temperature was measured by a device called a thermeter, a modern successor to the neurocalometer introduced by B. J. Palmer (Daniel David Palmer's son) in 1924. Starting from the base of the skull, the doctor carefully moved the two-pronged, handheld device slowly down the spine, recording temperature differences between one side of the spine and the other. When the temperature is lower on one side, chiropractors claim, nerve interference may be indicated. In Ken's case, Dr. Roberts found four vertebrae where these differences existed and noted their location on Ken's chart. Other chiropractors sometimes include what they call "applied kinesiology" – simple muscle-strength testing – as part of their chiropractic analysis. By testing certain muscles of the body, they say, they can tell if a related organ or tissue is weak and trace that weakness to a misaligned vertebra.

Finally, Dr. Roberts brought Ken into the X-ray room and took two pictures of his neck to determine the nature and extent of the suspected misalignment. The pictures confirmed the earlier findings: there was a major subluxation of the second cervical vertebra of the neck that was putting pressure on the nerve. Dr. Roberts said this was contributing to Ken's stiff neck as well as his morning headaches, especially when he had slept on his right side. The chiropractor also explained that other subluxations further down the spine were attempts to compensate for the major misalignment in the neck and that they could be corrected as well.

A ten-week program of adjustments was drawn up, which was typical of nonemergency but chronic cases such as Ken's: two adjustments a week for four weeks and one per week thereafter. (Other patients, such as recent accident victims, might begin with five adjustments per week, while patients with minor subluxations might start with one.) At the end of the tenth week, Ken's progress would be evaluated, and he might need preventive maintenance only once a month thereafter. Chiropractors often recommend preventive care long after the original subluxations are corrected. Because chiropractic is based on the body's natural ability to restore and maintain good health, they maintain that regular adjustments are necessary to keep the nervous system free from interference and the organism in good health.

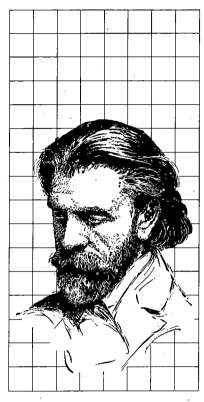

B. J. Palmer, son of D. D. Palmer and also one of the first chiropractors. Furnished by the Association for the History of Chiropractic.

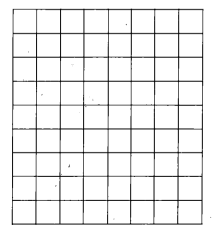

Ken's First Adjustment

After making appointments for future visits, Ken was ready to receive his first spinal adjustment. Dr. Roberts began with other temperature readings along the spinal column and wrote them in the record book. He then asked Ken to lie down on the table on his stomach, with his head turned to the right. At this point Ken tensed up a little, expecting a great deal of pain from the adjustment, but Dr. Roberts reassured him. Carefully applying light pressure on Ken's neck below the ear, he gave a sudden rapid downward thrust that made an audible "click." He did the same thing to the upper back and had Ken, still in a prone position, cross his left leg over the other before giving the sacrum (or lower back) a rapid thrust. Although he felt a tingling sensation in his head immediately after the adjustment, Ken was surprised to have felt no pain at all. After a few minutes of rest, he got up from the table, stretched and went home.

Over the next ten weeks, Ken received a total of 14 chiropractic adjustments and began feeling better than he had since high school. This experience prompted Ken to ask how often a patient should be adjusted. There is no standard rule to follow, he was told. Schedules for adjustments have been known to vary from twice an hour (usually in an emergency situation where a high fever is present and the patient's life is in danger) to two or three times a week (for a patient with a chronic subluxation). After the initial problem is brought under control, preventive care is scheduled once or twice a month. Some chiropractors suggest adjustments be discontinued as soon as symptoms disappear, but the majority believe that preventive maintenance should involve a long-term commitment.

Dr. Roberts had given Ken a pamphlet on the second visit. It described an exercise program to help strengthen his spinal muscles and avoid subluxations. An extra-firm bed was recommended to replace Ken's old sagging mattress. The doctor also taught him the proper way to lift heavy, bulky objects to reduce the chances of subluxating the spine. Finally, Dr. Roberts encouraged Ken to improve his diet and suggested he read several books on nutrition and food preparation. He claimed that the better our diets, the less chance we have of subluxating the spine due to the effect of toxins and overrefined foods. Dr. Roberts was a straight chiropractor who confined his practice largely to spinal adjustments. As mentioned earlier, many other chiropractors might have offered Ken heat treatments, acupressure and nutritional counseling in addition to his chiropractic adjustments. Adjustment techniques vary as well. Some chiropractors prefer more dramatic methods such as that developed by B. J. Palmer, which features a dynamic thrust and something called a "rapid recoil." Others choose slower, less abrupt techniques.

A Note about X-Rays

Most chiropractors take X-rays at one time or another as part of their regular examination procedure, although their use of the pictures varies considerably. Some chiropractors use them rarely, limiting radiation to specific areas of the spinal column. Others frequently use full-spine X-rays (which photograph the back from the base of the skull to below the pelvis) to get an idea of how the entire spine is affected by vertebral subluxations.

Although most patients feel uncomfortable about being X-rayed, an X-ray can determine if any contraindications to chiropractic care exist. For example, a hairline fracture of the second cervical vertebra may escape the scrutiny of a chiropractor during the initial examination. If an adjustment were given, the vertebra could break apart and injure a delicate vein or artery. Chiropractors claim that X-rays also give them a better understanding of the nature and extent of the vertebral subluxation and enable the practitioner to make a more exacting adjustment. If you are concerned about increased radiation risk, ask for smaller X-rays focusing on specific areas of your spine. If it is advised that you have follow-up X-rays a month later, question the request until you are satisfied that the pictures are necessary and not just routine procedure. If you are concerned about the dangers of frequent radiation, you may want to select a chiropractor who does not require it as a prerequisite to care. Also, reject any practitioner who advertises free X-rays. Radiation should never be used as a lure.

Do Chiropractors *Really* Help?

Finally, given the controversy that chiropractors inspire, we feel a little blunt editorializing – lightened by a little science – is in order: you either love chiropractors or you despise them. Or you don't know them.

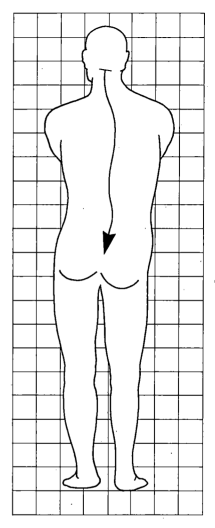

When the body is out of alignment, pain and disability can result. Here the left hip is carried too high, destroying the body's balance.

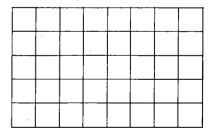

CHIROPRACTIC   185

That is perhaps an absurd statement to make about a healing art, but we've found that it's generally true. Most MDs have nothing but scorn for chiropractors, and many medical societies actively – one might even say viciously – attempt to deny chiropractors the right to practice. They constantly refer to chiropractic as an "unscientific cult" that has no basis in proven fact and is "therefore highly dangerous."

What apparently keeps the profession alive and gives it the vitality to fight back against the MD establishment is the testimony of thousands of people who swear by chiropractors and enthusiastically relate anecdotes wherein their troubles were solved by chiropractors after MDs failed to help.

Most people base these opinions of chiropractic on personal experiences. Several people we know have told us that their experiences have been excellent. Others were very disappointed and came away convinced that the chiropractor made them return to the office numerous times for manipulations which did nothing but induce pain. Others criticize chiropractors because at least some of them seem to be too eager to take X-rays.

The government conducted a study that they hoped would appraise the true value of chiropractic, but they discovered that the physicians involved in the study could not communicate with the chiropractors and vice versa. They simply did not talk each other's language. So it must be admitted that nearly all the evidence concerning the value of chiropractic is purely subjective and anecdotal in nature.

A Scientific Study

One exception to this evidence is a survey conducted by Robert L. Kane, M.D., and his associates at the Department of Family and Community Medicine of the University of Utah College of Medicine, who compared the effectiveness of physician and chiropractor care in 232 patients with back pain.

The patients were identified by scanning workmen's compensation records. The Utah researchers contacted and interviewed 232 persons who had been treated for back or spinal problems. Of these, 122 had sought the services of chiropractors, while 110 went to physicians. (Workmen's compensation in Utah permits the injured worker to select his therapist from among physicians, osteopaths and chiropractors. This ruling differs from state to state.)

The interviews revealed that patients who used chiropractors were slightly more satisfied with the care they received, more pleased with their improvement, and more quickly returned to their former status (*Lancet,* June 29, 1974). The differences were not very great, but the numbers clearly show chiropractors ahead by a slim margin.

They found, too, that in spite of the medical profession's disdain for chiropractic, more and more people are turning to chiropractors for assistance.

While those patients who were treated by a chiropractor required almost twice as many visits as the MD-treated patients, the average duration of their treatment was significantly shorter – 6.5 weeks as opposed to 9.3 weeks for the latter group. (Physician-treated patients average one to two visits a week, compared to two to three visits weekly for those seeing chiropractors.)

Evaluating each patient's disability and improvement with therapy, Dr. Kane and his associates concluded that "the intervention of a chiropractor in problems around neck and spine injuries was at least as effective as that of a physician, in terms of restoring the patient's function and satisfying the patient." Chiropractic patients scored an average of 0.92 on the Utah researchers' ratio of improvement scale, slightly ahead of the MD-treated patients' average score of 0.86.

On the other hand, there was a tendency for MDs to get the more serious cases, so the better record of the chiropractors must be seen in this light. Perhaps it would be fair to call it a tie – but also a "moral victory" for the much-maligned chiropractors.

High Marks for Chiropractors

In the area of personal relations, the chiropractors rated higher scores than the MDs. As many as 6.5 percent of the patients were dissatisfied with the MD's ability to make them feel welcome. On the other hand, no patient found any fault at all with the chiropractors in this area. Chiropractors also rated higher scores than the MDs in ability to explain the problem and the treatment in terms that the patient could easily understand.

CROSS-COUNTRY SKIING

If you live in a spot that suffers from the slings and arrows of outrageous winter, that doesn't necessarily mean that you've got to postpone all of your exercise plans until spring brings back the warm weather. Cold weather offers plenty of exercise opportunities.

When the snow piles up on the ground, you can enjoy yourself and get some excellent exercise breezing through the white landscape instead of staying shut up indoors, slowly developing cabin fever.

The way to do it is by learning how to ski cross-country.

Cross-country skiing, also called Nordic skiing and ski touring, has an undeserved reputation as something difficult and complicated. That's far from the truth.

"I was 42 before I saw a pair of skis up close," says Lou Polak, president of the Ski Touring Council, an organization of about 150 skiers, most of them in their sixties. "I wouldn't call myself robust, and I'm no more coordinated than the average guy. It's just walking. Anybody who can walk can go ski touring."

Ski touring takes almost no time to learn. "If you make up your mind that it's as simple as walking, it can be picked up in an hour," Mr Polak says. "After that, it's just a matter of developing confidence."

The basic movement of Nordic skiing is called "the diagonal stride." As one skier put it, "It's simply a matter of learning how to glide on one ski and then the other, while coordinating your arms and legs."

A friend can teach you or you can take a lesson, which might cost from $5 to $8 for 60 to 90 minutes. That's all the preparation you need to ski over rolling terrain. Skills, such as climbing and turning, come with practice.

"When you start skiing, it seems different and awkward," says Tom Perkins of Jackson, New Hampshire, president of the National Ski Touring Operators' Association and a teacher of ski instructors. "But after a day or two, it begins to feel like dancing. Ski touring is really neat, and it's not long before you accustom yourself to getting around."

There's no reason to be afraid of an occasional tumble.

"People learn that falling is not necessarily a bad thing," Mr. Perkins says. "I fall all the time. It's not all that far to the ground, and the snow is forgiving.

"Eventually you get a feel for the snow and for changes in the landscape." Then, he says, skiing becomes a magical sport. "It's a wonderful thing. Your body feels so good when you ski."

Feeling physically good is just one of the rewards of ski touring. "Another great thing," Mr. Perkins says, "is that you get to look at the world in winter. That's something most people never do. They stay indoors when it's cold, and that's unfortunate, because winter is a beautiful time of year, and cross-country skiing is a wonderful way to see the outdoors."

A Complete Exercise

Of all forms of exercise, Nordic skiing might be the most complete. Because you use both your arms and legs, and because you're usually carrying heavy clothes and equip-

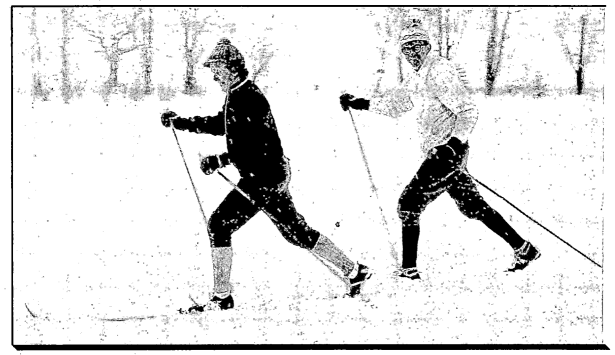

Cross-country skiing can be an invigorating aerobic exercise.

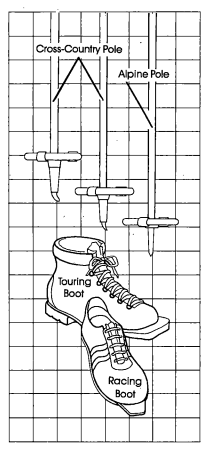

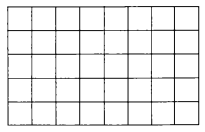

Cross-country ski equipment differs greatly from the gear used for other types of skiing. Cross-country poles have curved tips, unlike straight-tipped Alpine (downhill) poles. The top boot in the picture is a cross-country touring boot, much heavier than its cousin, shown below, a racing boot.

ment, you get roughly twice as tough a workout as you would jogging or walking at the same speed.

"Nordic skiing is excellent aerobic exercise," according to Edward G. Hixson, M.D., chief physician to the U.S. Nordic Ski Team that participates in the Olympics. "First, it's very good for the heart and lungs. It's more strenuous than running, but you don't have to go real fast.

"Second, it's a relatively painfree exercise. There are no aches and pains, there's no pounding on the pavement. Your heel doesn't take any shock, and there's not as much stress on the knees as in running."

Skiing is also a great way to lose weight. A person at rest burns about 100 calories per hour. But, Dr. Hixson says, an expert Nordic skier burns up to 1,000 calories an hour. The average skier would fall somewhere in between, depending on how fast he skis. Nordic skiing is also great for people who hate the cold. Skiers sweat even in subfreezing conditions.

Then there's that ineffable "skier's high," a cousin of "runner's high." Canadian marathon runner Jacqueline Gareau, who knows both kinds of highs, talks about Nordic skiing's "special atmosphere." Cross-country skiing "gives me a special feeling," she says. "Perhaps it's not what you would call ecstasy, but it's not that far off."

Inexpensive Recreation

You don't need much in the way of equipment to become a Nordic skier. For your first outing you can rent skis, boots and poles for less than $10 a day. That way you can find out if you like it. Once you're hooked, you can be outfitted for less than $150. An equivalent package for downhill skiing, by comparison, costs roughly $400 to $450. Nordic skiers also evade the expensive lift tickets that downhillers must buy.

Also, you don't need a lot of special clothing to go ski touring. The important thing is to wear several thin layers of clothes rather than one bulky jacket or sweater. Wool clothing is the best choice because, unlike cotton, it keeps you warm even when it's wet. Bright clothing keeps you visible in the woods, and wool mittens will keep your hands much warmer than gloves. It's also a good idea to wear a hat or hood. There are lots of optional clothes for Nordic skiers, such as nylon gaiters to cover your ankles and shoes, or knickers for freedom of movement, but they aren't required.

You burn calories so fast on skis that taking food along

is a must, especially for an all-day outing. Most people carry a sack of "gorp," a mixture of natural snack foods such as raisins, nuts, carob chips, sunflower seeds and dates.

A potential skier also needs some off-season exercise. A booklet, "Cross-Country Skiing for Old Americans," published by the United States Ski Association, recommends exercising the arms and shoulders as winter approaches. Two ways to do that, the USSA suggests, are exaggerating your arm swing while walking, or taking a brisk stroll using your ski poles.

However, compared to downhill skiing, Nordic skiing requires less arm strength, and it's also many times safer. Dr. Hixson says that, according to his figures, cross-country skiers injure themselves only one-twentieth as often as downhillers. Nordic skis are safer largely because only the skier's toe is attached to the ski. A downhill skier's toe and heel are clamped to his ski.

If a cross-country skier injures himself, it's often due to two common mistakes. Physicians at the Dartmouth-Hitchcock Medical Center in Hanover, New Hampshire, studied 11 injuries to Nordic skiers and found that many of them occurred because the skier tried to go down an icy hill and/or allowed the tips of his skis to cross in front of him. Avoiding these mistakes should minimize the risk of injury (*Journal of the American Medical Association,* January 23, 1978).

Two professors at McMaster University in Ontario, Canada, think that ski touring is safe enough to help heart disease patients rejuvenate their cardiovascular systems. Neil D. Oldridge, Ph.D., and J. Duncan MacDougall, Ph.D., say that doctors can prescribe Nordic skiing for their cardiac patients, but that such skiers have to take the following precautions: (1) no racing or sprinting; (2) making sure to exercise in the off-season; (3) staying home when it's very cold and windy; (4) slowing down when out of breath; (5) skiing with others; and (6) sticking to fairly level terrain (*The Physician and Sportsmedicine,* February, 1981).

Where to Ski

For many people, the best part of ski touring is getting away from it all. Unlike a downhill skier, a Nordic skier doesn't have to rely on ski lifts or prepared slopes. He can ski wherever there's snow. Some people ski right out their back door. Other people bushwhack through the untracked woods where only skis, snowshoes or wild game can go. On the other hand, when a blizzard paralyzed the city of New York a few years ago, some urbanites simply skied to work.

For the beginner, open rolling terrain is the best place to start. City parks are ideal for this, and so are golf courses. Two warnings about golf courses: stay off the fragile greens and tees, and be sure to get permission before setting out. Skiing on snow-covered hiking trails challenges even the best Nordic skier. A winding, rolling trail can turn skiing into a thrilling bobsled ride. Unused meadows and fields and old logging roads are good also.

From about 2500 B.C., which is roughly the date of the oldest ski ever found, to about 1973, Nordic skiing was relatively undiscovered as a sport. Today, ten million pairs of cross-country skis are in use in the U.S. One benefit of its rising popularity has been the establishment of major ski centers and trail networks just for touring.

About 150 of these centers belong to the National Ski Touring Operators' Association, and there are an estimated 400 additional centers. These ski centers have up to 80 miles or more of what are called "groomed" trails, which means that even before the crack of dawn a road crew uses special equipment to blaze a trail and save you the chore of breaking snow. Nordic centers are becoming as numerous as downhill resorts, and the two are often found together. Rentals are usually available.

All of this has made ski touring very easy to get into, and, once on skis, most people's anxieties about winter quickly melt. As one ski instructor told us, "People who learn to ski don't feel threatened anymore. As you get older, you often dread the thought of the cold and the snow, but this gives you an opportunity to get outside. Ski touring makes you look forward to winter."

DANCE THERAPY

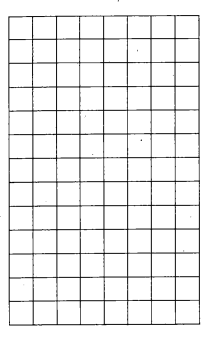

Dance therapy is a very new treatment for mental and emotional problems. Although the good idea that grew into this impressive practice came to someone in the late 40s, it wasn't until 1970 that dance therapy as defined by its professional organization, the American Dance Therapy Association (ADTA), was accepted by medical schools and universities as a reliable form of psychotherapy. And it wasn't until very recently – some exasperated dance therapists might even say "the day before yesterday" – that their type of work was deemed safe for so-called normal, not-particularly-serious and short-term mental disturbances. Previously it was judged fit for use with chronic and seemingly hopeless cases only. Anyway, the theory behind dance therapy says that we wear our actions like a suit of clothes. Sometimes the way we move, the way we habitually do things, disguises what we are thinking and feeling, just as clothes often hide the person we actually are. Yet, sometimes our actions express what we think and feel better than our words – again, the way clothing frequently does – a complex broth that has been boiled down into the gravy of "body language." But there is *always* a direct connection between inner conviction and outer activity, and that's why dance therapy is used with patients who cannot talk to a counselor or who have great trouble communicating with those around them, such as autistic children and schizophrenic adults. If the patient cannot tell us what is wrong, goes the theory, perhaps we can guess by looking at how and when he or she moves. So dance therapy is a study of our cloaklike movements that seeks to both diagnose and treat mental troubles through our physical actions. It uses knowledge of how we walk, sit and stand (among other things) to determine what's wrong, and it prescribes movement of both new and old kinds as a way of releasing the stress and tension that may be part of illness.

All this sounds pretty uniform, as if all dance therapists do things in the same way, but that's not true. Although we shouldn't have been, we were surprised by how personal a thing dance therapy is. When we talked to a practitioner of

Dance therapy began in primitive societies. They used dance to express fears, exorcise demons and to try to cure illness.

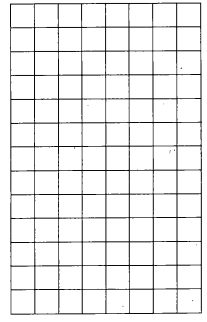

the art, we learned that because each patient is different, each treatment is apt to be different. What's more, because most therapists allow their patients a voice in how their recovery proceeds, each session is different from every other session. The sessions, in fact, are often improvised on the spot, fashioned from material drawn from the patient's immediate needs, the therapist's evaluation of his or her problem and the understanding both of them have of where they want to go in the days ahead. Because all of this is true, we decided to present dance therapy first through the eyes of one therapist and only then move on to a more generalized view of the whole profession. For our general knowledge we went to textbooks and articles in professional journals. For a personal look, we talked to Dianne Dulicai, M.A., D.T.R., head of the creative arts and therapy department of Hahnemann Medical College, Philadelphia, Pennsylvania, a registered dance therapist and an influential teacher of her skills.

Our first question to Ms. Dulicai was a request to talk about the beginnings of dance therapy and its early innovators. Her answer was one that we'd heard in other places but which had new authority with her. She said, "I guess dance therapy really began with the primitive societies that used dance as a way of expressing fears, exorcising demons, and, yes, attempting to cure illness. Although no one, of course, knew what was going on, I suspect that the seeds of dance therapy were there a long time before anyone ever tried to describe them." And we could believe it, because Ms. Dulicai's heritage is American Indian, and her interest in the field began with a career as a professional dancer and the remnants of Indian ritual dances in her childhood. People began to recognize what was happening in these primitive societies during the Second World War, she continued, when hospitals were jammed with returning soldiers suffering from mental illnesses that their staffs had not seen before and could not hope to treat. Volunteers stepped in to ease the situation, and volunteers and patients seemed made for each other. This was in the days before mental patients were routinely sedated, and there was the simple need to give the soldiers something to do. Since many of the volunteers were professional dancers, they turned to dance activities, and another perfect match occurred. The men were suffering from shell shock and other nervous disorders. Many could not communicate with those around them. The dancing, however, seemed to help, and it did so without requiring that patients talk to doctors. These volunteers were not trained therapists, and so they often used pure dance. But it worked. Soon pioneers like Marian Chace at St. Elizabeth's Hospital in Washington D.C., Blanche Evan in New York City and Trudy Schoop in California, working independently, began to investigate their successes in hopes of learning why dance had worked. Their efforts defined dance therapy and led to the establishment of the ADTA in 1966.

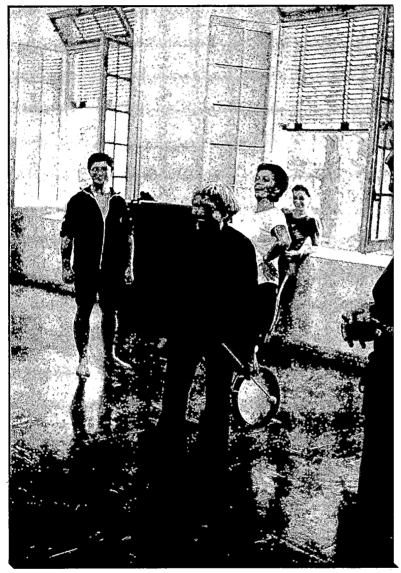

Trudy Schoop with patients.

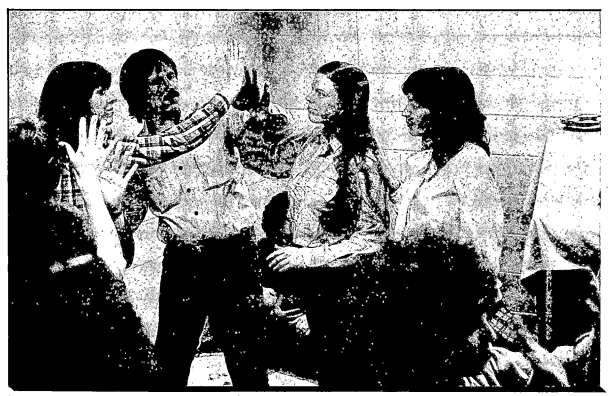

Instructors and staff explore in a movement therapy class at Hahnemann Medical College.

Next we asked Ms. Dulicai to expand on the limited definition of dance therapy we had. The process, she said, changed very rapidly from an art form used for relaxation to a therapy when it was discovered that "there was something in the interacting movement of two or more people together that produces a healing result." At first, this was simply the intuition of the pioneers, but by the 60s, as films and videotapes of therapy sessions were studied, researchers saw that this healing interaction was a fact. In the decade after its founding, the ADTA defined dance therapy as "the psychotherapeutic use of movement, . . . a process which furthers the emotional and physical integration of the individual." What this means is that dance therapists want to make your suit of movement clothing as unconfining as possible; they want to alter your cloak of behavior so that it parts easily to reveal your emotions and convictions. Most of all, they hope to avoid the bind that has you behaving one way and believing another. Some practitioners, Ms. Dulicai claimed, prefer the term "movement therapy" to distinguish what they do from both dance exercise and dance artistry, but most have stuck with the traditional term. Of course, there are certain health benefits from activity of this kind, especially for children (who are very vigorous in it) and older folks (who may not get any other exercise), but the major goal here is self-awareness. Dance therapy makes us more aware of our bodies – more accepting of them, actually – and more attuned to the effect we have on others and that they have on us. This, in turn, brings an ability to handle social situations, and *that* carries with it some desirable personality traits: an openness, a desire to communicate both good news and bad, and a self-confidence and sense of security that the world is a place to explore and expand rather than an excuse to conceal and hide.

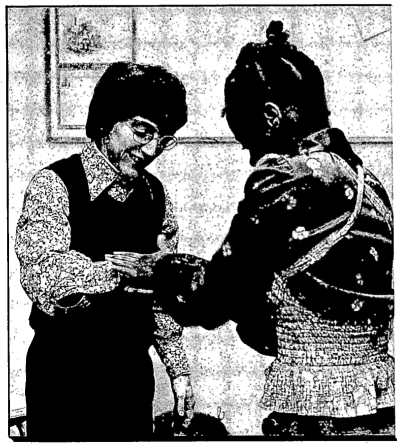

Movement therapy treats all parts of the body.

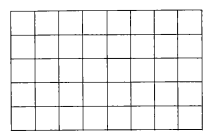

Dance therapy helps many older folks accept the changes age brings to their bodies. It can offer social contacts and possibly improve memory, concentration and the ability to analyze problems.

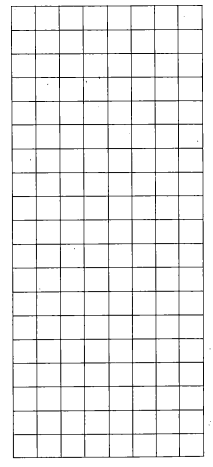

Who gets dance therapy? When is it appropriate? With whom is it most successful? Up until five years ago, we were told, a person probably wouldn't receive dance therapy unless he or she were hospitalized in a state or federal institution and were seriously and chronically ill. Then, it was used only to reach terribly disturbed adults and many children because of its nonverbal approach; a therapist didn't have to speak at length to a patient to help him or her. It was thought too new and too unproven, however, for use with less serious cases, and it was almost never used with educated, middle-class people. The nonverbal aspect of its methods was seen at first as a limitation rather than a new way of doing things. Since then, the application of dance therapy has taken off. It is still used for the very ill and for those who cannot speak to those who want to help them: victims of chronic mental disturbance, the retarded, the physically disabled, and – most successfully – autistic children, people who may never be "cured," that is, made whole and normal, but who seem able to achieve as full a life as they can through dance therapy. For these conditions, dance therapy's mode of treatment and its willingness to take whatever abilities the patient has and to move him or her as far as he or she can go seem perfectly suited. But in the last five years this therapy has been extended more and more often to the less serious troubles that we all encounter in life. Yes, it is used with children, but now it's turned on the full range of things that come up in youth clinics: anorexia nervosa, hyperactivity, the psychosomatic aspects of asthma, the pain and stress of juvenile arthritis and diabetes. In fact, Ms. Dulicai's students get jobs working in almost all psychological areas. They work with both normal and abnormal kids in public schools. With special education teachers, they employ movement to help children overcome specific learning disabilities, and with classroom teachers and daycare supervisors, they prepare programs of supportive growth and development for kids without problems. For younger children, they work in hospital pediatric wards to ease the stress of long stays away from home and the burdens of serious illness. And they work in something new, a program called "Families at Risk." It handles almost anything that can go wrong within a family group, from friction in the initial bond between mother and child, to problems with nursing, and on to the sometimes bumpy interactions between parents and siblings as everybody grows older. But it doesn't end there. Just as often, they get jobs in similar situations with adults: in mental health clinics dealing with everything from depression to very serious disturbances; in pain centers, where people are taught to adjust to both the physical and emotional demands of pain; in hospitals, with heart patients and sufferers of high blood pressure who must learn ways to manage and reduce the stress that often accompanies their complaints. Finally, just as dance therapy clicked with children years ago because it seemed fun and nonthreatening, it is now a hit with old people for the same reasons. It provides certain benefits of regular mild exercise for them. It helps release the tension generated by the confinement often experienced late in life. It helps many older folks accept the changes age brings to their bodies. When done in a group, it offers social contacts that they otherwise might not have, and its individual therapies improve memory, concentration and the ability to analyze problems.

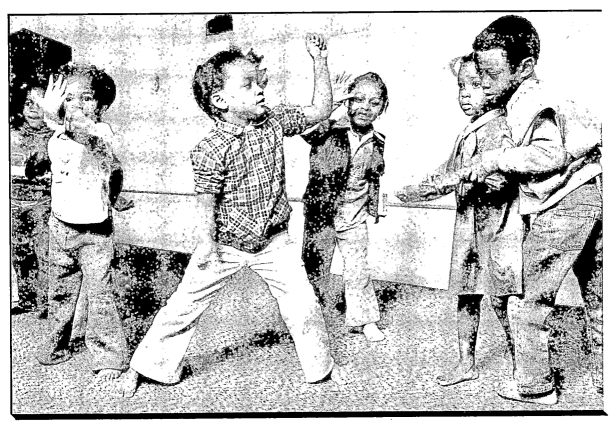

Children's learning abilities grow in response to movement.

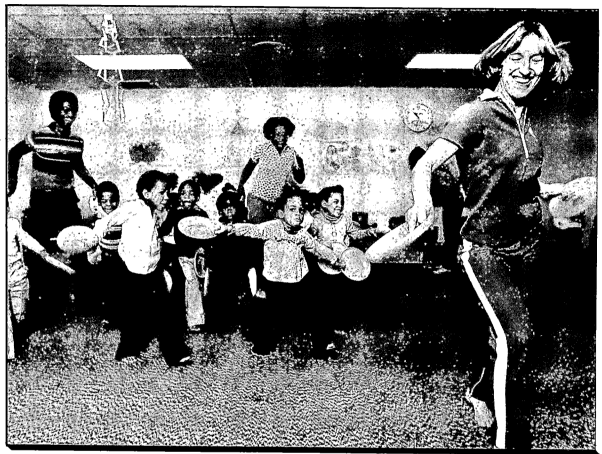

Dance therapy releases tension in youngsters.

Okay. That all sounds pretty good – and very reassuring. How do you get in touch with a dance therapist? And after you find one, who – better, what – is he or she apt to be? In the big cities of the East Coast and the huge "city" that stretches from Los Angeles to San Francisco on the West Coast, you may find one in the telephone book, for there are therapists in private practice in both places. But if you do, make sure he or she has "D.T.R." after his or her name. For that matter, a dance therapist found *anywhere* should be entitled to those initials. They mean "Registered Dance Therapist" and signify that the bearer has the education and work experience necessary to be certified as a therapist by the American Dance Therapy Association. And *that* means that he or she has:

- At least five years of dance training;
- A master's degree in dance therapy from an ADTA-approved school, a curriculum including courses in the theory and practice of dance therapy, methods of movement analysis, anatomy and physiology, and human behavior;
- At least three months of supervised clinical work;
- Six months of independent clinical work as a student; and
- At least two years of full-time employment as a therapist.

In most places in the country, however, you won't find those initials in either the phone book or private practice. You'll have to depend on a large medical institution having a dance therapist on its staff, and, more often than not, you won't be able to go directly to one even then. You'll have to be referred to a dance therapist by a more traditional counselor, a psychologist or psychiatrist. Which is good news and bad news. The good news is that health insurance plans will sooner pay the fees of a nontraditional therapist if he has been recommended by an MD or Ph.D. The bad news is that even with an explosion in the use of movement therapists in the past five years, many conventional mental health people still don't know about them or, in some cases, don't approve of what they do. There are still battles to be won, Ms. Dulicai says.

If these battles haven't been won in your area, if there are no DTRs in the phone book or the large hospitals nearby and if no doctor or psychologist will refer you to one, there is still a way to go. The American Dance Therapy Association will send you the names and addresses of the registered members who work in your community, and you can contact one of them on your own. The place to write is the ADTA, Suite 230, 2000 Century Plaza, Columbia, MD 21044.

Oh, about cost. It's hard to talk about the cost of any kind of treatment in a book like this, because it will be read throughout the country, and medical fees differ greatly from place to place. But Ms. Dulicai said that a good rule of thumb is that a skilled dance therapist will charge what a skilled counselor with a Master's of Social Work might ask for his or her services. A few phone calls told us that $30 to $35 for an hour-long session would be the average cost – more in big cities, less away from them. A more important factor than the per-session rate in determining cost, however, is the length of treatment. How long does it take for dance therapy to work? It's impossible to say, of course, because each person and each set of problems creates its own schedule, and many dance therapists allow patients to establish their own pace in treatment. Like Ms. Dulicai, they help their patients set goals for the therapy, goals that will be constantly reviewed and changed as the work progresses, and the nature of these objectives and the speed with which they are achieved determine the length of their treatment. Still, when we pushed her, Ms. Dulicai said that minor, everyday problems could usually be eased in three to four months of once-a-week sessions, while more serious troubles would, obviously, require much more time to bring under control.

Having learned as much as we could about the general practice of dance therapy, we got to the best part of the interview. We asked Ms. Dulicai to describe how she got a series of treatment sessions going with a new patient. She offered not only that information, but she also took us through, in a play-by-play sort of way, some videotaped sessions. She helped us see several kinds of movement and behavior through a therapist's trained eyes. What we discovered both surprised and amazed us.

Ms. Dulicai's sessions always begin with some very fundamental things, the first of which is a medical history of the patient – medical *histories,* actually. She wants as complete a chronicle of a patient's past illnesses and injuries as she can get, a record of the drugs and treatments he or she has taken and is taking, plus a picture of any previous emotional problems the patient has had. She also wants much the same information about the patient's family and some rather specific knowledge of any life situations that may impinge on his or her condition. Is the patient married or single? Is his or her family intact? Are the patient's parents alive? In other words, she tries to collect all the factors that may be contributing to the present difficulty. But once she has them, she makes very sure that the difficulties aren't physical rather than mental in nature. She recommends that each patient visit an MD for a physical and asks that a report be sent to her. Many apparently emotional symptoms, Ms. Dulicai has found, are actually the tail ends of physical illnesses.

After these preliminaries, Ms. Dulicai and her patient sit down to talk. What, she asks, do you want out of this therapy? How do you want your life to change? After they establish these goals, they make a contract which, in its simplest form, might stipulate, "We'll meet once a week for six weeks, and then we'll reevaluate. Have you gotten what you want out of therapy? Are there other things you want to consider?" The point here is to give the patient a sense of control, a feeling that he or she has escaped the helplessness and dependence that mental turmoil can bring. And, to this end, the contract is taken very seriously. For example, when we arrived at the hospital, Ms. Dulicai was seeing a patient, a young woman who had had trouble forming and keeping intimate relationships all her life. Her goal for treatment was to get rid of that handicap, and every session in her contract period contained something aimed in that direction. In fact, Ms. Dulicai said that she would not move from that issue unless her patient came in with an urgent new subject she wanted to put in its place.

Once the terms of the contract are set and its goals established, the exclusively verbal part of treatment ends, and its dance or movement segment begins, a portion that could get started in either of two ways. If the patient is fairly articulate or knows exactly what he or she wants from therapy (or if the therapist believes strongly in this approach), the work might commence immediately – that is, without a period of diagnosis. With the woman who had trouble with intimacy, for example, Ms. Dulicai said that she had begun by talking about the patient's first intimate relationship, the attachment to her mother. The woman had had trouble remembering those times, and they had tried some movements together that therapists have found can trigger such recall: being held, rocking, being swung around, pushing, pulling. These movements evoke what insiders call "kinesthetic memory," the muscle's memory of some former activity, and they can both get the therapeutic process started and convince the patient that there is something to this form of counseling. An experience of kinesthetic memory can be the final proof necessary to demonstrate that our actions are directly connected to our thoughts and feelings.

The other road a therapist might take after making a contract with a patient – if that patient is not terribly verbal or the therapist does not believe in plunging ahead intuitively – is into a formal diagnostic tool called "movement analysis." Using the terms provided by Labananalysis (or some other system), he or she will describe the patient's movement, posture and "body language" in great detail. To do this sort of thing, Ms. Dulicai and her colleagues use a form that has them looking at several large categories – how the body and its parts are held and move, how the patient

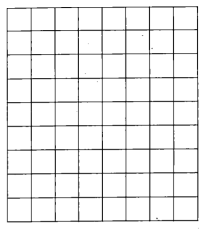

Dance therapists treat action as a language through which it is possible to read messages about deeply hidden feelings and desires.

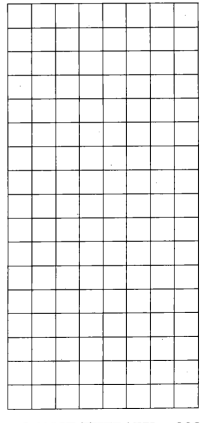

moves from place to place and how much effort he or she requires to act, to name three – and countless smaller details, each as it relates to a person's habitual movement and behavior. They record their observations of each of the form's categories by jotting down its frequency in the subject's activity; for instance, in the time given over to diagnosis, did the patient hold his or her upper body erect and rigid constantly? Almost always? Frequently? Occasionally? Or rarely? What comes of this athletic accounting is an assessment of the client's "movement repertory," a term that means his or her collection of usual actions and postures. What the therapist wants to know is: does the client do most of the things other folks do under similar circumstances? Are there things he or she can't or won't do? Do certain actions seem preferences? Would the client's life be *physically* easier if he or she learned a few new tricks? And would it be *emotionally* healthier if the client could make certain other changes?

This sounds simplistic, but it's not. Ms. Dulicai showed us a tape of her initial contact with two youngsters who had recently lost their father – brothers seven and ten years old and in trouble at school. As the meeting progressed she had them rolling on the floor, rocking about, lots of things they enjoyed. She found, however, that as the maneuvers got more complex the little boy grew less inclined to do them. She wasn't quite sure why until she asked the kids to be as "small" as they could be. This the younger kid loved. But when she asked them to be "big," he refused, and she concluded that the misbehavior problems at home and at school were part of an unwillingness to do the "growing up" that he felt his father's death required. Another tape we saw contained the first gathering of a family group of six with their therapist. The parents thought they were at the hospital to have the youngest child's behavior problems looked into, but it was evident even to us that the troubles spread beyond the little one. The family was understandably nervous in the strange clinical setting, but most of the members seemed reasonably calm. Two of the kids, though, including the youngest, were very fidgety, and when Ms. Dulicai pointed it out, we saw why. The others were unconsciously using them as safety valves for *their* nervousness; they appeared to be *looking* their own jitters into the kids and out. The poor kids had become the family's scapegoats.

Of course, this diagnosis didn't end with these simple observations, but you get the idea. Actions are regarded as a language through which it is possible to read messages about deeply hidden feelings, desires, even social processes. One of the most surprising things about dance therapy is that treatment doesn't necessarily begin after this diagnostic period is over, however long and complex it may be. Treatment has been going on *all through it.* There is practically no line between diagnosis and treatment in dance therapy, because both are movement, pure and almost simple. A retarded man on another videotape was asked to stamp his feet in sequences demonstrated by his therapist; she wanted to determine his range of motion and his ability to follow directions. But the very act of stamping was a form of expression that he may not have experienced before. And doing it with another human being was a kind of social interaction he seemed to delight in. This simple act contained both treatment and diagnosis. Still another recorded session we saw told the story of an exchange student who came to Ms. Dulicai feeling depressed but unable to talk about it. The girl was a trained dancer, however, and through sessions of folk dancing – dancing from her native country – with her therapist she could "speak" about her sense of culture shock, of separation from things she knew and valued, and of loss. Again, diagnosis and treatment were inseparable.

Which brings up the most fascinating thing about dance therapy – at least to us. There are no protocols in its practice, no patterns or set routines. Almost no traditional choreography. When you go to your family doctor with a vague complaint, he or she always does the same things. Records symptoms. Takes temperatures and pulses. Knocks knees. Kneads chests and stomachs. And then asks questions, leading to other questions. What the doctor's doing is going through a systematic process of elimination in hopes of finding out what's wrong. It's important that the doctor go through these classic steps – leaving nothing out, carefully respecting the standard order – because he or she doesn't want to overlook anything. Not so with dance therapy. Each treatment program is different, because each "vague complaint" is different. In fact, each session is different, because new aspects of the problem present themselves each week. So there can't be sets of exercises for one problem and established dance steps for another. The therapist must make up each meeting on the spot, calling upon all available knowledge about the patient, human movement and its interpretation as he or she goes along. And that's incredible, we think!

DRUGS AND EXERCISE

We all know what a weaving car means – another drunk driver meandering down the highway, ready to self-destruct at any minute. It would be comical – if it weren't so dangerous. Drunk driving is a serious problem.

Alcohol is a drug that scrambles your coordination. The idea of getting behind the wheel with a haze of booze between you and the windshield is absurd.

Well, when you exercise, you're driving your body instead of your auto. And drugs affect how your body is going to motor down the exercise highway (though their effects may not be as obvious as those of alcohol).

In the best of all possible worlds, all exercise would be done without any drugs in your body. But most of us exercise in the real world of asphalt roads, gyms and swimming pools, and we do things differently there.

We may have no choice about some of the drugs we take. If you're taking a prescription drug under a doctor's direction, you can't stop taking it just because you want to exercise. But you should be aware of how that drug is going to influence your exercise. That way you can make allowances for the drug's effects.

First let's look at alcohol, a drug that will do nothing but bad things for any kind of activity. Alcohol is considered a recreational drug, a substance that people take for "fun."

Booze Dries You Out

While it's obvious that getting sloshed will not help your running, swimming or whatever, some people advocate beer as a refreshment during and after endurance events like marathons.

But alcohol is a depressant that's bound to drag you down. You may feel an initial rush from your first sip of beer, but those drafts will soon inhibit the functions of your central nervous system. Your reaction time will suffer, and your coordination will go out the window. That's why the American Dietetic Association says that "although alcohol is a ready source of energy for muscular work, its use by athletes is not recommended."

Alcohol may seem like an adequate and pleasurable thirst quencher after a long run or a hot tennis match, but that appearance is only a disguise.

The alcohol actually has a diuretic effect, which in the long run will make you lose more fluid than the suds supply. This effect can dehydrate you.

According to Nancy Clark, sports nutritionist for Boston's Sports Medicine Resource, Inc., "Drinking beer inhibits the release of the antidiuretic hormone (ADH), which retains water in the body. Instead of replacing fluids, you will urinate more frequently and lose body fluids."

Other drugs besides alcohol can have a depressant effect on your nervous system. These include sedatives and tranquilizers such as Seconal, Nembutal, Amytal, Luminal, Valium, Librium, Thorazine, Miltown, Equanil and Tofranil. (These are brand names of some of the most commonly used sedatives.)

Abram Hoffer, M.D., Ph.D., a psychiatrist in British Columbia, says that "when you take tranquilizers, you shouldn't do high-reflex sports like hockey or tennis. Your reaction time will be slowed and you won't perform as effectively as you would without the drug.

"But taking these drugs isn't bad for jogging, running or walking. Many of my patients who take tranquilizers walk eight to ten miles a day."

Many other kinds of drugs also make it necessary to modify your exercise.

A drug such as Inderal, which is taken to control high blood pressure, slows your pulse. Of course, if you're taking Inderal under doctor's orders, you can't stop taking it without medical advice. Just keep in mind its pulse-dampening effect. Under the influence of Inderal your heart may not be able to beat rapidly enough to keep up with extremely vigorous exercise. You'll poop out sooner than you would normally.

Antibiotics can also trip up your exercise program. Stephen Paul, Ph.D., chairman of the department of pharmacy economics and health care at Temple University, warns that some antibiotics cause digestive problems. "Some of the penicillins," he told us, "can cause diarrhea on the run. If you're taking ampicillin or moxicillin, you might find it hard to finish a long bike ride or long run. Of course, not everyone will react the same way.

"Some of these antibiotics may also increase your sen-

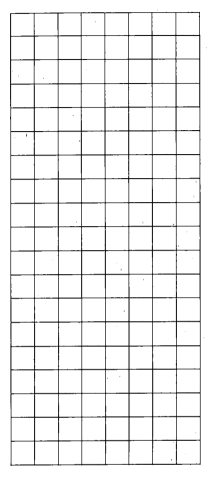

If you take medication and are involved in a heavy-duty exercise program, you must remember that the drugs you take affect your performance and endurance.

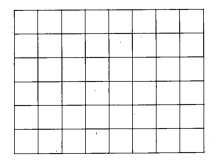

sitivity to the sun, so some people who are on them may get badly sunburned if they're not careful. Sunscreens like PABA (para-aminobenzoic acid) may not be effective for them, so they should try to stay out of the sun."

The Caffeine Zip

Many exercisers and athletes drink coffee before a workout or competition, and for good reason. Caffeine improves concentration and enables muscles to more rapidly turn the body's supply of fat into fuel. A study by David Costill, Ph.D., director of Ball State University's Human Performance Lab, showed that caffeine enables bicyclists to pedal longer and harder before exhaustion (*Medicine and Science in Sports,* Fall, 1978).

A problem with caffeine is that, in the parlance of drug users, you "crash." If your exercise routine lasts longer than the effects of the caffeine, you're going to find yourself losing steam in the midst of a workout or competition.

A particularly insidious family of drugs that affect athletic performance is that of amphetamines. These drugs mask fatigue and increase aggressiveness. Football players often take them before games because these little pills turn them into unfriendly people. That's an advantage during a rough pro football game, but it's not going to win many friends for the average person.

If you're on medically prescribed amphetamines for any reason, we recommend that you stay away from endurance activities. These drugs can interfere with the body's fatigue-alarm system.

Amphetamines, known colloquially as "speed," can make you unaware that a part of you is hurting, or that you're overtired or overheated. Since you can't feel that you're overdoing it, you run the risk of pushing yourself past the point of no return.

Aspirin, an Anti-Inflammatory

Another drug often mixed with exercise is aspirin. Since aspirin reduces both pain and inflammation, many people use it to exercise in spite of an injury.

But aspirin can backfire. Pain is often a signal that a part of you needs a rest. If you take aspirin and continue to exercise, you also take a chance of turning a mild injury into a serious one.

Taking aspirin can also upset your stomach, and a bad stomachache can stop your exercise program in its tracks. The stomach upset caused by aspirin could also be a precursor to stomach bleeding.

So if you are taking medication for any reason and are involved in a heavy-duty exercise program at the same time, remember that the drugs you are taking are going to affect your performance and endurance.

You may have to cut back your exercise program to accommodate your drug. If you have any questions about how much exercise you can do, ask your doctor. He should be able to give you a rundown of the drug's side effects.

But if you're still using a recreational drug like alcohol before or during exercise, you should cut it out! The best exercise is natural exercise – and the natural good feeling that goes with it.

FASTING

Fasting is a questionable way of losing weight or dealing with health problems. While many people swear by it, many medical people warn against this extreme method. To clarify the issues, we've included a question and answer section on the subject, incorporating the most common queries about fasting.

Q. *One of my friends told me about fasting and suggested that I try it, but I'm still puzzled. Is it all right to fast?*

A. That depends on why you want to fast and how you go about doing it.

Most people think of fasting as eating nothing for a period of time, or consuming nothing but water. That type of fasting is used by physicians as a tool in the treatment of patients who are allergic to certain foods or chemicals and who may have symptoms ranging from sneezing and coughing to depression and schizophrenia.

While the patient is on the fast, which may last for up to five days, his allergic symptoms usually disappear. When the patient is allowed to eat again, he may have an immediate, severe reaction to the offending food.

Another type of fasting is the modified fast, which is used under a physician's care for the treatment of massive obesity – a dangerous condition that can lead to diabetes or heart attack.

During a modified fast, a patient may eat nothing each day but a protein and carbohydrate supplement, a multivitamin tablet and a potassium supplement. In one such program, more than 500 patients were placed on a modified fast for about 30 weeks, and 78 percent of them lost more than 40 pounds.

Some people go on one-day fasts, making certain that they drink at least two quarts of water during the day. Others simply substitute fresh fruit and vegetable juices for solid food. They feel that fasting for a day gives their body the opportunity to detoxify itself – to rid itself of the pollutants it has unavoidably accumulated from food, tap water and even air.

Other claims made for fasting are that it may help you live longer, help you heal yourself faster when you're sick, help relieve your arthritis and make you more alert.

But fasting is not just a bowl of cherries. It can be dangerous for people with such medical conditions as diabetes, kidney disease or heart disease. Children shouldn't fast, nor should pregnant women.

Fasting can also have unwelcome side effects. Nausea, hair loss, dry skin, muscle cramps, fatigue, depression, bad breath, liver problems and loss of interest in sex are a few. Some researchers even think that under certain circumstances fasting can increase your risk of getting stomach cancer.

The point is that fasting is not something to be taken lightly. If you decide to try it, check with your doctor first.

Q. *Can I lose weight quickly by fasting and doing intense exercise at the same time?*

A. You might lose weight quickly, but you would be taking a big risk. The combination of fasting and demanding exercise (such as jogging) can be a dangerous combination. Marathoners who have been on extremely low calorie diets have had cardiac arrhythmias and have died during running.

When you fast, you deprive your body, and of course that includes your heart, of the nutrients it is accustomed to utilizing. If you simultaneously put extreme demands on your body, like running, you chance having your body quit on you altogether.

Q. *Aren't the liquid protein diets okay to use? Don't they keep you supplied with enough protein to keep you going?*

A. No, they're not okay. In fact, they may be more dangerous than eating nothing at all. First of all, they supply you with poor-quality protein – the amino acids are not in the proper balance that your body needs. Second, they don't give you the right amounts of potassium, phosphorus, magnesium and copper. These imbalances can kill you! A study in the *New England Journal of Medicine* (September 25, 1980) warned that "data demonstrate that a liquid protein diet is frequently associated with potentially life-threatening arrhythmias."

Q. *I'm starting to think that any kind of fasting is too dangerous to do. Should I never fast at all?*

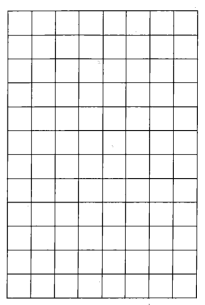

Long-term fasts are potentially dangerous and should be done only under close medical supervision. But there's probably nothing wrong with an unsupervised short-term fast of one or two days.

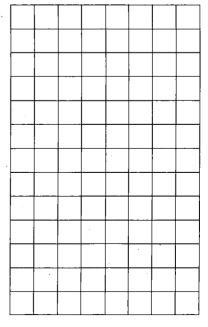

A. Long-term fasts are potentially dangerous and should only be done under close medical supervision. But there's probably nothing wrong with an unsupervised short-term fast of one or two days. Psychologically it can be helpful if you've been trying to diet and lose weight but you can't seem to loosen your ties to the dinner table. Fasting may give you some helpful perspective on the problem by giving you some distance from your consumption problem.

If you do try a short-term fast, there are a couple of things you should remember. Drink plenty of liquids. Don't let yourself get dehydrated. And don't try to do vigorous exercise. Some light to moderate walking is fine. But don't overdo it. Not eating puts you into a stressful situation. Don't add to the stress.

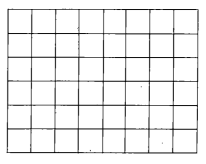

FATIGUE AND STAMINA

Sometimes you have to reexamine your ideas about your body. They may seem like *common* sense, but they don't make *body* sense. Take the problem of fatigue and energy, for instance. Your common sense might tell you that you have only a certain amount of energy to use, so you'd better conserve it in any way you can. And that includes not exercising. But nothing could be further from the truth! Exercise actually provides you with more energy; it's *inactivity* that wears you out.

Fatigue is often the result of too little physical activity. But lack of exercise is only one cause of fatigue. Lack of proper nutrition is another.

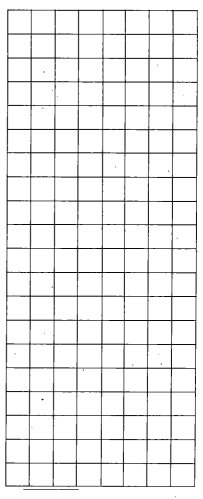

Exercise: His Cup of Tea . . . and Coffee

Here's a case in point. A writer friend of ours does a lot of work at night. Occasionally, when it gets late and he still has work to do, he'll find himself starting to nod over his typewriter.

"I used to drink a lot of coffee to keep myself going," he told us. "But I found that the more coffee I drank, the more I would need the next night if I wanted to stay up. I could see that I was getting into a vicious cycle of never-ending coffee cups.

"I tried switching to tea, but that proved to be the same as coffee. Once again, I was drinking more and more. The only difference was that I had substituted tea for coffee. And that was no improvement at all.

"The big problem was that I was sitting down for long stretches of time. I only got up to go to the stove to make tea or coffee. Or to go to the bathroom after my third cup. I was in a real rut, feeling dragged out and crummy. The coffee and tea weren't helping, and my work started to suffer as a result. That was when I discovered a new use for my exercise bicycle.

"I'd always been into jogging and I had an exercise bike down in the basement that I used when bad weather made it impossible to run. But one time, late at night, I decided to spend half an hour on the bike because I had missed my afternoon run. I figured that after 30 minutes on the bike, I'd be bushed and have just enough energy to crawl into bed. Boy was I surprised!

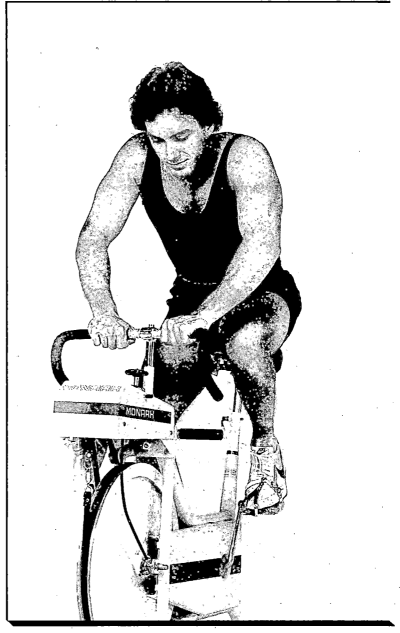

Exercise bicycles develop your aerobic capacity.

"The ride on the bike woke me up. And that was the opposite of what I thought would happen. The stimulation of working up a sweat gave me another hour of solid work at my typewriter.

"A couple of months ago I gave up tea and coffee altogether. I got tired of all that caffeine. Now when I need a lift, I drink a little fruit juice and work out on the bike. It works as well as the caffeine ever did. And I feel better the next morning."

Our friend's discovery doesn't qualify him as the Edison of exercise, though. He was beaten to the punch by Hippocrates, the famous physician of ancient Greece, who said that "inactivity wastes" and "activity strengthens." A more contemporary doctor, Ray C. Wunderlich, Jr., M.D., of St. Petersburg, Florida, echoed that statement in an interview. "Fatigue is often the result of too little physical activity," he told us.

But during the interview Dr. Wunderlich used a word that would have sounded strange to Hippocrates: *aerobic* activity. If you've read our chapter on aerobic exercise and dance, you know what he was talking about. Jogging, cycling, walking. Any activity you keep at for 20 minutes or more that speeds up circulation and floods muscles and tissues, including weary brain cells, with oxygen. And as our friend found out, an activity like typing doesn't qualify. That's because it's *an*aerobic – a short burst of action that doesn't push oxygen into every cell. Taking out the garbage, lugging laundry up steps, chasing the bus and other frenzied bursts of daily life are in the same category. They leave you frazzled, not fresh. And constant frazzle can lead to chronic fatigue.

But lack of exercise is only one cause of fatigue. Lack of proper nutrition is another.

The Antifatigue Nutrients

If you have chronic fatigue, there's a checklist of nutrients you should consult. Even a slight deficiency in any one of them could put your vitality under the weather. The first item on that list is magnesium.

Magnesium sparks more chemical reactions in the body than any other mineral. In a severe deficiency, the whole body suffers. You stumble instead of walk, feel depressed, have heart spasms. Doctors are trained to recognize these and over 30 other symptoms of a severe deficiency. But they aren't trained to recognize a mild deficiency of magnesium. It has only one noticeable symptom: chronic fatigue.

"A deficiency of magnesium is a common cause of fatigue," says Dr. Wunderlich.

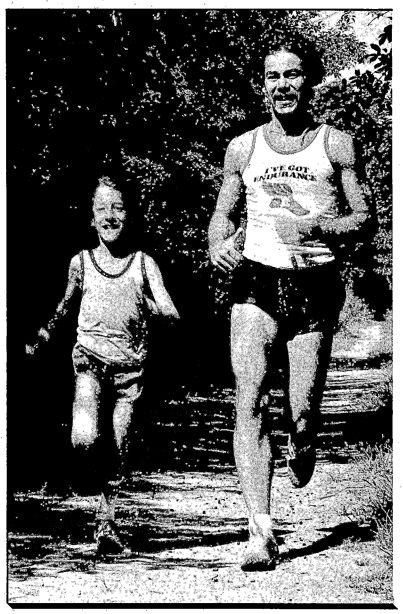

Vigorous exercise boosts energy levels.

But that fatigue can be cured easily.

In a study of magnesium and fatigue, 200 men and women who were tired during the day were given the nutrient. In all but two cases, waking tiredness disappeared (*2d International Symposium on Magnesium,* June, 1976).

Tiredness is hard to define. But, in many cases, it means tired muscles, muscles that feel leaden or drained of energy. A lack of magnesium, which helps muscles contract, can cause that tiredness. So can a lack of potassium.

Potassium deficiency is a well-known hazard among long-distance runners and professional athletes. The mineral helps cool muscles, and hours of exertion use it up. If it's not replaced, the result is chronic fatigue, even for a highly trained athlete. "When you lack potassium," says Gabe Mirkin, M.D., runner of marathons and coauthor of *The Sportsmedicine Book* (Little, Brown, 1978), "you feel tired, weak and irritable."

But a potassium deficiency and the weakness that goes with it aren't limited to athletes. In one study, researchers randomly selected a group of people and measured their potassium intake. Those people with a deficient intake of potassium – 60 percent of the men and 40 percent of the women in the study – had a weaker grip than those with a normal intake. And, as potassium intake decreased, muscular strength decreased (*Journal of the American Medical Association,* October 6, 1969).

You could probably put up with a few days of weakness. But after a few months you feel terrible. "In chronic potassium deficit," wrote a researcher who studied the mineral, "muscular weakness may persist for many months and be interpreted as being due to emotional instability" (*Minnesota Medicine,* June, 1965).

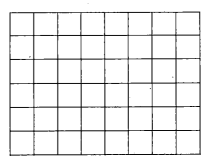

In chronic potassium deficit, muscular weakness may persist for many months and be interpreted as being due to emotional instability.

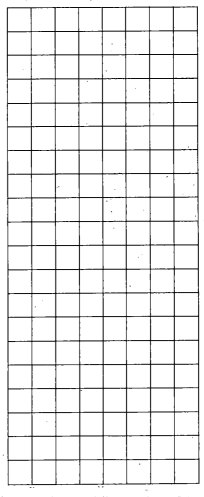

"The Housewife Syndrome"

Could a teary, depressed and irritable housewife be nothing more than the victim of a potassium deficiency? Yes. One physician dubbed the problem "The Housewife Syndrome." It looks something like the following . . .

Twenty pounds of laundry, but you don't have an ounce of strength. The kids want a maid, your husband a lover, your mother-in-law a saint, but all you want is a good night's sleep. You wake up tired and go to bed exhausted. For you, life is a chore.

If you can't take any more, check to see if your diet provides enough potassium and magnesium.

A doctor chose 100 chronically fatigued patients – 84 women and 16 men – and put them on a supplementary regimen of potassium and magnesium. Of the 100, 87 improved.

"The change was startling," writes Palma Formica, M.D., of Old Bridge, New Jersey. "They had become alert, cheerful, animated and energetic and walked with a lively step. They stated that sleep refreshed them as it had not done for months. Some said they could get along on 6 hours sleep at night, whereas formerly they had not felt rested on 12 or more. Morning exhaustion had completely subsided.

"Almost all patients have undertaken new activities," she notes. "Six who had not worked outside the home before obtained part-time jobs. Two of the pregnant patients continued to work for a time. Several of the husbands called and expressed appreciation of the physical improvement and consequent increase in emotional well-being of their wives."

Some of those patients had had chronic fatigue for over two years. Yet it took only five to six weeks of magnesium and potassium therapy to clear up their problem (*Current Therapeutic Research,* March, 1962).

But not all cases of chronic fatigue are caused by a lack of potassium and magnesium. In fact, many are caused by a lack of iron.

Iron helps form hemoglobin, the substance in red blood cells that carries oxygen from your lungs to the rest of your body. If that oxygen supply is reduced, you have the blues: apathy, tiredness, irritability – the symptoms of iron-deficiency anemia. But even if your blood tests show adequate levels of hemoglobin, you may still have an energy-crippling iron deficiency.

You Can Be Iron-Deficient but Not Anemic

"A deficiency of iron may be present when blood hemoglobin falls within normal limits," says Dr. Wunderlich. "This syndrome of iron deficiency without anemia," he continues, "is an exceedingly important cause of fatigue."

Iron deficiency creeps up on you. Periods drain iron. Pregnancies sap it. Reducing diets cut down your intake. Before you know it, every cell of your body is dragging.

One study shows just how slow you go compared to

somebody who's not iron-deficient. Researchers studied the "physical work capacity" of 75 women, some anemic, some not. The anemic women could stay on a treadmill an average of eight minutes less than the nonanemic group. None of the anemic women could perform under "highest working load" conditions. All of the nonanemic group could. During a work test, the anemics' heartbeats rose to an average of 176 per minute, the nonanemics' to 130. Levels of lactate, a chemical in the muscles that is linked to fatigue, were almost twice as high in the anemic group (*American Journal of Clinical Nutrition,* June, 1977).

But relief from iron deficiency is simple. Replace the iron.

Workers on an Indonesian rubber plantation were paid by productivity, and researchers found that those who were anemic earned the least. But after two months of iron supplementation, the previously anemic workers had normal levels of iron and earned the same amount as those free from anemia (*American Journal of Clinical Nutrition,* April, 1979).

In a similar study, researchers gave a group of anemics iron for 80 days, while another group with anemia received a placebo, a fake iron pill. Before the iron supplementation and again after 80 days, both groups took a "step test," repeatedly stepping on and off a small bench.

In the first test, the anemics who were to receive iron had an average heart rate of 154 beats per minute. After receiving iron, it was 118. During the final step test, they also had 15 percent more oxygen delivered per beat than the placebo group. And their lactate levels after the final step test were about half the placebo group's (*American Journal of Clinical Nutrition,* September, 1975).

Iron deficiency is, of course, caused by lack of iron. But anemia – too little hemoglobin – has other nutritional causes as well.

"The commonest cause [of anemia] is iron deficiency, but folate deficiency . . . can also be a cause," says a report in *Lancet* (February 21, 1976).

Blood Needs Folate, Too

The report goes on to cite a study in which women received either iron alone, folate alone, or iron and folate together. Only 26 percent of those who received a single nutrient had a rise in hemoglobin, while 96 percent of those who received iron and folate had a rise.

The B complex vitamin folate is a must for the creation of normal red blood cells. Without enough of this nutrient, red blood cells are too large, strangely shaped and have a shortened life span. A lack of healthy red blood cells means less hemoglobin, which in turn means less oxygen is delivered to the body. The result is lethargy, weakness, fatigue.

A psychiatrist found that four of his patients with "easy fatigability" and other symptoms had low levels of folate. He supplemented their diet with the nutrient. As folate levels rose, fatigue disappeared (*Clinical Psychiatry News,* April, 1976).

But all the folate in the world won't do you any good unless you get enough vitamin B_{12}. Folate stays trapped in a metabolically useless form until B_{12} releases it. B_{12}, however, is more than folate's understudy. It plays an important role of its own. It can relieve tiredness.

Twenty-eight men and women who complained of tiredness but who had no physical problems were given B_{12} and then asked to evaluate its effect. For many of the 28, the vitamin not only made them feel less fatigued but also improved their appetite, sleep and general well-being (*British Journal of Nutrition,* September, 1973).

The checklist is almost complete. It needs vitamin C.

Miners in Czechoslovakia who received 1,000 milligrams of vitamin C a day reported less fatigue and faster reaction times after taking the vitamin (*Review of Czechoslovak Medicine,* vol. 22, no. 4, 1976).

And a study of over 400 people who filled out a questionnaire that asked them to list their vitamin C intake and their "fatigue symptoms" showed that those who took over 400 milligrams of vitamin C a day had less fatigue (*Journal of the American Geriatrics Society,* March, 1976).

Vitamin C may relieve fatigue by cleansing the body of pollutants, such as lead and cadmium.

A doctor in a Swiss village found that his patients who lived close to a busy highway passing through the town had twice as much fatigue (and insomnia, depression and digestive disorders) as those living 50 or more yards from the road. He treated these patients with vitamin C, vitamin B complex and calcium. Over 66 percent got relief.

So remember, staying fatigue-free is a two-sided problem. High energy levels depend on what you eat and how active you are. With regular exercise and good nutrition, you can be full of life.

FEET AND FOOTWEAR

Y ou look down on them. You squeeze them, squash them, pound them into the ground, and when they start to give you trouble, you curse them. To put it bluntly, you walk all over them. Just about the only thing you don't do to your feet is what you should do – treat them with respect.

Aching feet are more likely to elicit chuckles (if they belong to someone else) or wry appeals for sympathy (if they belong to you) than serious attention. Corns, bunions, hammertoes and the lot are easier to complain about than to correct. What's worse, the disregard with which you contemplate these down-to-earth organs is likely to be shared by your doctor.

"There's a tendency to ignore feet," says Melvin Jahss, M.D., chief of the Orthopedic Foot Service at New York's Hospital for Joint Diseases and Medical Center, and founder and past president of the American Orthopedic Foot Society. "Doctors pay little attention to 'minor' things like aching feet, but they can cause a lot of problems. When your feet hurt, you hurt all over."

It's a fact that foot miseries have a way of "infecting" the whole person. Aching feet can make it hard to feel anything but tense and irritated. "If your feet are bothering you, you're going to subliminally pull away from the source of pain," says Elizabeth H. Roberts, D.P.M., New York podiatrist and author of *On Your Feet* (Rodale Press, 1975). "You'll throw your posture out of line. And the more out of line your body is, the greater the stress and fatigue. When you're slumped over, your digestive tract won't function well – it will be cramped for space. You're likely to develop lower back problems, knee problems."

Most important, perhaps, is the damage that bad feet can inflict on your plans for a full, active life. "You'll cut down on your social life," says Dr. Roberts. "You're not going to want to play tennis, go for long walks, do the things that make for better respiration, that keep your body agile, that keep you feeling young."

By making walking or running a painful experience rather than a pleasure, a simple bunion, plantar wart or blister can stop your exercise program in its tracks.

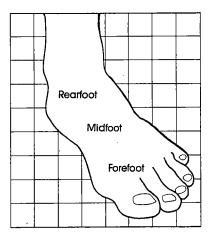

Going barefoot is better than wearing improper footwear. Poor shoes can throw the foot out of alignment and cause injury.

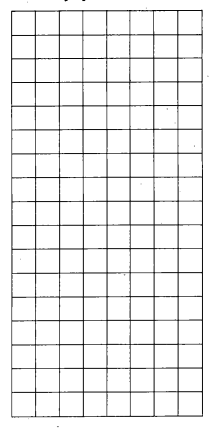

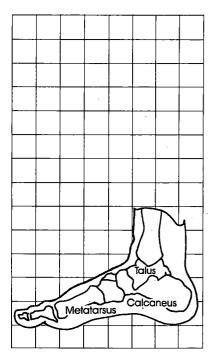

The foot contains a complex arrangement of bones because it does a complex job. It supports you when you're standing still and also carries you to your destination when you're on the move.

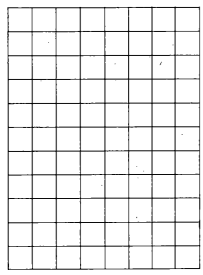

A Lot to Go Wrong

It seems no exaggeration, in fact, to call the feet the foundation of good health.

If so, it seems a particular shame that so many foundations are in such poor repair. Some 80 percent of us suffer from aching feet at some time or another; according to surveys, it is the third most common medical complaint. And these complaints are not always trivial. At the Hospital for Joint Diseases, says Dr. Jahss, some 20 to 25 percent of all surgical cases involve the foot.

Why is the foot so vulnerable to ache and injury? For one thing, it is a very complex organ, a structure of 26 bones (one-eighth of all the bones in the entire body), 56 ligaments and 38 muscles. With each step you take, the whole ensemble must shift and flex properly to carry your weight. There's a lot to go wrong.

What's more, this complex structure takes a heavy dose of wear and tear. By the time the average person is 35, one's feet have carried him or her some 45,000 miles. "When you walk, each step puts your entire weight on each foot," says Dr. Jahss. "Pushing forward, raising your heel as you step, you may concentrate a force greater than your weight on a localized area – if you weigh 150 pounds, for instance, the ball of your foot may carry 200 pounds. Do this 1,000 or 2,000 times a day, and you're really beating the soles of your feet on the ground. If you hit your head against the wall 2,000 times, it would be sore. That's what happens to your feet – the bones, the ligaments hurt after a while."

Being farthest from the heart, the feet generally have the poorest circulation in the body, and the circulation diminishes with age. As a result, infections and inflammations are slow to heal. (And the warm, moist climate created by shoes and socks, incidentally, provides perfect growth conditions for bacteria and fungi.)

The natural shocks that feet are heir to may sound severe enough, but if they belong to modern man, the abuse is compounded. While it's a treat to beat your feet on the Mississippi mud, it's no fun to pound them on pavement, which is exactly what most of us do.

"We're the first animals to walk upright, on two feet, and it's possible that our feet are not built to bear as much weight as we give them," says Neal Kramer, D.P.M., a Bethlehem, Pennsylvania, podiatrist and a member of the

American Academy of Podiatric Sports Medicine. "When we walked on soft grass, there was no problem. But now we spend most of our time on hard surfaces, and our feet have to absorb a lot more shock."

If you stay off your feet whenever possible, they will become even more vulnerable, experts say. A sedentary way of life makes feet weak. Encased in shoes all day, your feet remain immobile, denied, for the most part, the exercise they would get if you went barefoot. "Certain foot muscles are far less pronounced than they were in bygone days; they just don't get a chance to develop," says Dr. Kramer.

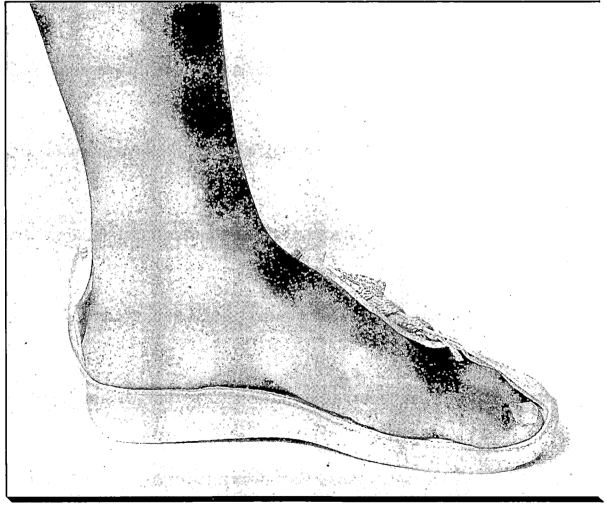

Running shoes give feet cushioning and support.

The Wrong Footwear

When you get to the bottom of many foot problems, in fact, what you'll find is a pair of shoes. Too many people give style and appearance disproportionate weight when choosing shoes – at the expense of their feet. Cinderella wasn't the first woman to try to win her prince by jamming her feet into tiny footwear, nor was she the last. The price has been high.

"If you put your hand into a glove that kept squashing it, your hand would bother you – and it doesn't have to bear the weight the foot does," says Dr. Roberts.

Under the constant pressure and friction of ill-fitting shoes, your foot defends itself by producing the dead, toughened tissues of a callus. A corn, made up of the same tissue and formed in the same way, projects downward, into the foot, concentrating pressure into a point of pain. Shoes that press down on the toes can produce ingrown toenails or a painful thickening of the nail over the big toe.

According to Dr. Jahss, some shoe styles are particularly liable to cause difficulties. "About 85 percent of the foot problems I see are in women," he says. "This is because of the style of women's shoes – they don't conform to the foot. High heels make the whole foot slide forward; it jars in the front of the shoe. The higher the heel, the more weight is carried on the ball of the foot, which can cause a callus. If a woman has a wide forefoot, it will be especially jammed, and raise the danger of deformities like corns, bunions and hammertoes."

Other styles are associated with other problems. Platform shoes, according to physicians, can cause painful bleeding under the big toenail. And tight boots can actually cut off circulation. By distorting the normal way in which the foot strikes the ground and carries weight, ill-fitting, ill-designed shoes can cause damage to muscles and joints. Bunions, which are inflammations of the joint where the toes meet the foot, are often due, at least in part, to shoes that force the big toe into an unnatural angle. High heels, worn habitually, can shorten the Achilles tendon, making the wearer susceptible to injuries.

How to Shop for Shoes

There are general principles that apply to any shoe purchase, whether you're shopping for running shoes, basketball shoes, walking shoes or high-fashion footwear.

To give your toes a chance to spread out naturally, your shoes should be about one-fourth of an inch longer than your longest toe. They should be high and wide enough not to squash your toes. The shank, which is the part of the shoe between the ball of the foot and the heel, should be wide enough to accommodate the bottom of the foot. Ideally, there should be no more than a two-inch difference between the height of the heel and the sole. And the sole should be flexible enough to bend with your foot and thick enough to absorb some of the shock of life on concrete.

"The shoe should conform to the foot, not the foot to the shoe," says Dr. Jahss. "Children's shoes conform to their feet, so we don't see children with the foot pains and complications that adults have. If adults wore kids' shoes, they'd be fine."

Give an eye to material when you buy shoes. Because they retain heat and moisture, some nonporous man-made materials are more likely to promote fungus and bacterial infections than naturally porous leather.

Different Shoes for Different Exercises

There are a few more things to look for when buying a shoe to exercise in. We're going to talk about three different kinds of shoes that you'll be shopping for if you start an exercise program: shoes for walking, shoes for running and general-purpose sport shoes for court sports like basketball.
Walking. Make sure your shoes are well cushioned, with soles that are thick enough to deal with the punishment of hitting the sidewalk over and over. A solid oxford is well designed for walking, says Dr. Kramer, and good hiking boots are also fine. He particularly recommends running shoes. They're good for walkers for the same reason they're good for runners: a sophisticated design that includes solid cushioning and support for the foot.
Running. When you run, you subject your feet to a force equal to three times your body weight. That's why choosing a good running shoe is very important. Otherwise, you won't get very far down the road before you run into an injury. Don't take a chance on a bargain shoe without a brand name; stick to well-known brands.

A running shoe's sole should be flexible. You should

be able to bend the shoe easily along the area under the ball of the foot.

The heel "counter" – the part of the shoe that wraps around the heel – is another important running shoe feature. The counter should be firm to protect your Achilles tendon and the rear of your foot.

Shop for running shoes in a store that specializes in running equipment and has a large supply of shoes and a knowledgeable staff. A wide selection of footwear will give you a better chance of finding a shoe that meets your needs. A well-informed salesperson, hopefully someone who does a lot of running, can give you advice on what kind of shoe will be good for your body and foot type.

Modern running shoes don't need to be broken in. They should feel comfortable the first time you put them on. If they don't, you shouldn't buy them. At the shoe store, you should actually do a small amount of jogging in them to see what they feel like. Take a spin through the aisles or around the front of the store to get a good idea of how they fit. Some stores will let you run around the block.

Court sports. Many people wear running shoes to play other sports. That's a mistake.

When you run, you move forward, and a running shoe's design provides protection for forward motion exclusively. Other sports, however, are not so simple. When you play basketball, racquetball or tennis, you change direction frequently, and running shoes don't have good stability for sudden movements to the side.

Generally, shoes for court sports should be well cushioned and have good durability. They shouldn't bind your feet, but they should fit snugly enough so that when you pivot or change direction suddenly, your feet do not slip around inside the shoes. If the shoes are too loose, they're going to cause blisters. (If you end up with shoes that are a little too big, wearing thick socks or two pairs of socks will prevent most blisters.)

Your shoes will last longer if you give each pair a 24-hour rest after wearing them. That lets them dry out completely between wearings. So, if you have a favorite pair of shoes, buy another identical pair – same make, same size. Alternate them, and you'll get more wearings per pair than you would if you wore the same pair every day.

HEADACHES

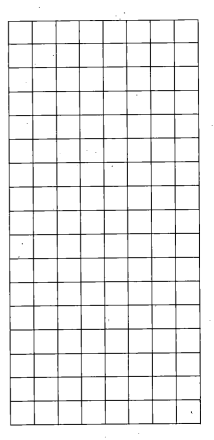

Headaches are a bit like explosives. They come in different sizes and strengths. There are the Fourth of July firecrackers, and then there are the TNT blockbusters. The garden-variety tension headaches that many of us occasionally experience pale in significance before the megaton blasts of pain delivered by the migraine and its less well-known relative, the cluster headache.

While migraine often singles out women as its victims, cluster headaches are much more likely to strike men. "The pain of a cluster headache is perhaps the most intense pain that a man will ever know," says headache expert Seymour Diamond, M.D., in his book *More Than Two Aspirin: Hope for Your Headache Problem* (Follett, 1976). He points out that many men weep because of the pain, while others roll on the floor in agony.

Cluster headaches get their name because they occur in groups. Each attack may last for only 30 minutes to two hours, but is part of a barrage of up to four or more headaches daily. Pain is usually confined to one side of the head and centers around the socket of the eye, which waters profusely. Runny nose and sweating are also common. Cluster headaches may strike every day for weeks or months and then disappear – only to return several months later.

"Some men will literally beat their heads against the wall to escape the pain," says Dr. Diamond. "I had one patient, a young man, who pleaded with his father to knock him out so that he would no longer suffer the pain. I've even heard of some victims who became so distracted by the pain that they considered suicide."

Despite that dreary outlook, however, some cluster victims are finding relief, and in a very improbable manner. Not with drugs or pain-numbing narcotics, but through programs of regular, vigorous exercise.

A regular running program can benefit people with migraine headaches, according to Dr. Appenzeller. He's seen several patients find relief by jogging seven to nine miles daily.

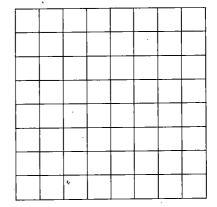

15 Years of Pain

One such case is described by Ruth Atkinson, M.D., and Otto Appenzeller, M.D., Ph.D., in the November, 1977, issue

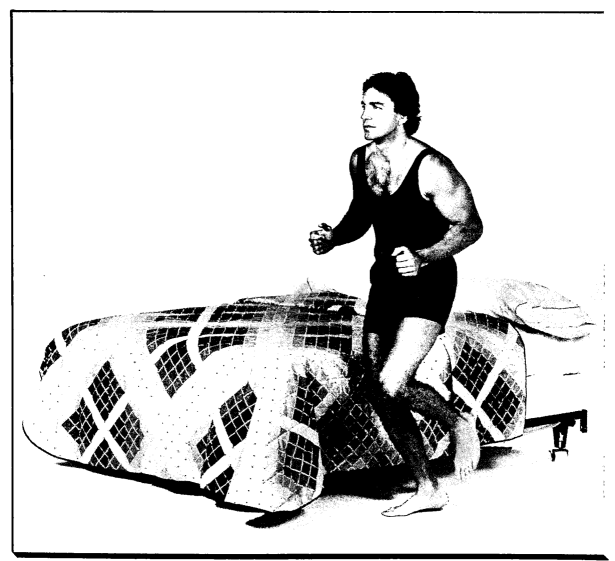

Running in place can help relieve headaches.

of the journal *Headache*. Both Dr. Atkinson and Dr. Appenzeller are associated with the neurology department and headache clinics at the University of New Mexico School of Medicine in Albuquerque. The patient, a 56-year-old senior administrator for a government agency, had suffered severe headaches beginning in 1961. Since October, 1975, the pain had become a *daily* occurrence.

"It is excruciating and feels as though a finger were pushing out my eyeball from the upper rear of the orbit," he complained. "At least 65 percent start when I am asleep and awaken me when pain becomes strong enough. During an active cycle, two headaches per night are common, and I have had as many as five per night between 10:30 P.M. and 6 A.M."

Antihistamines, painkillers and other drugs were ineffective in controlling the symptoms.

Then the man stumbled upon a curious pattern: "The headaches occur during quiescent periods an hour or two after lunch or dinner, when I am reading, watching TV or having casual conversation. They have never occurred when I am working around the house, during backpacking, skiing or playing tennis . . .

"Because I never had headache during physical activity, I tried running one evening in July, 1974, when I felt pressure starting to build in my head. I ran 220 yards in 25 seconds, and within three minutes all pressure had disappeared, both nostrils were clear and no pain developed. A headache awoke me later that same night and I ran in place until my heart rate was 120 per minute." Within a few minutes the pain was gone.

The patient has continued ever since to successfully counter his frequent headaches with exercise. "Usually one running session is enough, and the pain stops within five minutes."

There is possibly an added benefit to the therapy. As Dr. Atkinson points out, the man's "fine physical condition may in part be attributed to the exercise he gets in attempting to control his headaches."

A regular running program can also benefit people with migraine headaches, according to Dr. Appenzeller. He's seen several patients find relief by jogging seven to nine miles daily at a speed of seven to nine minutes per mile. "I have 18 patients who suffered from migraines. After reaching this level of activity, they are headache-free and medicine-free," he told us.

Dr. Appenzeller, who is a frequent marathon runner himself, believes such a program would be good for just about anyone whose health permits it. If the results of his study are any indication, you'll lose weight, feel better and, he predicts, "you will be cured of all headaches."

What makes exercise so effective in silencing headache's heavy artillery? No one is really sure, but there are plenty of theories.

Dr. Appenzeller speculates that endurance training such

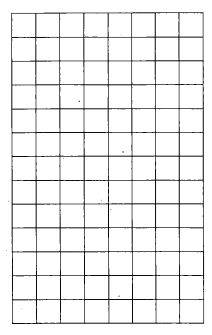

Extra oxygen may be another key to solving the cluster headache mystery. That's exciting, because vigorous exercise such as jogging delivers more oxygen to the body.

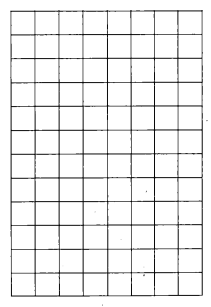

as running, cycling and swimming may spur the body to produce an important enzyme. That enzyme might prevent blood vessels in the brain from expanding and painfully pressing against nerves.

Such swelling, or vasodilation, as doctors call it, is believed to be the cause of vascular headaches, which include migraine and cluster. Tension headaches, on the other hand, usually involve the tightening of head and neck muscles in response to stress or worry.

Of course, exercise may help relieve the latter kind of headache pain as well, by reducing tension and inducing a relaxed bodily state.

Extra Oxygen May Do the Trick

Extra oxygen may be another key to solving the cluster headache mystery. In a letter to the *Journal of the American Medical Association* (January 16, 1978), Jerold F. Janks, O.D., a San Francisco optometrist, describes how oxygen helped him.

"I have been a victim of cluster headaches for the past 12 years," he confesses. "The intensity of pain is the same regardless of sidedness, but for some reason the left-sided clusters, in addition to involving the eye, ear and neck, also involve the left upper molars, the left side of the soft palate, and the left side of the Adam's apple."

Janks tried many medications without success. Then, five years ago, he visited a neurologist who suggested that if all else failed he might try oxygen.

Janks put an oxygen tank with breathing mask next to his bed and started using it during attacks. The result? "I am still a cluster statistic but not a victim," he reports. Breathing oxygen "totally aborts the headache in less than ten minutes." With another tank in his car and one at the office, Janks says, "I have reduced my cluster headaches from episodes of devastation to mere inconvenience."

The Body Can't Store Oxygen

That's intriguing, because vigorous exercise such as jogging *also* delivers more oxygen to the body. As Kenneth H. Cooper, M.D., points out in his landmark fitness book *Aerobics* (M. Evans, 1968), "The key to endurance is oxygen consumption.

"The body can store food," Dr. Cooper says, "*but it*

can't store oxygen. . . . The problem is to get enough oxygen to all the areas – all the small hidden, infinite areas in this wonderful mechanism we call the human body. . . ."

When we run, he says, the lungs process more oxygen and the heart pumps it via the blood more effectively. In short, "the training effect increases maximal oxygen consumption by increasing the efficiency of the means of supply and delivery." As a result, the body is literally saturated with oxygen. And that's when some problem-headache victims finally experience relief.

As Dr. Cooper notes in his follow-up volume *The New Aerobics* (M. Evans, 1970), "A few readers of *Aerobics* claimed that exercise helped, and in some cases, relieved them of their problem with migraine headaches. I can't scientifically document such a statement, and therefore report it only as an observation."

There may be still another contributing factor, however, that makes running and other aerobic exercises so effective against headaches.

As Dr. Appenzeller sees it, "Endurance training requires a great deal of discipline and perseverance; it leads unquestionably to a change in perspective and behavior. I believe these changes in outlook and personality are the most important causes of improvement in vascular headache patients after endurance training."

Dr. Cooper says much the same in *Aerobics:* "The training effect [of jogging, cycling, etc.] may change your whole outlook on life. You'll learn to relax, develop a better self-image, be able to tolerate the stress of daily living better." That's the kind of uplifting formula that could stop the average tension headache dead in its tracks.

Big headache or little headache, it seems that exercise is one avenue to pain prevention that's worth exploring.

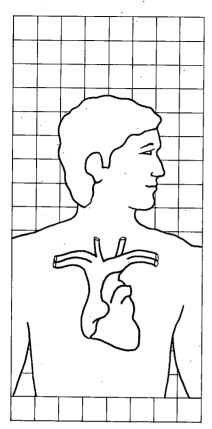

Although it never gets a vacation, the heart usually performs admirably—if you treat it right.

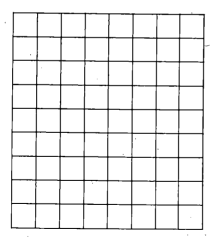

THE HEART

Make a fist. Now open and close it about once a second as you read. Does your hand quickly start to get tired? Does your forearm begin to cramp? Can you imagine doing that all day and night without any rest? Out of the question, you might say. Well, your heart is about the same size as your fist, and that opening and closing motion is exactly what it's doing right now and does day and night, about once a second, pumping blood without complaint. Most of the time you're not even aware that it's working to keep you alive. That's a pretty impressive task considering that it gets done in most people's chests continuously for 70 or more years.

And the heart not only beats for that long, it also takes a beating! As Michael DeBakey, M.D., and Antonio Gotto, M.D., two doctors who established a National Heart and Blood Vessel Research and Demonstration Center at Baylor College of Medicine in Houston, tell us in their book *The Living Heart* (McKay, 1977):

"It is indeed extraordinary to think that the heart must operate for 70 years without ever being permitted to rest or shut down for extensive repairs. It staggers the imagination to think of the wear and tear that the heart valves, those critically important parts of the cardiovascular machinery, must sustain in opening and shutting with considerable hydraulic pressure 2.5 billion times in a lifetime. The magnitude of these forces is apparent to a surgeon when replacing a defective heart valve with a *prosthetic device* consisting of a silicone ball in a steel cage. Some of these hard silicone balls become pitted, rutted and battered out of shape after only three or four years of being pounded by the blood."

Your Heart Needs Your Cooperation

Don't put your fist down yet! Now imagine that you are using a squeegee hand pump to move water from one bucket to another through a plastic, flexible tube, the same way the heart pumps blood through your arteries. You have to keep squeezing the hand pump to keep the water moving. You'd use both hands if you could, but we've tied one of them behind your back. Not only that, but there are people standing around who used to help you with your water pumping task, but now they're doing everything they can to make it harder for you. One of them, Mr. Hardening of the Arteries, is squeezing on the tube, making it narrower so that it is almost impossible to get water through it. Another evil doer, Ms. Cigarette, is pinching your nostrils, forcing you to breathe through your mouth, as she blows smoke in your face, making you choke, cough and splutter. At the same time, Mr. Nervous Personality is standing by your ear and hollering at you in a harsh, domineering voice, "Hurry up!"

Sounds unpleasant, doesn't it? If you had to work under those conditions, you would probably complain to the National Labor Relations Board. But those kinds of tortures are exactly what many people force their hearts to endure. And then they wonder why their hearts go crazy, running at funny rhythms or quitting altogether during a massive heart attack.

The heart is not an island unto itself, beating and pumping the blood through your body without regard to other events within its internal environment. The kind of life you live, the amount of exercise and the kind of exercise you get, the foods you eat, even the emotions that you feel – all of these things affect the heart.

Our picture of the beleaguered squeegee pumper parallels the kind of conditions that Robert A. Miller, M.D., chairman of the Coronary Care Committee at the Naples Community Hospital, Naples, Florida, describes in his book *How to Live With a Heart Attack and How to Avoid One* (Chilton, 1973):

"A 40-year-old man has narrowing of his coronary arteries by arteriosclerosis, but he has never had symptoms from the disease; it hasn't progressed far enough. On a particular day he is tense and anxious over a business deal. He smokes an unusual number of cigarettes. The carbon monoxide in the cigarettes combines preferentially with the hemoglobin in his red blood cells, and the blood is able to carry less and less oxygen to his heart. His anxiety is stimulating his glands to produce more adrenaline. His heart beats faster and therefore requires more oxygen for nourishment. A certain critical point is reached, and the heart revolts against the abnormally low oxygen supply. The nervous system of the heart goes into rebellion, and the result is a total disor-

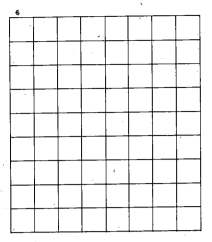

Many people force their hearts to endure torture, and then they wonder why their hearts go crazy, running at funny rhythms or quitting altogether.

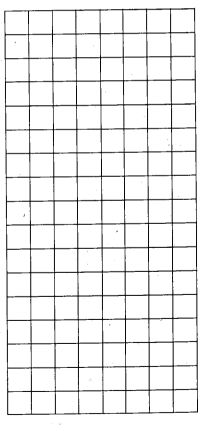

ganization of the heartbeat – known medically as ventricular fibrillation. Within five minutes the victim is dead."

How to Take Care of Your Heart

The most important component of the air that you breathe, as far as your heart is concerned, is oxygen. The heart muscle, just like all the other muscles in your body, needs a steady supply of oxygen in order to survive. Without it, the muscle tissue dies very quickly.

If you go back to our squeegee hand pump image, and the villainous Ms. Cigarette, you can see exactly what smokers are doing to their hearts – choking off their oxygen supply and making it more difficult for them to function. But people who lead a sedentary lifestyle and never exercise also lower their capacity to use oxygen (although they don't do it as drastically as do the smokers).

They do this because an unused body organizes itself around the principle of being able to do just enough to get by. If you spend all day, every day, sitting still at an activity like working at a desk and never exercising, then that is the level of activity your body and your heart will be capable of sustaining. It will have very little reserve for dealing with more strenuous activity. The situation is similar to living in a large mansion but using only one or two of the rooms and closing the doors to the rest of the house. The condition of the unused rooms deteriorates. If company suddenly shows up on Memorial Day weekend (your old school buddies, let's say) and you need a place for them to sleep, you're in trouble. You throw open the door to one of those unused rooms, and you're greeted by dust and mildew. Neglect, no matter how benign, results in decay. If you neglect your physical conditioning, it's the same as closing off the rooms to that house. You won't retain the use of what you don't use. You won't be able to cope with unusual demands.

Dr. Miller's 40-year-old smoker mentioned above, who dies under the strain of a harrowing business day, is an example of the disaster that can result from not having this reserve capacity. A little extra strain can put you in danger if you don't have that vital reserve. In the case of Dr. Miller's businessman, "the heart revolts against the abnormally low oxygen supply." If he had been a nonsmoker and had been physically fit from a good, long-term aerobic exercise program, chances are that he could have survived almost any stress and strain his job could have thrown at him.

One of the basic ideas of an aerobic exercise program is to gently push your heart to work at a level beyond what it normally has to do. This enables it to more easily handle average, day-to-day situations and gives it that reserve capacity to cope with extra stress. (For more information on this subject, see our chapter on aerobic exercise and dance.)

According to Sidney Alexander, M.D., a cardiologist and marathon runner who is on the faculty of the Harvard Medical School, "One of the major determinants of fitness [is] the efficient operation of the mechanisms necessary for bringing oxygen to the exercising muscles and burning it properly once it arrived there. . . . Cigarette smoking is the major cause of poor lung function in adults. Smoking severely injures lung tissues, interfering with oxygen uptake and carbon dioxide removal. Aging also reduces lung function. Some believe that a good fitness program may slow this deterioration" (*Running Healthy,* Stephen Greene Press, 1980).

Physical conditioning is a key tool for preventive maintenance of the heart, even for former heart attack patients who want to prevent the recurrence of heart trouble. For example, the Downstate Medical Center of the State University of New York has a program called the Cardiac Exercise Laboratory, which teaches heart patients and those who wish to avoid becoming heart patients how to exercise safely and effectively.

Recovering from a Heart Attack

It wasn't that long ago, recalls Richard Stein, M.D., director of the Cardiac Exercise Laboratory, that a program like his was unthinkable. "After a heart attack, the usual thing used to be: sell your business, retire, move to Florida. A lot of people," he adds with a wry smile, "were in the embarrassing position of being still around 20 years later – and very good at golf."

Now, he points out, doctors recognize that while heart disease may require some curtailment in activity, it rarely necessitates a complete withdrawal from active life. In fact, it is that fearful, protective attitude, rather than the disease itself, that often threatens to make heart attack victims into lifelong invalids.

"Taking a patient and throwing him out of a job and putting him into a very dependent position where every-

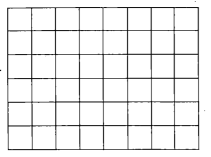

Physical conditioning is a key tool for preventive maintenance of the heart, even for former heart attack patients who want to prevent the recurrence of heart trouble.

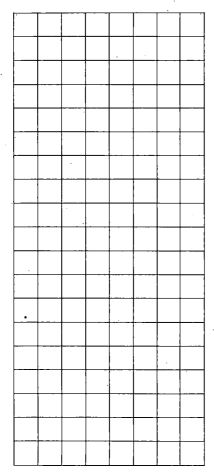

body picks up after him and talks softly in front of him – that turns him into a neurotic, sick cripple," Dr. Stein says. "It gives him less to live for."

The heart patients who work out under Dr. Stein's direction are more likely to start businesses than sell them, to play softball with their kids than to insist on silence around the house. With the caution of a scientist, Dr. Stein won't speculate on whether or not exercise prevents further heart attacks, but he will cite enthusiastically the human accomplishments of his program.

"We certainly have created a group of patients who are robust, vigorous, back at work, living full, meaningful lives, who have in no way had their lifestyle cramped by the disease," he says.

As little as 12 weeks after a heart attack, a patient may start the return to a full life by coming to the laboratory for evaluation. Unless problems like severe heartbeat irregularities contraindicate it, the patient is given a stress test – a brisk walk or jog on a treadmill while the EKG, pulse rate and blood pressure are watched carefully. "We assess how much exercise the patient can safely do. On the basis of that, we devise an exercise program for him to follow," says Dr. Stein.

Pedaling Back to Health

Here, an exercise program generally means an ergometer, a stationary exercise bicycle that can be adjusted to make pedaling strenuous or easy. Two more sessions at the laboratory train patients to use the ergometer, adjusting it to bring the heart rate up to the point where a positive training effect is produced (about 75 percent of the heart's maximum capacity).

Tested and trained, the patients take home an ergometer of their own and follow their "exercise prescription" three times a week, for at least a half hour each session. They come to the exercise lab every three months to have the performance of their heart monitored while they work out. "As patients get more fit, we up their prescription – increase the amount of exercise," says Dr. Stein.

What does a patient get for all this effort? One of the first and most important benefits, says Dr. Stein, is psychological – a victory over fear. "After you've had a heart attack, it's very difficult to push it out of your mind, convince yourself that you're well and concentrate on living. It's easy to become a 'cardiac neurotic,' an individual who's constantly concerned that the next moment he's going to have his pain and die.

"But if you work out on a bicycle three times a week, or go out and run around a track and work up a sweat, then this kind of problem is taken care of. You're proving to yourself that you can exert yourself and not die."

The change in a patient's outlook, according to Florence Frank, a nurse in the program, can be striking – and immensely rewarding. "People are so frightened when they come in here, and they're so happy when they've gotten into exercise," Ms. Frank says. "They no longer have to fear their daily activities, since they know they can do much more strenuous things. They learn they can live pretty much as they did before – prudently, but without fear."

There was a man in his early fifties, Dr. Stein recalls, who after a mild heart attack found a return to normal activity virtually impossible. Medically, he was doing quite well, but he complained of extreme fatigue. Several months after his heart attack, he had not yet resumed his sex life.

"Both he and his wife were extremely nervous about any activity, including sex," Dr. Stein recounts. "So we had the wife watch his stress test. We pointed out, at each stage, what kind of activity demanded an equivalent exertion: 'Now he's mowing the lawn,' we told her. 'Now he could be having sex; now he could be playing tennis. You can see that his heartbeat, his EKG are fine.' And the visual impact of the demonstration was enough to dispel their anxieties, allowing them to resume their sex life and making it possible for him to enter the exercise program."

In general, Dr. Stein says, statistics show that participants in the Downstate program have reaped substantial emotional and psychological benefits. Tests of life satisfaction, self-image and sense of well-being show dramatic improvement. "And we've seen a significant reduction in the amount of sleeping pills that patients need, a decrease in their use of tranquilizers," Dr. Stein says.

With regular exercise, he adds, heart patients don't just *think* they are capable of more activity; they generally *become* capable of more activity.

"It's called the training response," he explains. "If you ran up ten flights of stairs, your pulse would be, say, 180. But after running up those stairs every day for six weeks, your pulse wouldn't go higher than, let's say, 140. Your

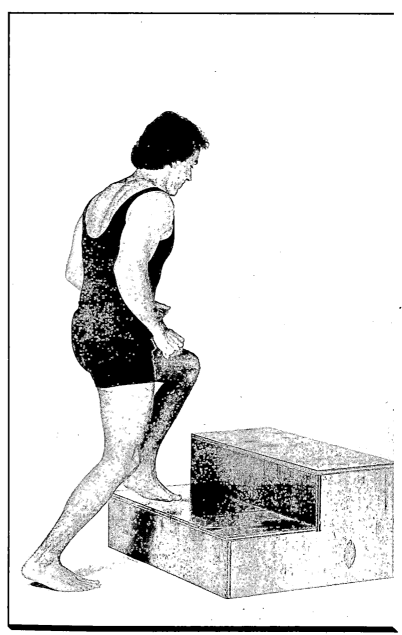

Going up and down a step is good heart exercise.

muscles would be doing the same amount of work and requiring the same amount of oxygen, and your heart would have to pump the same amount of blood. But now your heart has been trained to eject more blood with each beat, so it doesn't have to pump as many times. And at a lower heart rate, your heart itself needs less oxygen than it did before.

"So let's say a patient with coronary disease gets chest pains at a heart rate of 150. After training, he'll still get his pain at 150. But where two flights of stairs would cause him pain before, now he can go up four flights before reaching that point. He may be able to go through an entire day without that kind of physical stress. It's an improvement in efficiency; you can do more external work (like walking) for the same cardiac work. So you can tolerate more exercise."

Such physiological improvements, Dr. Stein says, mean that some 20 percent of the patients who stay in the program for over a year are able to cut down on the use of cardiac drugs. Many, he adds, report a decrease in symptoms.

Workouts at the Y

More impressive than statistics, though, are the participants themselves. "We have heart patients who are more fit than the average sedentary noncardiac individual," Dr. Stein says. "If you go over to the Y, you'll see people who have had heart attacks running vigorously for 30 minutes at a time."

At the 92d Street Y on Manhattan's Upper East Side, cardiac patients sweat and strain alongside healthy joggers, in a program directed by the Cardiac Exercise Laboratory. The Y is no hospital, but it has its own stress-testing center ("with equipment just as sophisticated as that in my laboratory," says Dr. Stein) and a staff that includes a cardiologist, a nurse and a nutritionist. A participant at the Y is given an individually designed exercise program, built around his or her preferences and needs. It may involve running in place, skipping rope, doing sit-ups or calisthenics or running. "We ask, 'What do you find fun? What turns you on?'" Dr. Stein says.

Participants also meet with the nutritionist for advice on improving their diet and with a social worker for counseling on how to reduce the stress in their life.

"About 45 percent of our people have had heart attacks," says Charles Bronz, health and physical education director at the Y. "They are treated the same as those people who enter the program for preventive reasons. We find that bringing the two groups together has a beneficial effect for everyone."

For heart patients, the benefits can be striking. "We had one 51-year-old man who'd had a heart attack and double bypass surgery," Mr. Bronz recalls. "When he first came here, all he could do was work out, slowly, on a bicycle. Now he's running. In five months, his endurance has improved by nearly 50 percent."

Another man had very severe angina, chest pains that reflect insufficient blood flow through the coronary arteries. "When he first started in the program four years ago, his 'run' was more like a fast walk. Now he's playing singles tennis. His endurance has almost doubled."

Training, Mr. Bronz points out, can help some heart patients perform feats that healthy men might envy. "We have one man, a psychiatrist, who'd had two heart attacks. He's doing particularly well. He even caught a mugger! Some kid grabbed his wife's purse; he chased him for two blocks and caught him!"

One thing that makes the Y program successful, apparently, is the friendly community setting. "People take an interest in each other," says Mr. Bronz. "If somebody misses a few sessions, they ask, 'Hey, where's John?'" Nurse Barbara Eisenstein and nutritionist Gail Levey are always available for participants who want information, reassurance or just friendly conversation.

At the Y, they recognize that after a heart attack, a patient's family may need as much reassurance as the patient does. "Often, children don't know how to act," says Dr. Stein. "'Shall I take out the garbage so Daddy won't have to?' they ask. 'Can I talk to Daddy about staying out late Saturday night, or is that going to get him upset and give him another heart attack?'

"So we have Family Day, and invite the family down to watch everybody exercise. Watching Dad put on a sweat suit, jog for 30 minutes and work up a good sweat – that goes a long way toward eliminating those fears. If you just *tell* them, 'Don't worry about your father,' it won't have the same effect."

Preventing the First Attack

Healthy people who want to prevent heart attacks also find support at the Y. Motivated, often, by the illness or sudden death of a close friend or relative, they sign up for rigorous stress testing and blood tests to determine the health of their hearts and arteries and the risk of future trouble. Those who pass the tests with flying colors are sent on their way, says Mr. Bronz. " 'Whatever you're doing,' we tell them, 'keep it up!' " Those with a medium to high risk of heart disease, about 10 percent of the people tested, are invited to join the program. Like the cardiac patients, they receive individually designed exercise schedules, advice from the nutritionist, stress counseling from the social worker and encouragement from the nurse. "That's why the program works so well; it doesn't just come at prevention from one aspect," says Ms. Levey. "It's comprehensive."

Participants, she adds, seem uncommonly receptive to nutritional advice. "Some come to see me periodically for counseling on weight loss, or to see if their diets are okay. I encourage a low-fat, high-carbohydrate diet, lots of whole grains and fresh fruits and vegetables, less beef and more chicken and fish. They are really open to change."

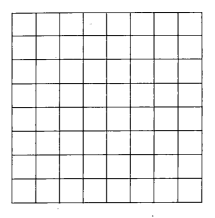

Exercise helps your heart by doing good things for the fat on your belly and the fat in your blood.

Ms. Eisenstein, whose years as a coronary care unit nurse have taught her the need for programs like Downstate's, is particularly enthusiastic. "Once someone gets into the physical aspect of the program, it becomes a way of life," she says. "It gives him a wholly different outlook, and it's all to the good."

That, in effect, is the fundamental idea of the Downstate program – to start both patients and nonpatients on the path to a healthier, more vigorous lifestyle. "All we try to do is form a lifetime habit of exercise," says Mr. Bronz. "We encourage people to be on their own." More than a few of his patients have, in fact, become "enthusiastic exercise addicts," Dr. Stein says.

But what about risks? Everyone has heard tales of stress tests interrupted by fatalities, and of apparently healthy middle-aged men found dead on the side of the running track.

One study that Dr. Stein likes to cite shows the likelihood of death or serious complication in the course of a stress test to be 1 in 200,000. In a good, modern center, he speculates, the risk may be even less. "We do very careful screening before exercise testing, we always have a physician and a nurse trained in EKG and cardiopulmonary resuscitation, and there's always a full set of cardiac arrest equipment. With better monitoring devices, we can pick up early warning signs of when to stop a test."

Exercise itself, Dr. Stein grants, does involve some increased risk for a heart patient. "We minimize it by bring-

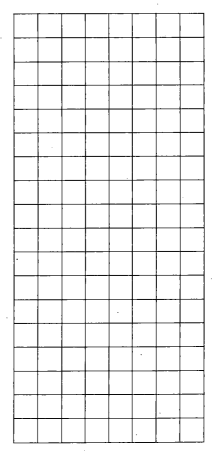

ing your heart rate higher, when we test you on the treadmill, than it will be when you train. And overall, we lower the *daily* risk of the individual by putting him in a training program. If you exercise enough to train, in other words, then running for the bus on a windy day will involve less physical stress than it would otherwise."

In the four years since the program began, he adds, "we've found out that people's hearts and bodies are much sturdier after a heart attack than we had thought. We're comfortable prescribing more exercise than we used to; we seem to do it safely."

Similarly, he says, much of the anxiety about running for healthy people is exaggerated. For a vigorous, active person under 40 without symptoms or significant risk factors like overweight or smoking, "a stress test may be an unnecessary precaution," according to Dr. Stein.

A sensible attitude is not, however.

"If you're in your late forties, a stress test would be appropriate every three or four years." And the "competitive nut" who pushes himself for the extra two miles, or ignores the heat of summer, may be moving into a high risk zone, Dr. Stein adds. "And if you feel an irregularity in your heartbeat or you start to have chest pains you've never had before, be prudent and see your doctor."

In with the Good Fats, Out with the Bad

Exercise also makes your heart more fit by reducing your fat – particularly the fats in your blood. These blood fats are called lipoproteins (they are actually combinations of protein and fat), and they carry cholesterol, a fatlike, waxy substance, through the body. There are two main types of lipoproteins – high-density lipoproteins (HDLs) and low-density lipoproteins (LDLs). When cholesterol is carried by LDLs, it tends to cause trouble, clogging up arteries and making the heart's job more difficult. But when cholesterol is associated with HDLs, it doesn't seem to accumulate; instead, it gets whisked away to the liver for storage or elimination.

A study of 41 male long-distance runners aged 35 to 59 showed blood fat distribution levels closer to that of younger women rather than of sedentary, middle-aged men – a reassuring find since, out of all age groups, young women are about the least susceptible to heart disease. The study, by the Stanford Heart Disease Prevention Program, looked at runners who averaged 15 miles per week for at least a year. According to the study, many of the subjects had only started their running programs within the last few years and were not lifelong athletes, providing proof that it's never too late to begin the fitness habit.

In the study, the runners were compared to control subjects – men of similar age who lived in three northern California towns. When blood tests for coronary risk factors were done on the two groups of men, the runners did better on every test. The runners had higher levels of HDLs, lower levels of LDLs, lower overall cholesterol levels and lower amounts of triglycerides (a common blood fat associated with atherosclerosis). All this led the doctors who conducted the study to conclude: "Vigorous activity in older men is associated with a pattern of blood lipids considered by most authorities to be conducive to heart health, and such activity is to be commended, at least from this point of view, in fit individuals." In other words, if you want to help your heart out, don't just sit there, do something!

HEAT THERAPY

I f you've ever soaked your tired feet in a basin of hot water or used a hot water bottle to fight an infection, you've already doctored yourself with heat therapy, and perhaps you've discovered how this simple remedy can make you feel better. Well, you're part of an ancient tradition *and* a modern medical trend. Today's doctors are starting to realize what folk healers have known all along – that heat therapy can be used to treat *many* diseases, including serious conditions such as arthritis and cancer.

A hot bath, for instance, seems to be a universal remedy for maladies like fatigue and muscular soreness. Hot water expands the body's blood vessels, bringing extra blood to nourish and relax tightened muscles. Throughout the ages, many people have used hot baths to fight muscle problems and related diseases. (For more information about the healing power of hot baths, see our chapter on water therapy.)

You can also use heating pads and hot water bottles to selectively heat parts of your body and treat local soreness. They come in handy for the treatment of certain running injuries and other stiffness caused by athletic injuries.

Wrapped in a Warm Cocoon

While a hot water bottle may also be helpful in alleviating arthritic pain, it is not the only heat therapy available to arthritics. Katherine Doetterl of Cheektowaga, New York, an arthritis sufferer for 30 years, wrote to tell us about her simple heat remedy – thermal underwear. Wearing the underwear during sleep provided "great relief and rest" from the painful condition, she said. She also wore it under pantsuits during the winter and experienced less pain in her joints during the cold weather.

Another unusual and effective heat remedy for arthritics has been documented by Earl J. Brewer, Jr., M.D., at the Texas Children's Hospital in Houston. A young Boy Scout under his care who was suffering from juvenile rheumatoid arthritis found he did not wake with the usual morning stiffness and pain when he slept in his sleeping bag. His grandmother, who had osteoarthritis, tried sleeping in one and also felt better.

After seeing the results, Dr. Brewer encouraged his arthritic hospital patients to try it. Some were so pleased with the results they continued sleeping in the bags after returning home.

Whether donning thermal underwear or zipping into a sleeping bag, the cocoon effect is the same. A uniform warmth wraps around the body, keeping it snug and warm all over. The dampness and cold that can irritate arthritic joints are kept at bay.

In some health problems, though, the body takes over and generates its own healing heat. "Give me a fever and I can cure any disease," said Hippocrates more than 2,000 years ago. But a number of researchers today still aren't certain that a fever is good for a patient. They believe it may be a harmful by-product of infection and not an ally against disease.

Matthew J. Kluger, Ph.D., at the University of Michigan, is a scientist who has tried to find out if a fever during illness is truly a natural healer. In his work, Dr. Kluger set out to see what happens when a cold-blooded animal – which relies on external sources such as the sun for its body heat – gets sick. Does it try to scurry to a hotter area? And does it get sicker if it can't find one?

First, Dr. Kluger took some desert iguanas and placed them in a simulated desert environment. He found that the lizards selected a normal body temperature between 100.4° and 102.2° F. But when the lizards became ill, they raised their body temperatures to between 104° and 107.6° F by moving to a warmer site on the "desert."

Dr. Kluger then took some infected lizards and placed them in either low, normal or high (fever) temperature chambers. At the end of three days, 96 percent of the lizards caged in the "fever chamber" were still alive. Only 34 percent of the lizards were alive in the normal temperature chamber, and less than 10 percent survived the coolest climate. The study, says Dr. Kluger, suggests that fever is a natural healing device and that people should allow their fevers (if moderate) to continue (*Natural History*, January, 1976).

While some researchers explore nature's heating mechanisms, others are investigating the mechanics of heat technologies that battle various ailments.

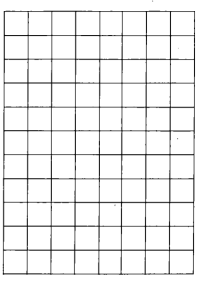

Dr. Kluger's study suggests that fever is a natural healing device and that people should allow their fevers (if moderate) to continue.

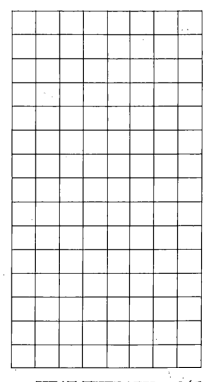

Ultrasound and Heat Therapy

Ultrasound is one of those new technologies. A form of energy similar to but higher in frequency than ordinary sound waves, ultrasound is used by physicians and physical therapists in hyperthermia, or deep-heating treatments. The therapy relieves pain and promotes healing in joints and muscles.

Doctors at Stanford University have also used ultrasound to treat patients with psoriasis, a chronic skin disease. Lesions were treated two or three times weekly for a total of six to ten treatment sessions. In most instances, the first treatment decreased scaling and redness. Over time, 60 percent of the infected patches completely regressed, and 30 percent exhibited a partial response to treatment (*Official Publication of the American Federation of Clinical Research,* April, 1979).

A Weapon against Cancer

Total body hyperthermia, another product of heat therapy technology, is being used by some doctors to fight cancer. During this procedure, the patient's entire body temperature is elevated in order to destroy or to diminish the size of the tumor. Donald Cole, M.D., of the Holistic Center in Floral Park, New York, and a member of the staff of American International Hospital, Zion, Illinois, has used total body hyperthermia on his patients for nearly two years. He believes that when a person has cancer, the entire body has to be treated in order to eradicate the disease.

"Surgery can't remove all of the cancer cells from the body. The entire body must be treated, not just one area, since cancer is a systemic disease," Dr. Cole told us.

Patients are wrapped in double thermal blankets filled with water, and their body temperatures are raised to 107.5° F for two hours. Some of the 200 patients treated have experienced a 50 percent reduction of the measurable tumor and are "noticeably better," says Dr. Cole.

A contrasting approach to total body hyperthermia is to localize the heating to just the cancerous area. Harry H. LeVeen, M.D., of the Medical University of South Carolina, has worked extensively in the use of radio frequency waves, which can be beamed directly at a tumor, heating and perhaps killing it.

In treatments lasting about three hours, the patient's

body temperature may rise to 102° F. At the same time, the radio frequency waves are raising the temperature of the tumor to between 110° and 115° F. While some patients are sedated, others are conscious throughout the procedure.

Fighting Disease Two Ways

When a person develops cancer, says Dr. LeVeen, the body undergoes several changes. We know the body recognizes that the cancer cells are different, and it will hold their growth in check for a while. But eventually the cancer suppresses and paralyzes the body's immune system. When this happens, the patient has nothing with which to fight the invading cancer. Second, the tumor itself has a poor circulation, and as it grows, it pushes the blood supply away and develops a new blood supply consisting only of capillaries, says Dr. LeVeen. But when local hyperthermia is applied to the tumor, both those abnormal body changes dramatically reverse. The capillaries in the tumor are destroyed, the tumor cells are killed, and a strong immune response is aroused in the patient.

Dr. LeVeen has treated approximately 175 cancer patients of different ages for more than three years. Most patients respond favorably, he reports, and some are cancer-free.

Further progress depends on the continuing research into heat therapy. Engineers at the University College of North Wales have designed "superb new equipment" for Dr. LeVeen that should make the success rate over cancer even more remarkable, he says.

Both Dr. Cole and Dr. LeVeen believe the use of heat therapy has been a significant breakthrough in the treatment of cancer. With new equipment and further research, scientists may prove, in cancer and many other diseases, what Hippocrates and common sense have told us all along: heat is a curing fire.

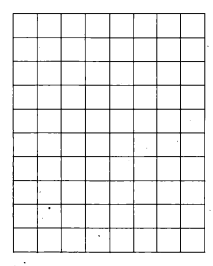

Hug's early meaning was to foster or cherish. Later it began to mean clasp or squeeze tightly with affection. That's when hugging really became something to do!

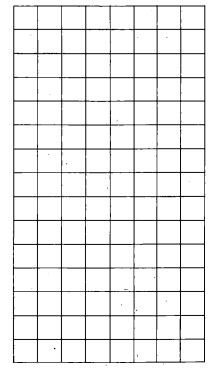

HUG THERAPY

by Kristina Davis, M.S.W.

I f you believe our ancestors stood upright for the first time in order to carry a heavier brain, you may not have seen the latest anthropological findings. Faded daubings on the walls of caves in southern France show pairs of human figures in various stages of uprightness – and embrace! It all started one summer day when two ancestors (maybe one of yours and one of mine) reached for the same ripe fruit in a primordial papaya tree. As they stretched toward that papaya, they lost their balances and grabbed onto one another to avoid a fall.

"Ah-hug," exclaimed one with shock and effort.

"Ah-hug," answered the other.

And that is how the first upright hug, and its name, came into being.

Like all fads, soon everyone was doing it, and as time passed, ah-hugging became the accepted way of greeting, despite the fact that walking on all fours made ah-hugging difficult and tiring. No sooner would one drop down from greeting an acquaintance when someone else would amble by, and the hugger would have to get back up on his hind legs again. It was simply easier, after a period of trial and error, to *stay* upright, and thus *Homo erectus* and the hug were born together.

Hugging Is . . .

Actually, the origin of the word "hug" is unknown and appears for the first time late in the sixteenth century, according to the *Oxford English Dictionary.* Its early meaning was similar to the German "hegen, to foster or cherish." The use of hug as a verb – to clasp or squeeze tightly in the arms, usually with affection – soon developed, however, and hugging became something to do! It became an active, engaging and most often affectionate act.

As early as 1773, the cheering, maybe even medical or therapeutic effect of hugging was noted by David Garrick in a description of Samuel Johnson, "who," he said, "gives you a forcible hug, and shakes laughter out of you, whether you will or not." We could call Mr. Johnson the first hug therapist, I suppose, but that would hardly be fair to all those men and women who have hugged their infants, children and each other down through the ages.

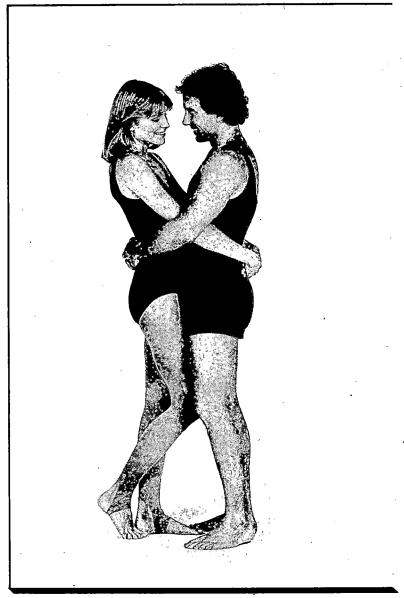

A hug shows someone that you love them.

Taking a cue from these early hug therapists and continuing the use of touch introduced in the encounter groups of the 1960s and early 1970s, many psychological counselors are expanding our definition of "hug" by hugging, patting and massaging their clients in the course of normal therapy. They are expanding their healing powers by adding touch to the powers of speech, listening and observation. They now see the client as a whole being, one whose skin can perceive care and reassurance just as readily as his or her eyes, ears and mind. In the medical field, hugging is also being used by nurses, health educators and doctors to calm and reassure people in the midst of health crises. And hugging is being offered to people in chronic pain as well. It has been found that this increase in pleasure allows them to forget their pain for a while.

Today, hugging is regarded by many mental- and physical-health workers, therapists, alcoholism counselors, child-care workers and divorce groups as a very intense way to communicate physically with another person and as a therapeutic tool that works best when used with the same care and sensitivity as any other form of therapeutic intervention.

The Proof Is in the Touching—or Lack of It

Why has hugging become a therapeutic tool? Hugging is so potent a form of touch because it takes us back to our earliest experiences of life, to a period before birth when our skin is surrounded by fluid in the womb. And immediately after birth, too, when touch continues to make a vital contribution to life and survival.

Research indicates that infants need to be hugged. Children under one year of age living in foundling institutions at the beginning of this century often died of a malady called "marasmus," or "wasting away." The then-conventional wisdom recommended the abolition of the cradle and suggested that picking up a crying infant only spoiled the child. As a result, infants in institutions were fed, kept clean and left in the insulated world of their cribs to die of a mysterious wasting away. More recently, of course, just the opposite has been the belief and practice. For instance, Rene Spitz, M.D., a professor of psychiatry at the University of Colorado Medical School, found that the practice of picking up and mothering hospitalized infants lowered their mortality rate.

What's more, an infant's sense of touch is its most well-developed sense. We come to *know* our world first as it touches us and we touch it. Research with animals indicates that separation from their mothers causes changes in the behavioral and physiological development of infant mon-

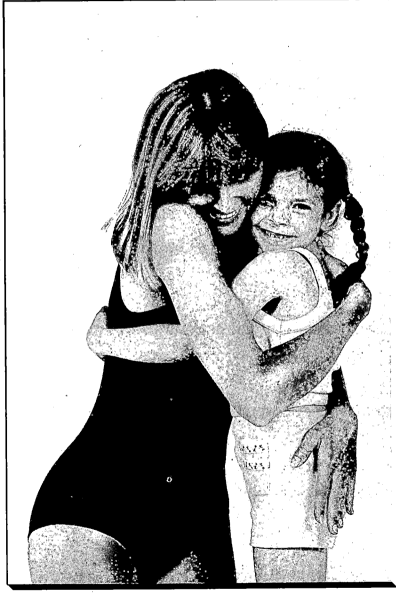

Children are great, spontaneous huggers.

keys. Martin Reite, M.D., of the department of psychiatry at the University of Colorado Medical Center, removed eight pigtailed monkeys from their mothers for ten days. Behavioral changes, such as frantic activity, loud protests and, later, disconsolate "slouching" and a decrease in play and habitual grooming were the results. Some serious physiological changes also occurred. The monkeys' heart rates increased after separation, their body temperatures rose, and there were disturbances in their sleeping patterns. When the infants were finally returned to their mothers, they cuddled a lot and slept more than they normally would (*Journal of Child Psychology and Psychiatry and Allied Disciplines,* vol. 22, no. 2, 1981).

Of course, we can't separate human babies from their mothers, but we can do the reverse; we can introduce more touch, more caring into their lives and observe the results. A study at Purdue University by Jeffrey Fisher, Ph.D., and colleagues did just that. Alternating during half-hour periods, checkout clerks at the university library were asked to touch the hand of students briefly as they returned library cards and then not to. Finally, students using the library were asked to answer questions about the staff. The questionnaire consisted of pairs of contrasting words for describing a subject's general feelings such as "happy" and "sad," "comfortable" and "uncomfortable," contrasting pairs to describe a clerk's performance, like "helpful" and "not helpful," and pairs describing the library environment in general. The results? Those subjects who had been touched, even those who did not recall it, chose more positive words to describe their feelings, the clerk's performance and the library environment (*Sociometry,* vol. 39, no. 4, 1976).

A Hands-Off Culture

So research *and* experience indicate the importance of hugging and touching. But whether we hug or not is influenced by the culture we live in. As with other touching behavior, hugging practices vary from culture to culture. For instance, in comparison with other cultures, like the Netsilik Eskimos, the Bush people of the Kalahari and the Arapesh of New Guinea, American and British parents hug, cuddle and hold their children very little! A common practice in these hugging cultures is the wrapping of an infant close to its mother's body in a cocoonlike sac, a practice which allows the baby to sleep and watch the world go by in constant contact with another human being. Americans, on the other hand, use toys to stimulate their children and often leave them alone in cribs or playpens for hours. Our more limited physical contact with our infants and their mountain of toys may explain, writes Ashley Montagu in *Touching, The Human Significance of the Skin* (Harper and Row, 1978), their need for consumer products as adults. It may also explain their difficulty in dealing with feelings toward other people.

What's worse, Bernie Zilbergeld, Ph.D., a psychotherapist in Oakland, California, believes we are trained from early childhood not to touch anything! In fact, he writes in his book *Male Sexuality* (Little, Brown, 1978) that "DO NOT TOUCH" has become a "familiar litany," one reinforced by how seldom our children see adults touching one another. He also feels that male children are touched in a caring way less than females. Herb Goldberg, Ph.D., author of *The Hazards of Being Male* (Signet, 1976), agrees, and he adds that when boys grow up, they are expected to do what they have not seen. They are expected to express affection physically, when they have been taught in childhood to deny this need for touching.

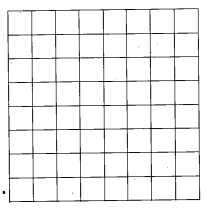

One way to understand your present attitudes toward hugging is to go back to your childhood and think about where and when you learned them. As children, many of us were trained not to touch anything.

The Hug Questionnaire

What did you learn about hugging and touching when you were growing up? One way to understand your present attitudes is to go back and find out where and how you learned them. The following are two exercises that may help you do just that.

Exercise 1. Write down in chronological order and in short sentences any experiences with touch that come to you. Begin with "I was born." For example:

> I was born, and then
> Mom cuddled with me when she read to me before bed, and then
> Dad spanked me that time I broke a toy, and then
> We had to hold hands crossing the street during recess.

Write whatever flows into your thoughts, and don't censor. Do *not* analyze, criticize or judge.

Stop when you have brought the sequence to the present or to the age of 21 or whenever you feel ready to stop.

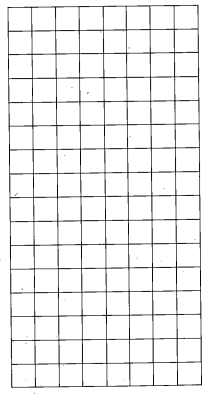

Ask yourself how you feel after completing these sentences. Do you feel a lingering sense of sadness at the memory of a friend or relative who comforted you with a hug years ago? Do you feel rage at a parent who punished you with physical force too often? Do you feel as blank as the page in front of you, suddenly unable to write down or feel anything at all? This blankness may mean you are not ready to explore this area at the moment. Try the exercise another time when you feel more secure and relaxed.

Now, read over what you have written without worrying whether or not you "passed." Read it aloud if you want to. What is your body's reaction to the reading? Pleasure? Relief? Anger? Sadness? Record these feelings. You might feel contradictory things, too. Let any insights about past touching experiences come to you by themselves. Reread your list from time to time or do the exercise again, writing down another sequence of touching memories.

Exercise 2. Get comfortable, away from noise, in a place neither too cold nor too warm, where you will not be interrupted. Close your eyes. "Feel" your breathing by placing your hands on your tummy. Breathe deeply and naturally, letting your abdomen rise as you inhale and fall as you exhale. Take about ten full breaths, and then picture a movie screen. The title of the movie is "You and Your Skin." Start with your earliest visual memory of touching. Pretend it is happening again. If anyone is speaking, hear what they say and listen to your responses. Let the visions float onto the screen by themselves. Continue until you feel ready to end your movie. Then let the screen fade away. Take a few deep breaths, gently shake yourself and slowly open your eyes.

What are you feeling? Do any insights come to you from what you have seen, heard and written? What did you learn about touching as a child? Who was or were your primary teachers?

Are you content with what others passed on to you about touching? Or would you like to "teach" yourself something different? Can you see yourself behaving according to these *new* attitudes? If you come in contact with children frequently, do you feel you are passing on healthy attitudes about touching? How does hugging fit in the scheme of things?

Is there someone you want to share the above experiences with? But do be careful about sharing yourself. Sometimes experiences lose their potency when they are shared.

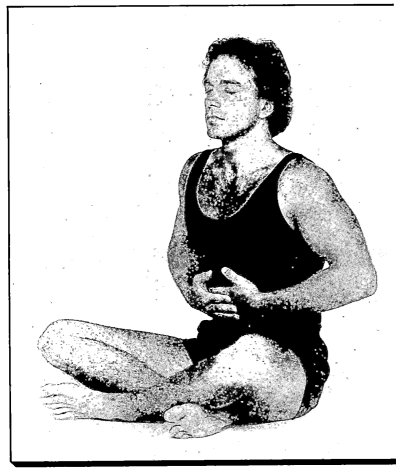

Awareness of your breathing is important.

Hugging for Medicinal Purposes

. . . Marie, a wonderful 66-year-old patient of mine, . . . had developed severe arthritis in her hands. She was very self-conscious about her physical condition and had become quite introverted. But when I gave her an excuse to break out of her shell, she didn't hesitate for a moment.

She would approach total strangers, and say "Hi, my name is Marie, and I know this sounds a little strange, but my doctor tells me that it may help my pain problem if I can get hugged four times a day. Here's my written prescription. Could you help me out? I need a hug."

She was never turned down (*Free Yourself from Pain*, Simon and Schuster, 1979).

Marie is one of the many chronic pain patients whom David Bresler, Ph.D., of the Bresler Center for Allied Therapeutics in Los Angeles and author of *Free Yourself from Pain* (Simon and Schuster, 1979), sends out of his office with the prescription, "Four hugs a day – without fail." He believes a patient can do a lot to relieve his own pain, and one method is to stimulate nerve endings with touch.

Hemoglobin levels in the blood are also affected by a "therapeutic touch," says a study by Dolores Krieger, R.N., Ph.D., professor of nursing at New York University. Since hemoglobin, which occurs in the blood, helps deliver oxygen to body tissues, Dr. Krieger decided it would be a good indicator of a person's state of health. Thirty-two nurses were trained in the use of "therapeutic touch," which Dr. Krieger describes as placing the hands on or just above a troubled area and leaving them there for a half hour. The motivation to help and heal a patient was a vital part of this healing process. Then she studied how their caring affected patients.

Sixty-four volunteer patients with a variety of ailments from hospitals in New York City were split into two groups. One group received normal nursing, while the other got "therapeutic touch" each day. The results? The hemoglobin – and presumably the health – levels of the "touched" group went up significantly, and the "untouched" group's levels did not.

If the simple laying on of healthy hands in a concerned and caring way can raise hemoglobin levels, what can an increase in *hugging* do for people who have health problems? Plenty, say Barbara Toohey and June Biermann, coauthors of *The Women's Holistic Headache Relief Book* (J. P. Tarcher, 1979) and *The Diabetic's Total Health Book* (J. P. Tarcher, 1980). They were first introduced to hugging when Dr. Bresler suggested that chronic headaches can be the way a person asks for love when he or she feels unable to ask for it directly. Ms. Toohey and Ms. Biermann tried hugging on headaches, and it worked.

The coauthors also discovered that hugging is great for diabetics. The feeling of self-worth a hug creates, they found, helps the diabetic accept himself or herself as a person worth caring for. Biermann, herself a diabetic, says, "You never forget the day you're told you are a diabetic. I felt changed and confused and overwhelmed. If the doctor had put his arms around me and hugged me, the physical connection with another human being would have reassured me I was not going to be rejected by others because of my health problem."

After a diagnosis of diabetes comes the task of educating oneself: what to eat, how to give oneself medication, how to deal with the reactions of others, and how to get through sugar-laden holidays and wine-filled social gatherings. Ms. Toohey and Ms. Biermann introduced hugging at the American Association of Diabetes Educators Conference in 1979 and suggested that nurses, dieticians and doctors hug their patients often. After all, even if they blush, it only helps the circulation! At the following year's conference, members reported that hugging was a "wonder drug"; it has no bad side effects, they said, and is especially good for defusing the anger and frustration that prevents some diabetics from moving forward in their lives.

The use of hugging does not need to be limited to the chronic pain or diabetes patient. With any health problem a patient may feel vulnerable, frightened, angry, frustrated and helpless. The patient usually needs to educate himself or herself, to make certain life changes. Hugging can give him or her the positive emotional state necessary to make these changes, and they, in turn, may aid the body in its healing process. Aaron Katcher, M.D., a psychiatrist at the University of Pennsylvania School of Medicine, once studied the life practices that seemed to contribute to the survival of heart attack patients. Pet ownership turned out to have a strong effect. Dr. Katcher suggests that the cuddling of pets has a soothing effect that reduces stress levels in heart attack victims.

Has hugging any preventive value? A study of rabbits on high-fat diets by scientists at Ohio State University and the University of Houston included this surprising result. One group of rabbits was cuddled by the research assistants, and another was not. The group that was cuddled had fewer atherosclerotic lesions than the uncuddled group, though both groups ate the same terrible diet.

Four Hugs a Day

One of the reasons hugging has the power to evoke strong responses is that we get so few of them. We may hug on special occasions like weddings or birthdays or holiday gath-

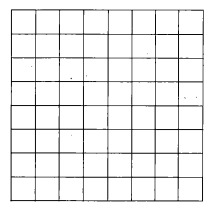

Skin hunger for hugs can be a real problem. We probably need at least three hugs a day to keep our hunger satisfied. Anything less is going to leave us malnourished. And the quality of the hugs is as important as the quantity.

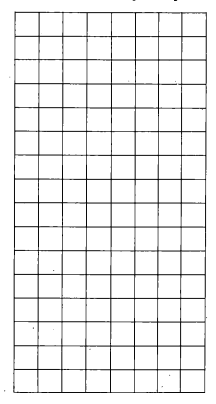

erings, but most of us do not hug daily, just to experience the skin pleasure of an embrace. As a result, family therapist Virginia Satir suggests we need at least 4 hugs a day for survival, 8 hugs a day to maintain our equilibrium and 12 hugs a day to grow. If you would like to hug more, the following section on the etiquette of hugging may help you get started.

Hugging Know-How and How to Hug

What could be simpler than hugging? You (1) open your arms wide, (2) step up to the person you want to hug, (3) wrap your arms around their body, (4) apply some degree of pressure for a desired length of time and (5) let go. Well, according to Sidney Simon, Ed.D., author of *Caring, Feeling, Touching* (Argus Communications, 1976), there are hugs, and there are HUGS! Simon believes skin hunger begins at home, and his book is a guide to help families begin touching. He believes that three hugs a day are the *least* we deserve and that less than three leaves our skin malnourished. But the quality of the hug is as important as the quantity, he says. Too many people give one of the five "nonhugs" Dr. Simon describes:

- The A-frame hug, in which nothing but the huggees' heads touch.
- The half-a-chest-is-better-than-none hug, in which half of the huggees' upper bodies touch while the other half twists away. The emphasis here is on twisting away rather than hugging.
- The chest-to-chest burp, in which the huggees pat each other on the back, defusing the physical contact by treating each other like infants being burped.
- The wallet-rub, in which two people stand side by side and touch hips.
- The jock-twirl, in which the huggee who is stronger lifts the other off the ground and twirls him or her around. If you are short, you get a lot of these.

Simon says these are all substitutes for the real thing, the "full body hug," which he describes like this:

> The two people coming together take time to really look at each other. There is no evasion or ignoring who it is they are about to hug. That is, there is no

(continued on page 264)

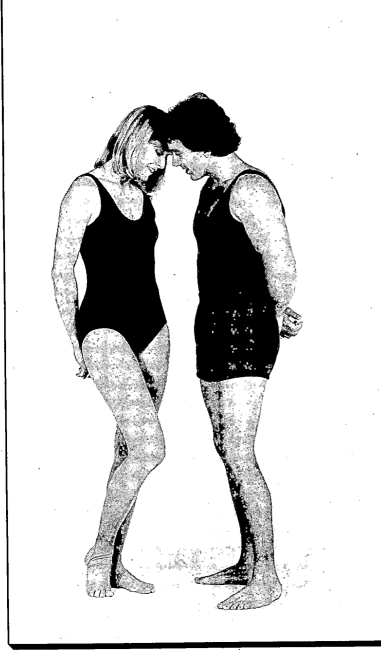

The A-frame hug.

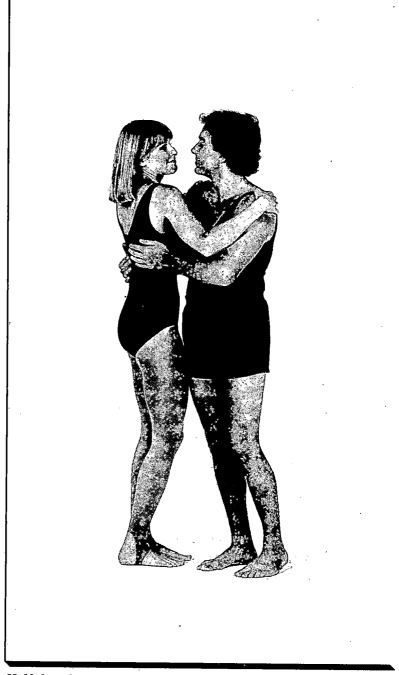

Half-chest hug.

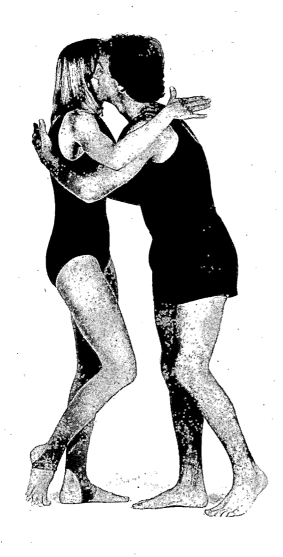

The chest-to-chest burp.

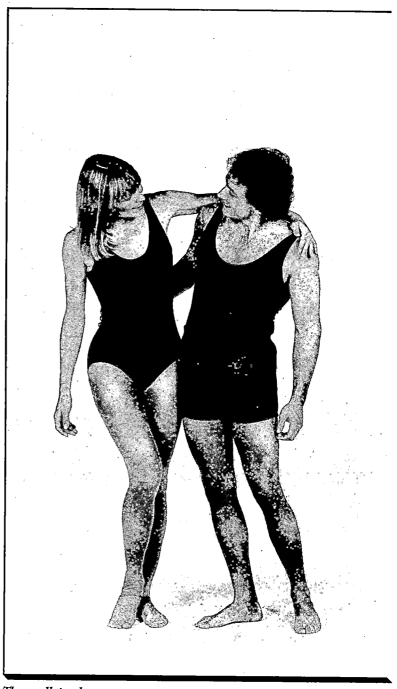

The wallet-rub.

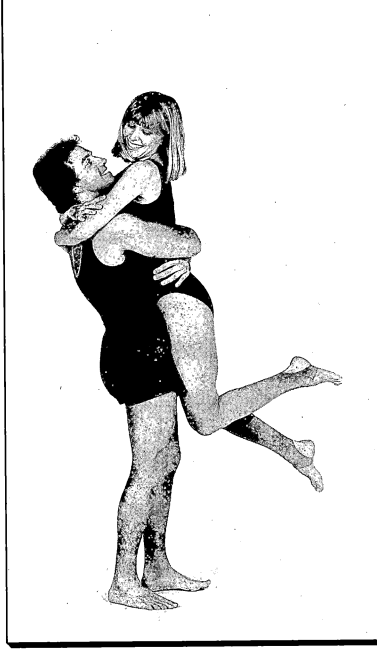

The jock-twirl.

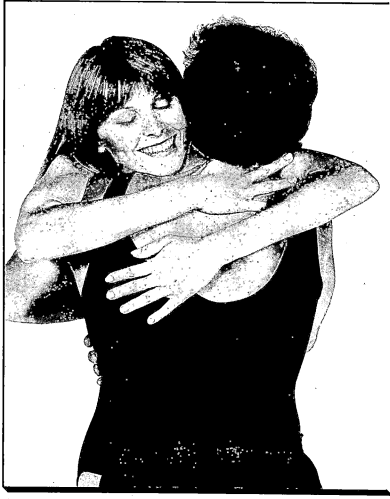

A proper hug touches all the bases.

one hug for *all* people. You try as hard as you can to personalize and customize each hug you give.

And if that means climbing on a stool or step so you can hug a taller friend, do it! Simon continues:

As you hold the person you unconsciously include and exude all the experiences and feelings you have recently shared, and memories of past experiences, as well. Above all, it is not routine or perfunctory.

In my experience of hugging, I find that not every person is ready for a "full body hug," and so I try to hug in a way that the huggee is comfortable with. But when I find a true body-hugger, the difference is noticeable. With a full body hug there is a sense of complete giving and fearless communication, one uncomplicated by words. Of course, I sometimes have to preface a hug with, "Are you huggable today?" or "Can I give you a hug?" If the answer is hesitant or negative, I respect that person's wishes.

Remember, one needs to be active to initiate frequent hugging. Still, most people find that after taking the first step, people they have hugged come back to return the favor. Hugging *is* contagious, and more people would hug if they felt they had permission to. When you hug, you are giving others that permission.

The rule to follow in deciding when to hug is to always listen to your body. Trust it. It is very wise. When you feel a hug coming on, tell the person you would like to hug about it first. Based on the person's reaction, you can then decide whether to go ahead or not. Simply becoming aware of the need to hug may require some practice because most people have learned to suppress it. If you have contradictory feelings, imagine the worst outcome the hug could have, and then decide if you are willing to risk it.

And when *you* need to be hugged, ask for one!

As you get in touch with the impulses to hug, you will also discover the people you want to hug. Is there anyone you think of immediately? Do not dismiss that person from your thoughts just because you think they might react badly. You cannot predict the future, and you cannot be sure how they will react. Are there people from your past you'd like to hug right now? Can you do anything about it now? Strangely enough, I have found that I can hug people I cannot talk to, because when we hug, we share a sense of each other's commonness, and our differences are put aside for that moment. You may want to take advantage of this quality of hugging and squeeze someone you feel tongue-tied with today.

Is there a special person you wish to hug but don't because you wonder what their response will be? Have a dialogue with them on paper. You may be surprised by what they tell you – as I was when I tried the exercise:

Me: Hi, Sam.
Sam: Hi, Kris.
Me: This is sort of hard for me, but there's something I want to talk to you about.

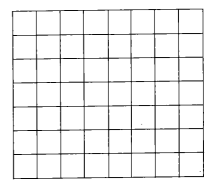

Most people find that after giving the first hug, people they have hugged return the favor. Hugging is contagious. More people would hug if they felt they had permission. When you hug, you give others permission to hug.

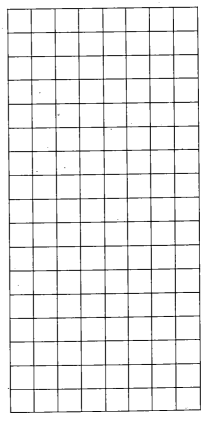

Sam: I get nervous when you start out like that, but okay, go ahead.

Me: I guess I don't always need to preface things so much. That's my way of gaining time. Anyway, I wish you'd hug me more.

Sam: Is that all?

Me: All? That's a lot. You don't hug me enough.

Sam: How often do you hug me?

Me: Hug you? I never thought about it.

Sam: Right, men don't need hugs.

Me: Wait a minute. You know I don't believe that.

Sam: Then why don't you hug me sometimes? Why am I supposed to be the one who always initiates things?

Me: I guess I didn't think about it that way. You're right. And if I want a hug from you, maybe the best way to get it is to hug you myself.

Sam: I can't wait.

Me: You don't have to. Here I come!

Whether you share your dialogue with the person in it or not, the practice may help you figure out an acceptable way to offer a hug.

A word of caution: since you cannot control the behavior of others, remember that when you hug, you are hugging out of *your* own desire to offer this gesture. Whether the recipient accepts or refuses it remains his or her choice, a choice tempered as much by past experience and cultural attitudes as by his or her feelings toward you.

Finally: Where to Hug

Dr. David Bresler tells his patients to ask someone in the supermarket for a hug if they cannot get one elsewhere. And if the supermarket is an appropriate place to hug, then so is just about any other place: home, work, school, church, a party, a conference, during intermission at the symphony or after a long airplane ride with an interesting seat companion. But ask yourself where *you* would feel most comfortable hugging. You may feel uncomfortable hugging at work and therefore may prefer a more intimate environment, such as at home with friends or at the church or synagogue. Begin by hugging in the situations you find the least scary. After you have some success (and you will), be more daring. You may even learn to hug employers, supervisors, principals and presidents.

HYPNOSIS

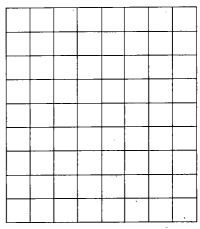

The ancient black-and-white movie flickers onto your TV screen. Scary music pours into the late night. Pretzel stuck to the roof of your mouth, you tremble on the edge of your living-room chair as a figure in a cape saunters before his seated, wide-eyed, beautiful female victim.

"You are getting sleepy . . ." drones the deep voice over the TV. The voice carries a vaguely Transylvanian accent. A gigantic gold watch swings on its chain. The girl's eyes follow it – back and forth, back and forth.

"You are getting sleepy . . ." once more drones the voice. "You are under my spell . . ."

That's how the villain of countless horror flicks gains control over his victims – through hypnosis. The hypnotic spell in those movies was used for evil; it was a tool with which a fiend hoped to gain control over the world – or at least control over the back lot.

Well, hypnosis *is* a powerful tool. But not in the way Hollywood has in mind.

Tapping Hidden Potential

Hypnosis is actually a way to use *healing* capabilities that under normal circumstances remain hidden and untouched. "The power that hypnosis has lies in its ability to stretch us to the limit," says Hamilton B. Gibson in his book *Hypnosis* (Taplinger, 1977). "Our capacities of endurance, strength, sensory acuity, memory and mastery of pain are seldom fully exercised because of the sheltered and protected lives which we lead in our technological society . . . the phenomena of hypnosis only appear to be uncanny because our ordinary assumptions about the nature of human behavior are not correct."

It is hard to define hypnosis. Some people refer to it as a form of disturbed sleep, but it is more than that. The hypnotic trance, while it may resemble sleep in some ways (thus the famous command, "You are getting sleepy . . ."), is actually closer to an intense concentration that blots out

Hypnosis is a way to use healing capabilities that usually remain hidden and untouched. It has been used to reduce the severity of asthma, arthritis, colitis, seizures, ulcers and hemophilia.

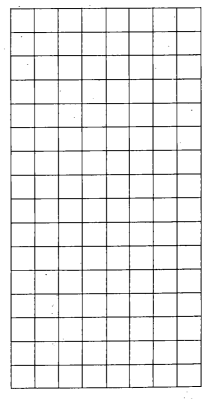

extraneous sensory information. You can think of it as being similar to the concentration you experience when you are involved with a very interesting book. If you are involved enough in a book, you may not even hear your name when someone else is talking to you.

Well, during hypnosis, the voice of the hypnotist most often takes the place of the all-absorbing book. The voice and its commands are the central focus that wipes out the rest of the real world and helps the subject reach into his or her unconscious mind.

"Hypnosis is not sleep," according to Herbert Spiegel, M.D., a nationally recognized expert in hypnotism. "Whatever sleep is, hypnosis is not. . . . Hypnosis is an altered state of attention which approaches peak concentration capacity."

In other words, you can think of your everyday state of mind as diffused light, like sunlight shining through hammered glass. During the normal events of your life, your attention is scattered, like that sunlight, among the distracting little tasks necessary to maintain your place in society – everything from remembering about dinner with the Joneses on Friday to calling the exterminator this morning.

Entering the hypnotic state is leaving all those distractions behind. You take that pane of hammered glass that breaks up the sunlight and replace it with a magnifying glass. Instead of a warm glow, you get a burning beam capable of penetrating into situations and problems that have taken root in your psyche.

All of your conscious "mind" energy can, through hypnosis, be focused on one particular spot, the same way a magnifying glass concentrates sunlight into a beam capable of igniting paper or wood.

Hypnosis has been used for relief from pain caused by fractures, chronic illness, migraine headaches, even as an anesthetic in minor surgery. It has been used with asthma patients, sometimes eliminating their symptoms altogether. There is evidence that hypnosis can reduce the severity of chronic illnesses such as arthritis, colitis, seizures, ulcers and hemophilia. Whether this is just a result of lowered anxiety in the patients or the result of some direct change in the patient's body chemistry caused by the hypnosis is not known.

Hypnosis has already been shown to be capable of altering cellular growth. It has been used, for example, to treat warts and to speed the healing of burns and wounds. Dabney M. Erwin, M.D., associate clinical professor of surgery at

Tulane Medical School in New Orleans, commonly uses hypnosis with burn patients. He has been using hypnosis for some 20 years, and he gives the impression there is nothing that extraordinary about it at all.

"If you hypnotize someone in a laboratory setting to think that one arm is anesthetized and the other is not," he says, "and apply the same heat to both arms, one arm blisters and the other doesn't.

"A major part of a burn is really the reaction of the central nervous system to heat. The mind sends out a message and the body responds. In the case of a burn, it's an inflammatory response. Consider it in slow motion, with a sunburn. When you first leave the sun, you're generally all right. It's only in the next eight hours that the swelling, pain, fever and blisters develop.

"If, in the first two hours after a normal burn, the person imagines that he wasn't burned, then he doesn't react.

"I've used hypnosis on headaches, asthma and warts," Dr. Erwin told us. "You can deal with anxiety, phobias, anything that involves the imagination. If the patient can expect something bad, he can expect something good."

Do-It-Yourself Hypnosis

Hypnosis is not just something that is done to you by someone else. It is also something that you can induce in yourself, if given enough practice.

You can train yourself to enter the hypnotic state by relaxing yourself and giving yourself signals that clear your mind of extraneous thoughts and sensations.

Self-hypnosis has been shown to help people fall asleep. Researchers in England compared the sleep-inducing ability of sleeping pills, hypnosis, self-hypnosis and a placebo on volunteer insomniacs. Some of the volunteers learned to put themselves into a trance by picturing themselves in a "warm, safe place – possibly on a holiday someplace pleasant."

When they had put themselves into a trance, the researchers told them, they would be able to give themselves the suggestions "that this would pass into a deep, refreshing sleep, waking up at the usual time in the morning, feeling wide awake."

The results showed that the subjects fell asleep faster by hypnotizing themselves than by using either the drug or

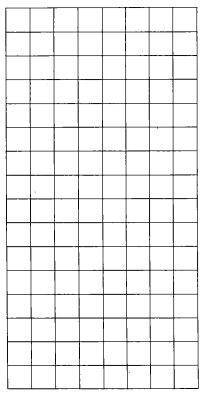

Unless you consciously train yourself to really relax, there's always a great deal of tension wrapped tight in your body. Your body is like a cloth that soaks up tension.

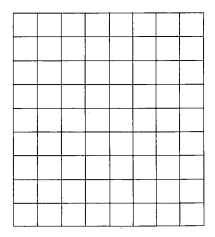

the placebo. None of the self-hynotized sleepers needed an hour to fall asleep, while a significant number in the placebo group and in the drug group did. More people in the self-hypnotized group fell asleep in less than 30 minutes than in the other groups (*Journal of the Royal Society of Medicine*, October, 1979).

In their book *Healing with Mind Power* (Rodale Press, 1978), Richard Shames, M.D., and Chuck Sterin point out four ingredients in hypnosis and self-hypnosis: *motivation, relaxation, concentration* and *direction*.

Motivation means that you have to really want to effect the change in your life that you are attempting with hypnosis. For instance, patients suffering severe pain often make excellent hypnotic subjects because the pain supplies a strong motivation for wanting the therapy to work. Increased desire for the therapy to work usually increases the possibility of the therapy's success.

Since hypnosis uses mind power, an unpleasant stimulus such as pain acts like high-powered fuel to get the mind moving toward a solution. Dr. Shames and Mr. Sterin give the example of a pregnant woman suffering a difficult labor as being an easy subject to hypnotize. Her high motivation made a trance particularly easy to induce.

Relaxation is the dust broom that clears the mind of interfering anxieties that might hinder the effects of hypnosis. "You must relax for two reasons," says Roger Bernhardt, Ph.D., psychoanalyst and hypnotherapist, in his book *Self Mastery Through Self Hypnosis* (Bobbs Merrill, 1977). "Relaxation, reaching its apogee in sleep, is an end in itself, a restorative balm to both mind and body. Furthermore, as employed in hypnosis, relaxation clears a pathway to the unconscious mind, where suggestions can more readily be accepted and acted upon."

Getting the Hypnotic Message

For self-hypnosis, Dr. Bernhardt recommends sitting in an easy chair, your feet up on a footrest, in a quiet spot where you know that you won't be disturbed. Sit back and take it easy. Think you're relaxed? Surprise! You're not.

"Oh, come on, sure I am," you might insist. Well, according to Dr. Bernhardt and other experts on relaxation, there's a great deal of tension still wrapped tight in your body unless you've consciously trained yourself to *really* relax. Your body is like a cloth damp with tension. You may not see the liquid it has soaked up, but it's inside it just the same. If you wring the damp cloth, you'll get a stream of water. Closely examine your muscles and you'll also find a residue of tension.

One easy way to aid your relaxation is to simply close your eyes. According to Dr. Shames and Mr. Sterin, this immediately cuts down on the amount of distracting stimulation that your mind has to deal with.

Dr. Bernhardt recommends alternately lifting and then dropping parts of your body in order to release hidden tension. For instance, as you sit quietly, raise your left foot a few inches off the floor, then let it fall back down. Do the same thing with your other foot. Each time, as you release your foot, focus on relaxing your muscles.

After you've lifted and dropped each foot, do the same procedure in your imagination. Picture your left foot rising and falling as you did before, but don't actually move it. Picture your right foot doing the same thing, but don't let it budge from where it's resting.

You can do the same thing with your arms and head to increase relaxation. If you are sitting with your head on a headrest, lift it forward a few inches before letting it fall back into its previous position. Then imagine the same motion without actually doing it.

Now doesn't that feel better?

Once you've done all the preliminaries and you are drifting on the seas of relaxation, you're ready to take the plunge into the hypnotic trance. The basic mental image to use for getting there is to imagine yourself in a place and situation with exquisitely pleasant connotations. As Dr. Bernhardt puts it, "In your mind's eye, picture yourself in a place where you have been or would like to go, some spot where you can be perfectly at ease and at peace with yourself and the world." The place you imagine can be a remote beach spot, waves quietly rolling in, or perhaps a mountain retreat caressed by cool breezes.

At the same time as you imagine yourself in the dream vacation of your choice (that trip you always dreamed of discovering behind door number 3 on the Great TV Contest Show), feel yourself moving downward, as if you were suspended from a high-flying parachute.

The combination of sinking down and relaxing aids you in your *concentration* – the harnessing of your mental powers to focus on the problem or situation you want to deal with. Dr. Bernhardt says, "Now as you picture yourself at the pleasant site of your own choosing, your body continues to float down, down into the chair. Your body is almost a thing apart from you now. You can leave it in place and remove yourself slightly from it. You can now give your body instructions as to how you want it to live."

The process of instructing your body on what you want it to do is the *direction*. Of course, this presumes a prior decision on your part about what it is you want to accomplish through hypnosis. The simple act of relaxation may be enough for you. In that case, you'll probably want to instruct yourself to feel calm, refreshed and energized when you come out of your trance. That kind of instruction, when you tell yourself about how to feel or what to do after you come out of hypnosis, is a *post-hypnotic suggestion*.

Hypnosis Can Wipe Out Bad Habits

Dr. Bernhardt advocates using hypnosis to eliminate bad habits, such as smoking or drinking. He feels that this is best accomplished by instructing your hypnotized mind with syllogisms. A syllogism is a three-step progression of logical statements. The first two statements lead you to the incontrovertible third state.

For instance, suppose you had two statements: (1) all roses are red, and (2) this flower is a rose. Your necessary conclusion would be: (3) this flower is red.

Syllogistic logic can paint the hypnotized mind into a corner from which there is no logical escape except the elimination of the undesired habit.

Let's say you want to give up smoking, but you're having a tough time of it, as do many veteran puffers. While you are hypnotized you tell yourself: (1) smoke is a poison that is polluting your body, and (2) you need your body to live. Therefore: (3) in order to live, you will protect your body by not smoking.

Mind Pictures Get Results

A good way to reinforce hypnotic suggestion, besides just putting the suggestion into words, is to visualize the results you are seeking. Word messages, even if they're in the form of Dr. Bernhardt's syllogisms, are usually not as persuasive to the unconscious as are pictures.

The two together, words and pictures, form a potent combination. It's like having the script of a movie and a print of it at the same time. When you're reading it and also seeing it, it's hard not to get the message.

Let's go back to our smoking example. You tell yourself the syllogism, and your unconscious mind starts to get the idea about what you're trying to accomplish. On top of the syllogism, you can add that every time you take a puff on a cigarette, you're going to feel as if you are breathing in the filthy exhaust of a dilapidated bus.

You can picture yourself standing on a city street corner, at a bus stop just as the bus pulls away. The 20-year-old giant jalopy groans and sputters, its wheels shimmying, and out of the back, as it lumbers down the block, emerges a cloud of brown gook. The cloud envelopes and chokes you.

And that's what your next cigarette is going to taste like, you tell yourself. Then, with this broken-down bus image as background, focus on how life without cigarettes will feel. Picture yourself on a mountaintop at sunrise – birds are singing, and you're breathing pure, fresh mountain air. This kind of positive image is a very important part of breaking your habit. It's an affirmative mental picture you can embrace in order to keep yourself on the right track.

Whatever your particular problem or situation is, you should invent an equally vivid picture to enhance the effectiveness of your hypnotic trance. You should visualize both the bad results of continuing your bad habit, as we did with the bus, and you should fantasize about the good results of changing your ways.

Coming out of the hypnotic state is as simple as entering it. You simply reverse the process. Instead of imagining that you are floating downward, as you did when you entered the hypnotic state, you imagine that you are floating upward, back to reality.

To ease your transition back to a nonhypnotic state, you can count backward from five to one. Before you do, though, it's a good idea to add the post-hypnotic suggestion that you will feel alert, refreshed and energetic when you emerge from your trance.

Wake up from the trance slowly; don't rush it. A slow awakening will help you emerge smoothly and leave you feeling better than an abrupt, shocking reentry.

Long-Range Solutions

Hypnosis will not solve your problems immediately. The process can't effect instant change in your psyche. Problems and habits take time to get implanted in your life, and it takes time to root them out. But don't let the lack of immediate success be discouraging.

Just the fact that you are using hypnosis to attack a problem shows that you, your mind and your body may have turned the corner in dealing with a long-standing problem. When you're using hypnosis, you're marshaling your mental powers in an all-out battle against what ails you, and what ails you is a part of yourself stuck in an annoying habit. (As Pogo used to say, "We have met the enemy, and he is us.")

Your mind and body form one unit and interact in ways that can't always be separately analyzed and dissected. The state of your mind affects your body, and that loop feeds back in the other direction. Hypnosis enables you to penetrate to the part of your mind which is usually hidden but which holds great potential for helping you take control of your life. When you ignore this part of your mind, pretending that it doesn't exist, either out of ignorance or fear, you turn your back on much of your hidden potential. Let's face it.

KNITTING

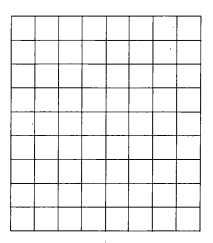

Her slim, white fingers disappear into a tangle of peach-colored wool. In the blur of activity, it is impossible to determine where her fingers stop and the even slimmer pair of pointed aluminum rods begins. She isn't merely knitting; under the guidance of Ona D. Bloom, she is knitting her way to health.

For 31 years Mrs. Bloom has been teaching and promoting needlecraft in her suburban Philadelphia yarn shop. "Knit your way to health" is her motto: it appears in letters as big as her name on the door of her shop and, inside, it is stitched, printed or scrawled on numerous placards that vie for wall space with boxes of yarn piled to the ceiling. Other placards remind the visitor, "Success is a journey, not a destination," and "Youth is the gift of nature. Age is a work of art."

Two women sit working at a comfortable table. One is putting the finishing touches on a two-piece sweater set; the other one is learning to master circular needles. Wearing a dress she knitted herself, Mrs. Bloom pours tea for a visitor, then jumps up to rummage through stacks of leaflets to find a vest pattern for a new customer.

Meanwhile, Mrs. Lee Voci looks up from her sweater to confide that "I have become much calmer in the four or five years I've been coming here. Ona is a fantastic teacher."

Knitting's calming effect is only one of its therapeutic benefits, says Mrs. Bloom. It also helps overcome arthritis and builds self-esteem. "When you work and you're creating, you haven't got time to think of your problems. Worries just melt away."

Knitting has a therapeutic, calming effect. When you work and you're creating, you haven't got time to think of your problems. Worries just melt away.

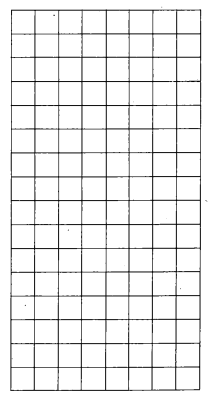

They Forget Their Pain

Wendy Borow, founder of the art therapy program at Boston Children's Hospital, agrees that "there is something inherently healing about being able to create." Arthritis specialist Morris A. Bowie, M.D., is even more emphatic. "It gives people a sense of satisfaction and alleviates stress. They

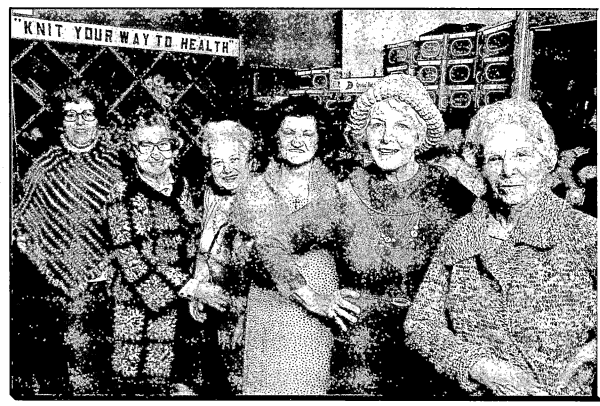

Members of Ona Bloom's class wear their hand-made creations and big smiles.

become so interested in what they are making, they forget about their pain."

In his Philadelphia practice, Dr. Bowie usually emphasizes weaving because it "helps exercise shoulders and elbows as well as wrists and fingers, which are generally the areas exercised in knitting. Knitting," he continues, "is fine for people who have trouble with their hands because it relaxes the tissues that are binding the middle joints of the fingers."

"I think knitting is a great help," says Judy Rivers, an Atlanta secretary. "Any finger exercise is good. I have arthritis in my hands and I type. The more I type, the better it is – it keeps the swelling down."

Not for Women Only

But knitting therapy isn't just for arthritics – or just for women. Mrs. Bloom has introduced many men to the craft.

"I taught one man who was a retired pipe fitter," she recalls. "You would think he couldn't do it because he had big hands – but they were agile!" Most of the men come out of loneliness.

"They can meet other people here and know they are not alone in their problems. My door is open to anyone," says Mrs. Bloom, whose lessons are free with the purchase of yarn. "I call these gatherings the 'I.M.I. Club.' That stands for 'I Made It,' which is what you say when everybody tells you how beautiful your sweater is."

Another member of the I.M.I. Club was a young man named Michael, "who is now working in the Houston oil fields. He started coming here after he got out of the service and crocheted such a beautiful sweater for his wife that the women in the group were jealous. I didn't actually teach Michael how to crochet," she recalled. "I just embellished what he had already learned from his grandmother. Michael told me he enjoyed doing it to relax."

And if you think any man who dabbles in needlecraft is a sissy, take a look at Rosey Grier and think again. The 300-pound, 6-foot-5-inch former defensive tackle for the Los Angeles Rams and New York Giants football teams does needlepoint as a hobby and lugs a bag of yarn along wherever he goes. Grier even wrote a book on the subject, *Rosey Grier's Needlepoint for Men* (Walker & Company, 1973). "Don't knock it till you've tried it," he advises.

It's a rare person she can't teach to knit, claims Mrs. Bloom. "It's a gift I have that comes from within. I enjoy helping and teaching people." She has even taught "touch knitting" to the blind. "It's not as difficult for them as you might think," she explains. "If you feel the row of yarn with your thumb, you know to purl. If you feel it with your middle finger, you know to knit." That's also something to keep in mind when knitting in dim light.

Mrs. Bloom is also ambidextrous and can teach right- or left-handed knitters. "It's a skill I learned when I fractured my right arm several years ago. I just tucked the knitting needle into my cast and went right on knitting."

Helping Bones to "Knit"

Others have also turned to needlecrafts while nature knits their breaks and fractures. When Mary Bernhardt broke her shoulder last July and was forced to wear a sling for six

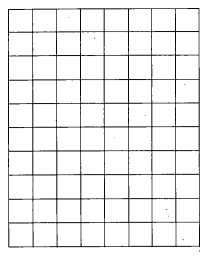

A lot of people feel the changes of the Relaxation Response while knitting. And the Relaxation Response, according to Dr. Herbert Benson, counteracts the harmful effects of stress and can add years to your life.

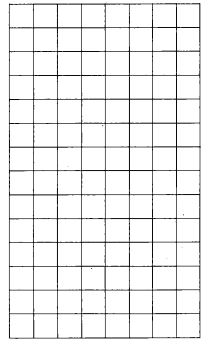

weeks, "I told my therapists I was looking forward to quilting over the winter, and they said, 'Great – if you can do it.' They told me it would be helpful. It worked very well and I'm glad."

Bertha Case says that the first time she returned to an afghan she had been crocheting when she broke her right shoulder two years ago, "I had a lot of trouble, but whenever I have any kind of trouble, I just try to keep going. It took me all day to make one four-inch block because I had to stop and rest after each row." Before her accident, she could turn out a dozen or so blocks in a day. Each afghan requires between 120 and 150 blocks.

"I've completed about five or six afghans since my shoulder's been broken," says Mrs. Case, who doesn't hide the fact that she'll be 80 in November. "I'm kind of proud of the fact that I can do what I do. It helps a lot to keep yourself busy. You just can't give up."

"My mother had a broken wrist, and her doctors told her crocheting would occupy her mind and her hands," recalls Philadelphia's Blanche Materniak. "They started her out squeezing balls."

Mrs. Materniak also knits and crochets; she has arthritis and finds the needlework "is good therapy for my hands and their circulation." An interesting side benefit is that it helps her with her housework. "You really push through the chores because you're looking forward to getting back to your knitting," she explains. "It takes away from the boredom of your day and gives you a real sense of accomplishment. Time doesn't hang heavy."

Boosting Morale

"Most of our knitters do this for therapy," agrees Evelyn Samuel, director of the Elder Craftsmen shop in Philadelphia. Her organization provides what she considers a real plus: a place where senior citizens can sell their handmade items. "It's a real boost to their morale."

John Hager has been teaching knitting on Friday afternoons at Elder Craftsmen for several years. He neither looks nor sounds as though he just turned 50. "How's that for its therapeutic effects?" he jokes. Like Rosey Grier, he picked up the needle on a dare – only in his case, he made it into a profession.

"My mother was operating a yarn shop in Doylestown, and a freelance designer was teaching an instructors' course in New York. Acting on a dare, Mom sent me." Mr. Hager was 24 years old at the time and embarked on a professional dancing career, but he had learned to knit as a boy, so he wasn't embarrassed by the caper. "I walked into a room full of women my mother's age, and they thought I was a yarn salesman until they saw how adept and serious I was. Later, I became like a son to them."

So serious was he that Mr. Hager and his 76-year-old mother, Norma, do custom knitting. He has found that teaching helps in his designing. "I suspected that by regressing to the beginner level, I could think of new concepts – and now I have. Still," he notes, "it is all really based on two basic stitches: knit and purl. And that's the reason it's therapeutic – because it's repetitive."

Herbert Benson, M.D., author of *The Mind/Body Effect* (Simon and Schuster, 1979) and the best-selling *The Relaxation Response* (William Morrow, 1975), which contains his widely acclaimed meditative instructions, agrees that "a lot of people feel the changes of the Relaxation Response while knitting." It fulfills the same basic requirements of "One, sitting in a comfortable position. Two, concentrating on a repetitive sound, word or action that absorbs attention. And three, passive disregard for other action."

The major benefit of the Relaxation Response, Dr. Benson says, is that "it counteracts the harmful effects of stress" and can add years to your life.

Knitting can, too. In a long-term study, researchers in Omaha taught creative arts to 30 volunteers, while another 21 acted as a control group. All the participants were over age 65. At the end of the instruction period, all but one of the senior citizens in the experimental group said they intended to stick with what they had learned. At the end of 11 years, 67 percent of the "creative" group were still living, as compared with only 38 percent of the controls.

The researchers concluded that "elderly persons found much satisfaction in a creative learning experience, the spread effect of which was to add greatly to the breadth and vitality of their interests and, apparently, to the number of their years" (*Journal of Psychology,* May 26, 1972).

So, when Ona D. Bloom says the sweater, afghan or shawl you start making now will do a lot more for your health than just keep you warm this winter, she isn't just telling you a yarn.

MARTIAL ARTS

There are a number of things that most of us accept. Things like "Don't eat raw dough!" Or "Don't bother a dog while it's eating!" Or "All Orientals are inscrutable!" Usually, however, when we investigate these truisms, our certainty and most of theirs fades. Now, we don't know much about raw dough or dogs, and we suppose that analyzing them would require rather more statistical sophistication than we possess. But Charlie Chan we *do* know about. If you can recall those wonderful B movies of the 40s and 50s, you'll remember that while Mr. Chan often *seemed* inscrutable, his ability to solve baffling crimes was not. The old Chinese gentleman's skill in piecing together hundreds of apparently unrelated details to produce a solution betrayed a supremely logical and orderly mind. His thoroughly Americanized Numba One Son, on the other hand, *was* most inscrutable. There was absolutely no thread of sense stringing the haphazard events of his life together, and his "gee whiz" brains seemed innocent of reason.

Which brings us, in a slightly roundabout way, to several Oriental exercise and health disciplines that some Americans practice but many others regard as – variously – inscrutable, incomplete or unfit for polite company. We are referring, obviously, to so-called self-defense systems like karate, judo, tai-chi, and tae-kwan-do. We'd like to suggest here that they make a lot of sense as fitness programs, because they offer the whole body a highly disciplined workout and, in some cases, even provide the aerobic benefits of a controlled breathing technique. What's more, most of them do not emphasize their offensive (or even defensive) qualities as much as their American purveyors would have us believe. Most scrutable Orientals practice these martial arts entirely for the sport, exercise and discipline they afford. They are *not* seeking dark alley arsenals.

Of course, we cannot tell you everything you need to know for getting started with the many forms of Eastern martial arts. In the ancient tradition, you need to apprentice yourself to a Master for that. What we can and are going to do is talk about the relative health and fitness benefits of four of the most popular and widely taught disciplines, and then let you seek specific how-to instruction on your own. From a welter of information we are going to play literary Charlie Chan and piece together an essay on some of the life-saving advantages of judo, karate, tai-chi and tae-kwan-do.

In keeping with our Charlie Chan motif, we are *not* going to start with our most complete piece of advice. Like Mr. Chan, we are going to start with a story, one told to us by Mark Bricklin, the executive editor of *Prevention* magazine, about tae-kwan-do and his bad back.

The Case of the Deadly Set Shot

"Everyone loves to talk about his or her diseases, and I am no exception. So let me tell you about my low back problem and how I cured it – by accident!

"The first time my back attacked me I was only about 12 or 13 years old. I had taken a 'set shot' with a basketball from the half-court mark, and I don't remember if a miracle happened and the ball went into the basket, but I do remember that I had to hobble home, crippled with pain. After several more such incidents, it seemed clear that I had inherited my father's bad back. His problem was quite serious, often laying him up for several days or more at a time, and necessitating, through the years, innumerable visits to doctors.

"At 14, I took up weightlifting and concentrated on exercises for the lower back – notably, one called the 'dead lift,' in which you squat down with the back held absolutely straight. Then, with fully extended arms, one palm facing frontward and one backward, you lift a barbell to the standing position. Logically, perhaps, such exercises should have destroyed me, but they didn't. At that point, my back was still in good enough shape to respond to these exercises with rapid development of very powerful muscles along the sides of the spine. Generally speaking, the more powerful these muscles are, the more they will support your spine and prevent discs from slipping around. Throughout my teenage years, I continued these exercises until I was able to deadlift about 250 pounds. During these years, while I was working out several times a week, my back didn't give me much trouble.

"In my twenties, I gave up weightlifting and every other form of exercise, and my back problem returned with a vengeance. About once or twice a year it would 'go out' on

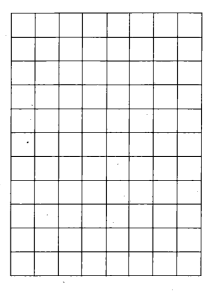

Six months after I took up karate, I suddenly became aware of an amazing fact: my poor, weak, vulnerable lower back had turned into stainless steel. I could carry anything!

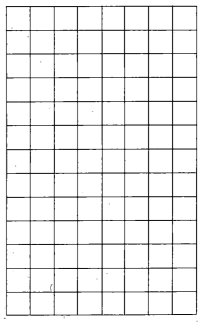

me, and as the years passed, these episodes became more and more painful and disabling. On various occasions, I visited a chiropractor, an orthopedic surgeon and several osteopaths, finding the greatest and quickest relief with the latter, who were able to snap my spine back into alignment whenever the occasion demanded.

"During this time, several doctors recommended that I do certain exercises, and I did do them – sometimes . . . for a while. The problem was that they didn't seem to do much good, even when I did them regularly, so after a while I just forgot about them.

"Finally, after spending most of one day moving furniture and then washing and polishing my car (like many other victims of low back pain, I just wouldn't *learn*), I got the worst attack of my life. I was limping around with my knuckles practically dragging on the floor, and I still vividly remember propping myself up on a tabletop with one hand to make a phone call to the first orthopedic surgeon I could find in the telephone book. I was in such pain that I insisted he be paged at the hospital even though I didn't know him. I must say, though, that he was remarkably nice about it all, perhaps recognizing the suffering I had. I described my symptoms, my history, and he said he was quite certain I had a slipped disc. He instructed me to lie down on a firm bed and stay there, with a heating pad under my back and a couple of pillows under my knees. Then, as I recall, several times a day my wife was to remove the pillows, grasp one of my legs and firmly and steadily pull it for a few moments. Then the other leg, and finally, both legs together. I was also to take aspirin for a few days to help relieve the pain.

"The improvement came quite quickly – in about two days, as I remember. In four days, I was just about as good as new, which surprised and delighted me.

"So now I knew what to do *after* I had thrown my back out. But I still didn't know what to do to prevent these terrible episodes.

Kicking Away Pain

"A short while later, for reasons having absolutely nothing to do with my bad back, I decided to take up karate – specifically, the Korean form of karate known as tae-kwan-do. Three times a week I worked out in a small gymnasium, for an hour and a half per session. About six months later I suddenly became aware of an amazing fact: my poor, weak, vulnerable lower back had turned into stainless steel! I could do *anything*, even carry heavy trash cans, without hurting myself. And most amazing of all, when I woke up in the morning, I never felt even the slightest twinge of discomfort as I rolled out of bed.

"Naturally, I tried to analyze why practicing karate had achieved this remarkable effect. Curiously, there was not a single exercise or movement that we did in karate that had much resemblance to the standard exercises I had been told to do to strengthen my back. We did not, for example, lie on our stomachs and raise our trunks while someone held our legs down. Neither did we ever do any kind of sit-ups. But what we did do was kick – and I mean *kick!*

"Korean karate, more than other forms of this martial art, emphasizes the use of the legs in self-defense. The Koreans feel there is no sense injuring your hand when you can use the heel or ball of your foot to do the job. So at every session, we practiced kicking endlessly. First, there were warm-up kicks with the leg held absolutely straight or as straight as possible, which loosened the massive, tight muscles in the back of the thigh. To complete the warm-up for these muscles, we would often hook our heels on a ledge about three feet high and then *gently* bounce forward. During our actual practice, we performed scores of front "snap" kicks, roundhouse kicks, side kicks, back kicks and leg sweeps.

"From a self-defense point of view, the purpose of all this was to give us sufficient control over our legs so that regardless of the position in which we were caught during an attack, we would be able to defend ourselves with our feet, striking the attacker anywhere from his knee up to his ear (after some practice, it is quite easy to stand directly in front of someone and deliver a kick to his ear).

"But as far as my *back* was concerned, I became convinced that all this kicking and stretching was what had done the trick. Why, I didn't exactly know, since I had the idea at that time that the way to help your bad back was to do exercises which made your back muscles *contract,* making them stronger. All I had done was *stretch* the muscles in the hamstring area and perhaps stretch my back muscles, too.

"It also occurred to me that while we never did sit-ups, when you pick up your leg to throw a kick, your stomach muscles are responsible for most of the lifting. And, in fact,

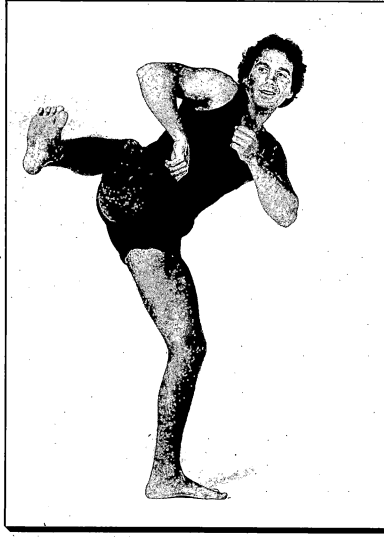

The martial arts are good body conditioners.

my stomach muscles had grown remarkably powerful, to the extent where I could be kicked (accidentally) in the stomach quite hard without feeling any discomfort.

"A few years later, my suspicions were confirmed when I read a book called *Orthotherapy* (M. Evans, 1971) by Arthur Michele, M.D., a former professor and chairman of the department of orthopedic surgery at New York Medical College.

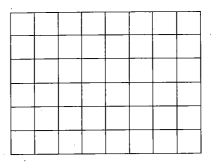

A Surgeon's Explanation

"Dr. Michele explains that the underlying cause of most back problems involves an extraordinarily large complex of muscles in the lower back known as the iliopsoas. He describes it as 'mainly a broad flat muscle in the lower back, but like an octopus, it has arms reaching out in many directions.' Its lower segments are attached to the pelvis, hips and thighbones, while its upper extremities go to every vertebra in the lumbar area of the lower spine, and even up to the lower thoracic (chest) vertebrae in the mid-back.

"All too often, Dr. Michele believes, one of the many arms of the iliopsoas is abnormally short – either because of a birth defect or, more often, because of contraction resulting from lack of stretching and use.

"The 'arms' of the iliopsoas have a grip on so many bones, joints and vertebrae, Dr. Michele explains, that a shortness of any one arm can result in a large number of symptoms – *which do not necessarily occur at the point of the underlying muscular problem.*

"These typical symptoms, he says, include pain or stiffness of the spine, slipped disc, actual fracture of the spine or degenerative disorders of the spine, arthrosis of the knee or hip, and even a pain in the chest and poor functioning of internal organs.

"Dr. Michele is convinced that many of his patients would never have had to limp into his consulting room or be wheeled into his operating theater had they followed a simple exercise regimen he has developed. Just as important – because the average person isn't interested in his back muscles until they desert him – Dr. Michele says that his exercises are equally potent as a cure, providing the spine has not become hopelessly degenerate. In fact, he says, after 35 years of orthopedic practice, he is certain that these exercises 'can bring about what seem to be near miracles' not only with back problems, but other related muscular-skeletal problems."

The points we'd like you to carry away from this success story are that (1) as long as Mr. Bricklin exercised (in *any* way) his "basketball bad back" was kept in line; (2) his venture in tae-kwan-do offered him much better exercise (and bad back insurance) than either basketball or weightlifting; and (3) the things Korean karate did for him were exactly the things Dr. Michele believes should be done to alleviate lower back pain.

Dr. Michele is convinced that many of his patients would never have had to limp into his consulting room or be wheeled into his operating theater had they followed a simple exercise regimen.

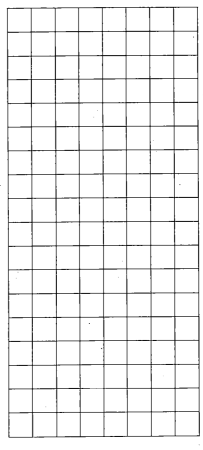

The Mysterious Benefits of Tai-Chi

With our story over, as Mr. Chan would say, please to move on to tai-chi, perhaps the most complete exercise program offered by the Eastern martial arts.

Tai-Chi Chuan, a unique system of exercise developed hundreds of years ago in China by Taoist monks, has recently been attracting the attention of American medical person- nel and physical educators. In hospital tests this exotic exer- cise has favorably impressed cardiologists as a form of activity that has potential in the treatment of heart patients. Accord- ing to the Chinese, who have a much longer experience than Americans with tai-chi, its practice for 20 minutes a day over a period of years can prolong youthful vigor and rejuvenate the body.

The 108 basic moves or forms of tai-chi use every part of the body. Hands, elbows, fists, legs, shoulders, head, but- tocks, feet, toes, sides of feet – even the eyes – are all brought into play in a pattern of continually flowing movement. The exercise is performed in a slow, almost leisurely manner, without any special muscular effort. And because it isn't strenuous, anyone from 8 to 80 can practice tai-chi at no risk to himself and with the promise of renewed vitality and longer life.

In China, tai-chi is viewed with great respect, and many Chinese claim that it has been known to lower high blood pressure and to alleviate joint diseases and gastric distur- bances. For most of its long history, the exercise was a jealously guarded secret of the Chinese elite, and the Com- munists, who took over all of the Chinese mainland in 1949, viewed it with suspicion. In their efforts to bring revolu- tionary thinking to the fore, they discouraged tai-chi, explain- ing that it was too traditional. Later, however, they had second thoughts, and in recognition of its therapeutic value, they began to encourage its regular practice.

Now tai-chi is part of the routine of millions of people in China, a fact that is illustrated by numerous documentary films. In the newsreels of President Nixon's visit there in 1972, for example, several of the films show solo and mass demonstrations of the art of tai-chi. Not only China but the Soviet Union as well has found value in this calisthenic. After a Soviet delegation to China saw and was impressed by tai-chi, it was carried back to the Soviet Union, where training classes have opened and several books on the subject have been published with the sanction of the government.

Tai-chi began to catch on in the United States in the 1960s. Although it was practiced secretly in Chinatowns all over the country before that time, few if any of the practitioners were interested in sharing their knowledge outside their own group. In fact, they often resented the activities of the Chinese tai-chi Masters – mostly recent immigrants from Taiwan and Hong Kong – when they started classes that were open to non-Chinese pupils. Like the Chinese aristocrats of centuries past, they believed that knowledge of the exercise should be reserved for a limited group.

In spite of such reservations, tai-chi began to attract devotees among non-Chinese Americans. At first, the tai-chi schools were limited to the East and West Coast, but they soon began to spread inland across the country. Now, along with acupuncture, the art of tai-chi is getting official attention from the medical community, and thousands of Americans are discovering this easy, "effortless" way to lasting health and long life.

No Strain but Lots of Gain

One test of tai-chi's effect on the heart was made recently at Montefiore Hospital in New York City. Lenore Zohman, M.D., chief of physical therapy, took an electrocardiogram on a well-known tai-chi teacher, Sophia Delza, the foremost woman instructor of tai-chi in the Western world. Although it is normally the case that exercise increases the heart rate, the cardiogram on Ms. Delza indicated that her heart rate was not changed when she practiced tai-chi. While laypeople might not be impressed, doctors appreciate the rare value of an activity that does not put stress on the heart, and they are alert to its therapeutic possibilities. According to Louis Brinberg, M.D., formerly a cardiologist at New York's Mount Sinai Hospital, "It will be interesting to see what can be done with tai-chi when used as an adjunct to the usual therapy of cardiac patients."

The value of tai-chi seems to stem as much from its psychological as from its physiological effects. The fact that modern medicine is finding more and more connections between mental attitudes and physical health may indeed help to explain the value of tai-chi, which is designed to have a calming effect on the mind and nervous system.

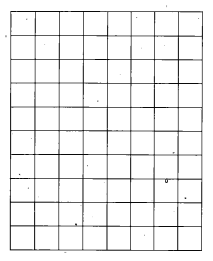

In China, tai-chi is viewed with great respect, and many Chinese claim that it has been known to lower high blood pressure and to alleviate joint diseases and gastric disturbances.

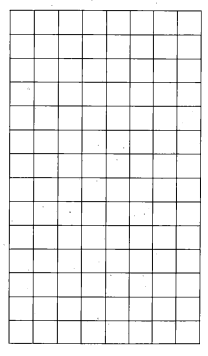

A Natural Tranquilizer

It has been quite conclusively demonstrated that tai-chi has a tranquilizing effect on the emotions. The overburdened executive, the harassed housewife, the uptight student, the anxious clerk – all might discover that a ten-minute break for a round of tai-chi can put them in a better frame of mind and help them to bear the pressures of everyday living without ulcers or nervous breakdowns.

Probably the most difficult tai-chi principle for a beginner to follow is the one of complete relaxation. Most Westerners attack daily exercise as though they were wrestling with a bear. They don't really enjoy doing it. Up and down, puff, puff, back and forth.

By contrast, tai-chi requires that you relax your facial muscles, shoulders, abdomen and thighs, and follow the shifting pattern of movements with a light, calm mind. Eventually you will experience a sensation almost like floating.

By their very nature, all of the movements of tai-chi are geared to encourage relaxation. The weight of the body shifts continuously from one foot to the other, and the movements are performed in circles, arcs and spirals. The end of each movement becomes the beginning of the next one, which conserves energy and produces a feeling of tranquillity and emotional security.

In order to perform the exercises properly, the body must move as a unit. This principle of unity in movement is one of the ways in which it contrasts most basically to Western calisthenics, which use various parts of the body independently. Robert J. Rogers, Ph.D., a Chappaqua, New York, psychologist, psychoanalyst and tai-chi practitioner, believes that tai-chi, "practiced correctly over a long period of time, creates a kind of protective psychological shield that helps a person combat stress, which is one of the main causes of disease."

The Baffling Case of *Chi*

At the heart of tai-chi is the Chinese concept of *chi,* a word of many meanings – air, vitality, spirit, breath, atmosphere and circulation. It is hard to define *chi.* One tai-chi expert calls it "biophysical energy generated by respiratory rhythm." Perhaps the best English equivalent is "intrinsic energy," or "vital force." Whatever *chi* is, doctors of Chinese medicine say it can be cultivated through practice of the exercise and stored in a spot called the *tan-t'ien,* located exactly three inches below the navel. Once stored, the *chi* can be circulated by the mind throughout the body. In an ancient Chinese treatise on tai-chi, the author states, "The mind directs the *chi,* which sinks deeply and permeates the bones. The *chi* circulates freely, mobilizing the body so that it heeds the direction of the mind. If the *chi* is correctly cultivated, your spirit of vitality will rise, and you will feel as though your head were suspended by a string from above." It is this "vital energy," as manifested through the tai-chi exercise, that accounts for the prolongation and rejuvenation of life.

Master William C. C. Chen, of the Tai-Chi School in New York City, was asked about the mystery of *chi* and replied: "It is certainly a mystery, but it works. Look at acupuncture; it has cured apparently incurable diseases, even though it is not yet clear how it works. All I can say is, if you practice tai-chi every day, you will eventually build up this inner strength or *chi.*"

At a demonstration in Madison Square Garden's Forum, Master Chen demonstrated the effectiveness of his *chi.* Four hefty volunteers, astride a motorcycle – weighing a total of more than 1,000 pounds – rode over Master Chen's stomach as he lay on the floor. Later these same volunteers took turns punching him repeatedly in the abdomen using full force. After several minutes the punchers became tired and gave up, but Master Chen just smiled.

The tai-chi postures that follow are just a few of the many which may be practiced.

When you perform these exercises, remember, the body always moves as one unit. This rule applies to all tai-chi movements. And when you move as one unit, you should notice that your body's awkwardness will be greatly reduced. In its place, you should experience a gracefulness that aids in your inner circulation of *chi.*

This gracefulness can be thought of as the outer expression of *chi.* You probably can't really experience the inner peace connected with *chi* without this outward grace. The external relaxation you radiate is a reflection of the inner peace you are creating. Awkward movements, on the other hand, will only disrupt the *chi*'s flow.

Move slowly, without any visible effort.

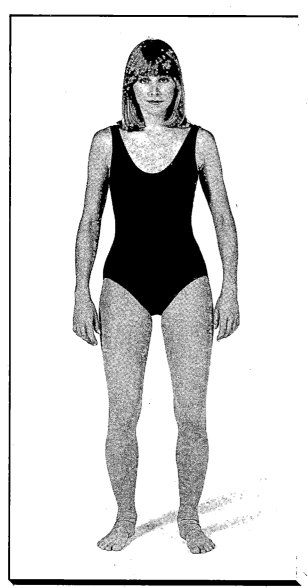 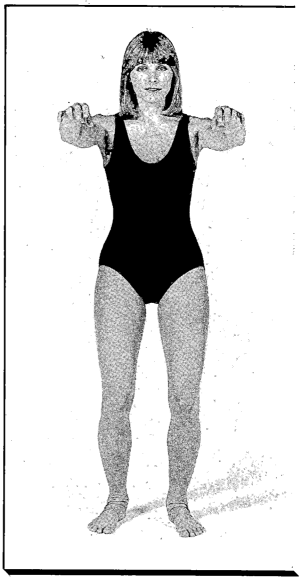

1. Tai chi beginning pose. Stand relaxed. 2. Raise arms to shoulder height.

Beginning of Tai-Chi

1. Stand relaxed, elbows and knees *slightly* bent.
2. Raise arms *slowly* to shoulder height.
3. Draw back your arms by bending your elbows.
4. Let your arms sink *gently* to your sides. You are again in the beginning position.

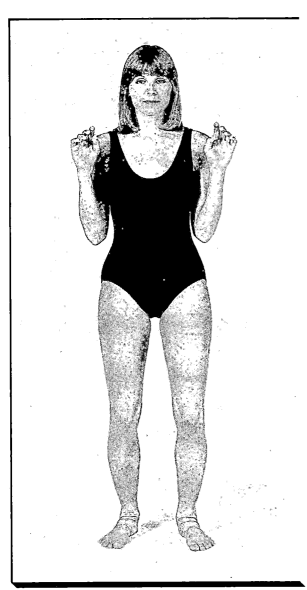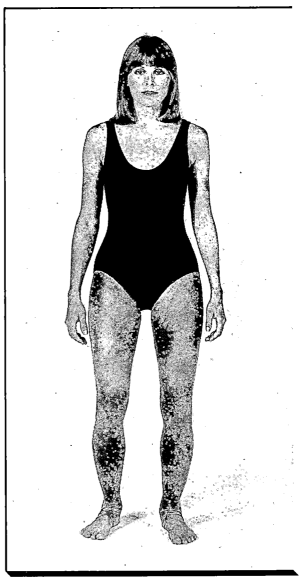

3. Draw your arms back. 4. Gently drop your arms down.

Note: Do not exert force, but let your arms rise as though they were floating up from water to the surface. In the same way, let them fall to your sides again without strain. Concentrate on total relaxation.

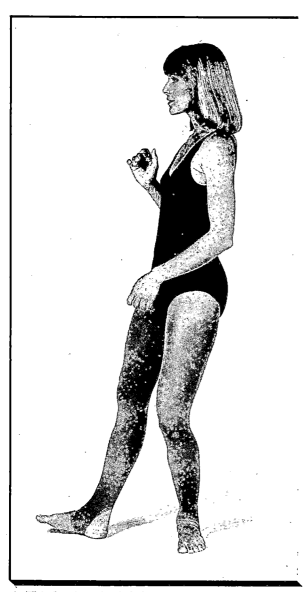 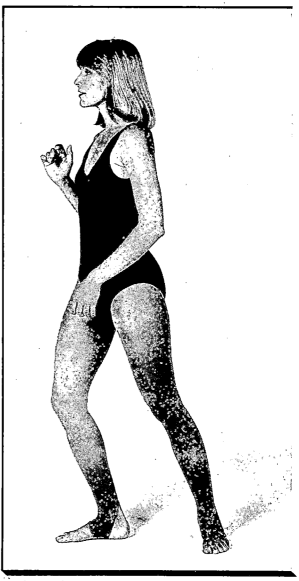

1. This begins the left hand ward off movement. 2. Shift weight to right foot.

Ward Off with Your Left Hand

1. This movement follows "Beginning of Tai-Chi." Shift your weight to your left foot, turn on your right heel, toes raised slightly, to your right.
2. Now shift your weight to your right foot. Left leg is relaxed.

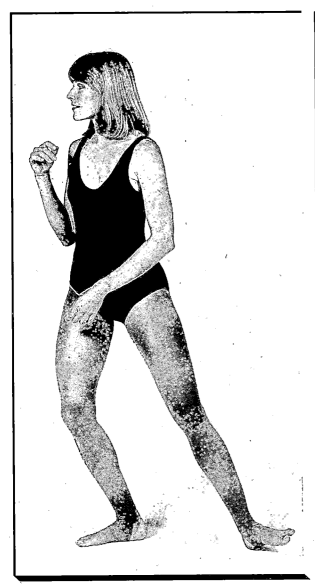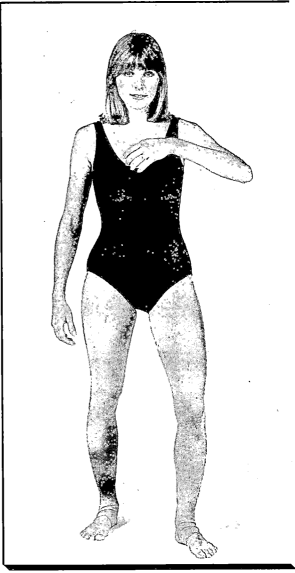

3. Step out with left foot. 4. Shift weight to left foot and pivot.

3. Step out with left foot, heel touching the floor slightly.
4. Shift your weight to your left foot and pivot to front. As you do, left arm rises, palm turned in, to chest height while right arm sinks gently to side. Follow by pivoting slightly to left and perform similar movements to "ward off with right hand."

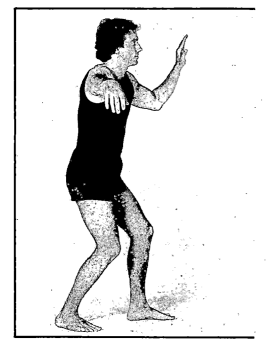

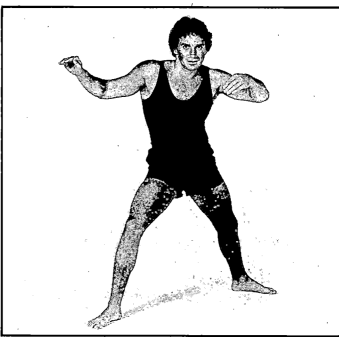

1. *This begins the squatting down movement.*
2. *Pivot to right; shift weight to right foot.*
3. *Squat down, left arm dropping gently.*

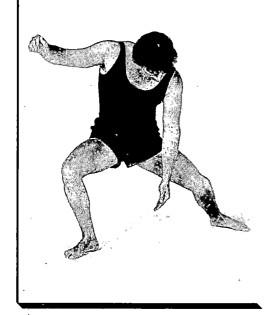

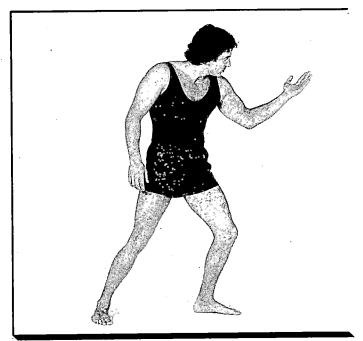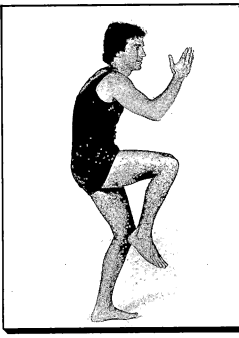

1. The stand on one leg pose begins with weight on left foot. 2. Lift right knee, and lift right arm. Left arm goes down.

Squatting Down

1. Stand with body weight on left foot, right leg relaxed, left arm palm out and bent at elbow.
2. Pivot to right, shifting weight onto right foot; arms and body move in one unit.
3. Squat down, left arm dropping gently in front of you, right arm extended with wrist limp.

Golden Cock Stands on One Leg

1. This posture follows "Squatting Down." From a squatting position, the weight shifts forward to left foot, body rising, with left arm, slightly bent, extending.
2. Lift right knee to waist height; right arm, with elbow bent, lifts upward in an arc, while left arm falls to side. Notice how left knee is slightly curved.

Note: Don't raise the knee too high or you will begin to feel tension. Let your eyes follow your hand. And remember to move slowly!

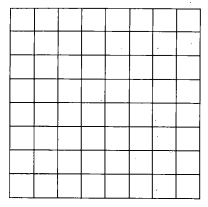

The essence of judo is getting hold of another individual, so it's great for people with personality problems, especially those who are phobic. It helps couples get over aggression that might otherwise not surface.

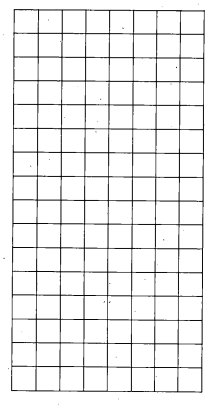

Some Nagging Questions

Most training in self-defense techniques, if religiously pursued, will give you *some* of the benefits of tai-chi and tae-kwan-do. The important question is: how good are the other well-known forms – like judo and karate – as general exercise programs? Do they tone the muscles the way tae-kwan-do does? Do they relieve tension the way tai-chi does? And are they as beneficial to the cardiovascular system as tai-chi and tae-kwan-do?

Well, most kinds of regular exercise that we know tone and build muscle. And we also know of one doctor who prescribes judo for aggressive patients. "Apart from keeping you fit, it's a good way to get rid of aggression," says Leslie Wooten, M.D., an English physician who at age 40 wears his black belt proudly and well. He even recommends his art for people who are shy. "The essence of judo is getting hold of another individual, so it's great for people with personality problems, especially those who are phobic."

"A kind of touch therapy" is how Dr. Wooten prefers to think of his curiously martial approach to marital strife. "It helps couples get over aggression that might otherwise not surface. And it stops them from being afraid to make contact with one another, which for many can be a real problem."

A flip to say good night. Or a flip to make up. "You're trained in judo to take aggression in a jolly way," he says. "If someone is better than you are, they throw you into the air, and as you hit the mat with a thud, you smile because it was a good throw." The forgiving attitude, Dr. Wooten is finding, can go a long way in holding together a household.

As for the fitness end, he points out that judo can prevent the clogging of arteries, a part of the body which otherwise can turn into a disaster area.

As a licensed instructor, Dr. Wooten finds himself throwing (and being thrown) quite a few times in an evening, "and so I can smile when someone comes belting into the office moaning and groaning at me." He finds such verbal aggression quite tame compared to the physical abuse judo teaches him to take.

"As a rather belligerent boy," Dr. Wooten took up the sport at age 16. "The belligerence slowly faded, though," he happily reports, "as the judo gradually became something of an art, a way of life to me. It's more gentle than it looks."

Karate and Your Lungs

Finally, is karate a good aerobic exercise? Does it provide the kind of workout for the heart and lungs that Dr. Ken Cooper had in mind when he coined the phrase "aerobic exercise?" Unfortunately, perhaps not as good as all those flailing limbs might suggest. Ten karate students were studied recently at the Applied Physiology Research Laboratory at Kent State University and, while heart rates attained during workouts were high enough for conditioning purposes (they averaged 168 beats per minute in response to the most vigorous type of training), the amount of huffing and puffing (oxygen uptake) demanded by the workouts was *not* sufficient for significant cardiovascular improvement.

Karate is normally practiced in sets of prescribed movements, called "katas." For the purposes of the Kent State study, students were made to go through these sets in either 30 or 45 seconds, and either continuously (15 in a row) or intermittently (being allowed a minute of rest between each). Highest heart rates and greatest oxygen uptakes were achieved, of course, during the continuous and more rapidly done routines, but not even these required enough breathing to make them recommendable cardiovascular exercise. The contrast between relatively *high* heart rates and relatively *low* oxygen uptake demanded by these exercises, in fact, led the researchers to advise against "kata exercise as an acceptable form of cardiovascular conditioning" for anyone with "compromised cardiovascular function" (at a high risk of heart attack).

The problem with karate seems to be that its movements are abrupt and involve mainly the arms. (Studies show that arm work raises heart rates more than an equivalent amount of work done by the legs, because the heart must work against gravity to supply the arms with necessary blood flow.) The safest and most productive exercises for cardiovascular conditioning involve prolonged fluid motions with muscle groups larger than just the arms (that is, the legs, or better yet, the arms and legs combined, such as in cross-country skiing). And the minimum prescription, remember, is three 20-minute sessions a week.

MASSAGE

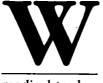

hen you massage someone, you're using a therapy as old as medicine itself. The ancient Chinese were well versed in massage techniques. And the ancient Greeks, including Hippocrates, used massage as one of their medical tools.

But somewhere between Hippocrates and the industrial revolution, Western medicine forgot about massage. So when the French brought back information about Chinese massage, the technique seemed brand new to Europeans. The foremost European popularizer of massage was not a Frenchman, however, but a Swede, Per Henrik Ling, who studied and taught massage during the early 1800s. Because of Dr. Ling's effort, basic massage is today called "Swedish" massage. Yet the actual massage strokes still carry their French names: petrissage (a kneading motion); tapotement (a striking motion or tapping of the skin); effleurage (gliding strokes). Yet massage really speaks a universal language: that of healing.

Viktoras Kulvinskas, a natural healer, lists these health benefits of massage in his book *Survival into the 21st Century* (O'Mango D'Press, 1975):

- Massage dilates the blood vessels, improving the circulation and relieving congestion throughout the body.
- Massage acts as a "mechanical cleanser," stimulating lymph circulation and hastening the elimination of wastes and toxic debris.
- Massage relaxes spasm and relieves tension.
- Massage, by improving the general circulation, increases nutrition of the tissues.
- Massage makes you feel good.

A Massage at Home

A relaxing massage, and all of its benefits, is as close to you as your hands. Massage makes a great gift for a spouse or friend. And after you do it to them, make sure that they do it to you.

Giving a thorough and effective massage isn't only easy – it's fun. You don't need any familiarity with formal anatomy to give a good massage. Nor do you need the Herculean hands of a burly Swedish masseur. And all that's required in the way of equipment is some padding to lay on the floor and some vegetable oil.

Do you have a few idle moments and a warm, private room? Then you're ready to begin learning the gentle art of massage. Read on, and enjoy.

The first instruction is: don't use your bed for massage. Surprised? A bed is too soft to provide firm support. So, instead of bouncing around on a Beautyrest, take two or three blankets, fold them lengthwise on the floor and cover them with a sheet. You can also use foam as a padding, or move a single mattress onto the floor. But whatever padding you use, make sure it's at least an inch or two thick, and it should be wide and long enough so that when your partner lies down, there's still room for you to sit or kneel to one side.

Also, you might want to turn off the overhead light; both the atmosphere and your partner will be more relaxed. Bright light that falls directly on the face will cause your partner to tense his or her eye muscles.

Keep the room warm, comfortable and free of drafts. George Downing, author of *The Massage Book* (Random House, 1972), cautions: "Nothing destroys an otherwise good massage more quickly than physical coldness." If your partner begins to feel cold, use a spare sheet to cover the body parts that you're not working on at the moment.

Now prepare the oil. Why use oil at all? Without a lubricating agent, your hands can't really apply enough pressure and still move smoothly over the skin. When applying oil, put about half a teaspoon into your palm and then spread it smoothly on your partner's skin. Keep the oil near you during the massage; a shallow bowl makes a handy container. Cover the entire surface area you're about to massage – arm, leg, hand or back – with a barely visible film. Massage professionals recommend vegetable oil (except for peanut or corn oil). Sesame and olive oil are the easiest to wash out of sheets and clothes. You can scent the oil, mixing in a few drops of essences such as clove, cinnamon, lemon, rosemary or camomile.

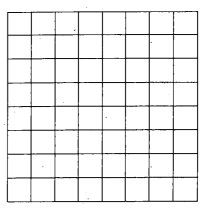

Massage acts as a mechanical cleanser, stimulating lymph circulation and hastening the elimination of wastes and toxic debris.

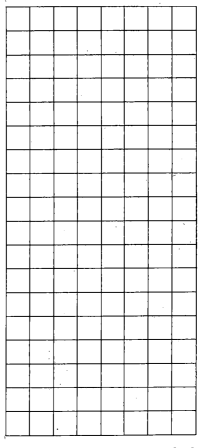

"Does That Feel Good?"

Before you actually use specific strokes, here are a few general hints. Keep your hands relaxed. Also, apply pressure. You'll probably discover that your partner wants quite a bit more pressure than you expected. But use the weight of your whole body to apply pressure rather than just the muscles of your hands.

Experiment with all the different ways of moving your hands that you can think of. Move them in long strokes. Move them in circles. Explore the structure of the bone and muscle. Move slowly, then speed up your tempo. Or use only your fingertips, pressing them firmly against the muscles or brushing them lightly over the skin. Gently slap. Or tap. Ask your partner for feedback. Is that enough pressure? Does that feel good?

While you're taking care of your partner, don't forget to take care of yourself. Keep your back straight whenever possible. And don't worry about how much or how little you do. You'll be moving and positioning your body in many new ways; if you don't take care of yourself, you'll end up with sore muscles. For now, concentrate on one or two body parts at a time.

Although we have the massage arranged in a particular order, you should start and end wherever you want. If you decide to work on more than a single part, apply more oil each time you move to a new area.

Finally, try to minimize the amount of turning over that your partner has to do. (It's easiest to work on the arms, hands, feet and neck while your partner is lying face up.)

Be Kind to Your Spine

Let's start with the back, for the back is the most important part of a massage. The spine is the stalk of the central nervous system, and often anxiety and nervous tension are caused by nothing more than tight, sore muscles around the spine. Loosening these muscles can, in the words of George Downing, bring a "deep sense of release."

First, straddle your partner's thighs. It's the easiest way to work on the back.

Now put your hands on the lower back with the fingertips pointing toward the spine. Move your hands straight

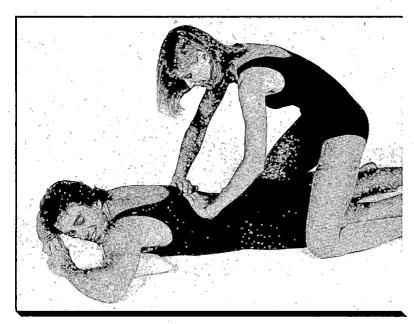

A back massage.

up the back. When you get to the top of the back, separate your hands and bring them over the shoulder blades to the floor, and then pull them back down along the sides. Do this stroke four to six times.

Now work with your thumbs on the lower back. Use the balls of your thumbs, and make short, rapid strokes away from you toward the head. Work close to the spine just below the waistline, first on the left side and then on the right.

Now put both hands on one hip with your fingers pointing straight down. Pull each hand alternately straight up from the floor, working up to the armpit and then back again. With each stroke, begin pulling one hand just before the other is about to finish so that there is no break between strokes. Do both sides.

Now move to the upper back. Knead the muscles that curve from your partner's neck onto his or her shoulders. Work these muscles gently between the thumb and fingers.

Now use your thumbs on the upper back, just as you did on the lower back.

Finally, take the heel of your hand and place it at the base of the spine. Gently press and release, moving little by little up the spine to the neck.

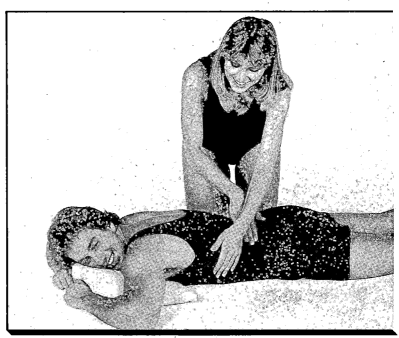

Massaging the side.

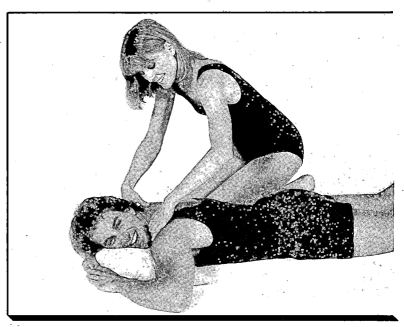

Kneading the neck muscles.

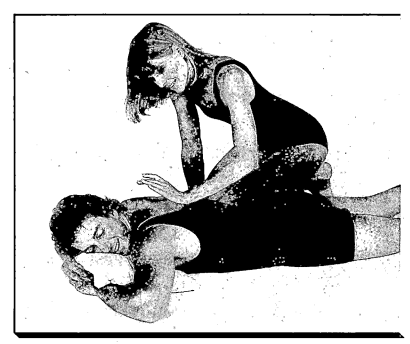

Use the heel of the hand along the spine.

A New Way to Touch

Now that you've finished the back, ask your partner to turn over so that you can massage the arms. But first, we'll learn a new stroke, one that we mentioned at the beginning of this section, an effleurage.

Place your hands together, one hand on top of the other with thumbs interlinked. When you move your hands, make your strokes long, flowing and unbroken, and put your weight on the heels of your hands rather than on the fingertips. This is an effleurage.

First, effleurage the entire arm from the wrist to the shoulder, taking your hands up over the shoulder and down the side of the arm.

Now massage the inside of the wrist with the balls of your thumbs. Work your hands downward until you have covered all the muscles lying along the inside of the forearm.

Now, place your partner's hand on his or her chest. Work from the elbow to the shoulder with the balls of your thumbs, paying particular attention to the muscles on the top of the arm.

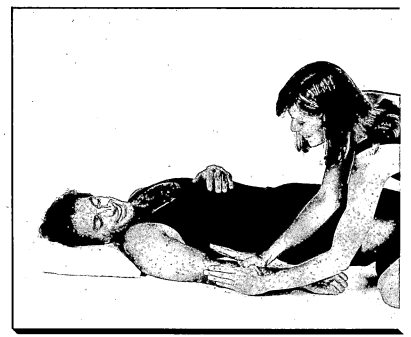

During effleurage, you link thumbs.

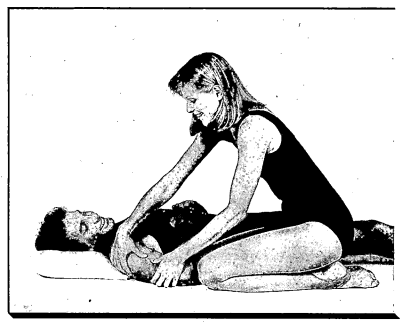

Massaging the upper arm with the thumbs.

Now explore and massage the shoulder joint with your fingers.

And end with another effleurage of the entire arm.

Soothing Strokes for the Browbeaten

Now let's go on to the head. Don't apply any oil to the face before you begin; just put a few drops on your fingertips. Massage the forehead just below the hairline with the balls of your thumbs. Start from the center of the forehead and glide both thumbs at once in either direction. Continue to the temples; now move your thumbs in a small circle. Repeat this stroke until you have covered the whole forehead – your last stroke should run just above your partner's eyebrows.

Cover the forehead with the entire left hand – heel toward one temple, fingertips toward the other. Press down. Now, using the right hand, slowly and evenly add more pressure until maximum pressure is reached (your partner will tell you if it's too much). Hold ten seconds, then release very slowly. Massage lore has it that this stroke can be used to cure a nagging headache.

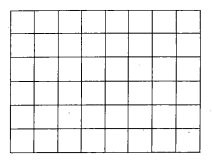

Massage can be useful in relieving fatigue and tension and is a wonderful way to express affection.

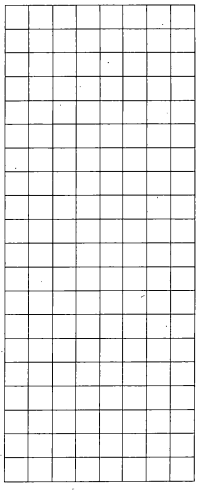

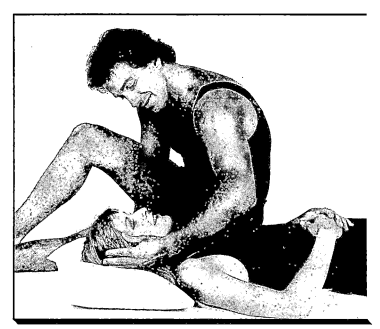

A forehead massage.

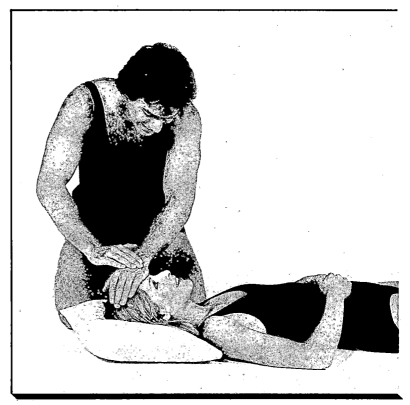

Pressing the head with both hands.

Now that you've smoothed your partner's harried brow, move on to the jaw, another area of tension on the face. Lightly grasp the tip of the chin between the tips of the thumb and forefinger of each hand. Follow the edges of the jaw until you have almost reached the ears, and then glide the forefingers into a small circle on the temples. Do this stroke three times.

Most of us have neck and shoulder muscles that are habitually tense – so much so that we don't even realize they're tight and bunched up. That's why loosening these muscles feels so very good.

First massage in egg-shaped circles just above the shoulder blades. Face your palms upward as you work under the body. Start at the outer shoulders, work in toward the spine, then back along the shoulders. You might want to change the direction, speed and width of your circles as you go.

Now work between the shoulder blades and the spine.

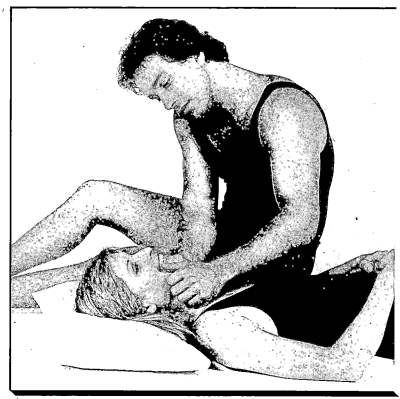

You can massage the chin between the thumb and forefinger.

Move your fingertips in small circles. Then put your hands under the back of your partner's head, gently lift it a little and turn it slightly to the left until it rests easily in your left hand. Massage the neck with your free hand. Then turn the head and work on the other side.

Take Your Body on a Vacation

Just by working with these simple instructions, you'll soon begin to realize massage's many benefits. Massage professionals say that massage often proves useful in relieving fatigue and tension and is a wonderful way to express affection.

They caution, however, not to do a lot of massage right away. Rather, they suggest, do a little at a time and gradually, if you care to, work up to a whole-body massage. Begin by working on those parts that are especially sore and stiff.

They also feel that massaging your children is a fine idea. Most parents touch only their child's hands or head or feet, but children, too, love to be touched all over.

But whether you make massage a daily event or reserve it for those special romantic evenings, rest assured that a tender touch is a gift that is a joy both to give and to receive.

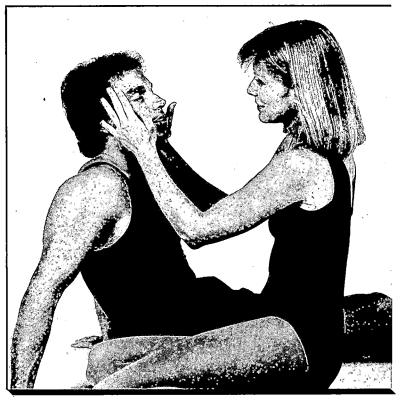

Use the palms on both sides of the face.

MUSIC THERAPY

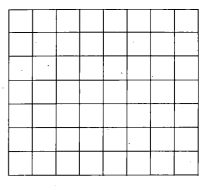

I n an apartment in New York City, members of the Western Wind, an *a cappella* vocal ensemble, were discussing why they sang – how they came to do it, why they loved it. At one point in the conversation – not a lull, really – the name of a song was mentioned, and several notes were hit, even as the random talk went on.

Suddenly, the six voices fused in song. The room reso-nated with sound, almost as if it were the musical instrument that produced this wonderful noise. You could see the members of the group straighten in their seats, listening to one another, opening their lungs to sing. The song dominated the moment; it filled the senses; it was a present, living thing that passed through the place in about a minute and then was gone.

In the brief hush that followed, it seemed amazing that something so magical could have occurred so naturally. But as Jack Thorp, the turn-of-the-century collector of cowboy songs, once wrote, "Singing songs, and making them, too, seem as natural to human beings as washing herself is to a cat."

As individuals, humans sing before they can form coherent sentences; as a species, we have sung since the dawn of recorded time. Homer's *Iliad* and *Odyssey* are believed to have been sung before anyone thought of putting them on paper. The ancient Greeks went so far as to define a person's humanity in terms of music. An educated and distinguished citizen was referred to as "musical," while a man who was ignorant and rough was said to be "without music."

Music and song have always been ties that bind us together in a common humanity. Of course, the modern world has disrupted this musical unity to a certain extent. We don't live in the same town and sing in church with the same people all our lives anymore. Because of advances in transportation and communication, we no longer automatically share the same cultural and musical heritage with our neighbors. The "old familiar air" has been replaced by the Top 40 hits, and tunes are sold like toothpaste.

Steven Urkowitz, Ph.D., a professor of English at the State University of New York Maritime College, who worked with the Western Wind on the dramatic, acting side of

Children learn to sing before they can even form coherent sentences.

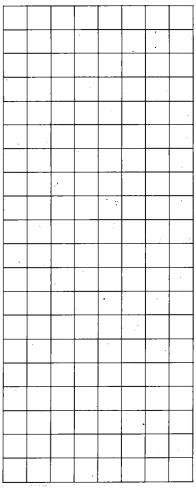

their stage performances, told us this trend disturbs him very much.

A Sense of Participation

"In traditional societies," he says, "there was much more singing than we have now. Today, most vocal music is a product. You buy records. You go to concerts. You consume singing rather than perform it. In Renaissance England they would have 5,000 people come to a service in the churchyard of St. Paul's Cathedral, and 5,000 people would all be singing complex hymns. It was a participatory act."

It's clear, though, that this sense of participation, or at least a longing for it, is still alive today, particularly in "ethnic" byways of the music business, such as black music and country and western.

In her book *Sing Your Heart Out, Country Boy* (Pocket Books, 1976), Dorothy Horstman tells how, in 1938, country singer Ernest Tubb wrote a song about the tragic death of his newborn son, Roger Dale, in a car accident. "It remains one of his most requested songs today," Ms. Horstman says, "more than 30 years later. Tubb says he knows of more than 300 children named Roger Dale in honor of his dead son. His devoted fans symbolically 'gave' their children to him to help replace his loss."

So there is obviously something about music and song that touches all of us, that makes us want to join with the singer and the rest of the audience in the common emotions songs reflect and express. Sometimes you can't even say exactly what it is the song touches in you, but the emotional attraction is so strong you can't resist it.

Ms. Horstman cites a rather extreme example of this kind of reaction when she quotes singer Jimmy Wakely: "I had a brother-in-law that was always knocking his wife around and drank a lot. I got to thinking that maybe one day she'd just have enough and leave, so I wrote a song called 'Too Late.' It was a smash. I went back to Oklahoma City, and I ran into my brother-in-law. And he said, 'Man, you never wrote anything as pretty as "Too Late" in your life.' I said, 'You *should* like it, you son of a — , it's the story of your life.'"

Some Things Can Only Be Expressed in Music

That mysterious ability of songs to tell the story of our lives – even if we don't really want to hear the story and have buried it deep within ourselves – has led therapists to use singing to treat both emotionally and mentally damaged patients. John M. Bellis, M.D., is a Connecticut-based psychiatrist who makes extensive use of bioenergetic therapy (he is director of the Connecticut Society for Bioenergetic Analysis) in his practice. Bioenergetics, a therapy pioneered by Alexander Lowen, M.D., sees a crucial connection existing between a person's state of body and his or her state of mind. Repressions of anxiety are believed to be reflected in the musculature of the body and cannot be relieved until the muscular as well as the emotional tension is banished. Obviously singing, the one form of music that uses the body itself as the instrument, is an invaluable tool in this kind of therapy.

"I see the use of the voice," Dr. Bellis says, "as one of the ways of playing with the frustrations and traumas of life, helping us integrate experience internally, on the feeling, affectual level, which can't, I think, be done with insight alone.

"Sometimes," he continues, "I find that people tell me, 'I've cried and I've cried and I've cried – what good does it do?' (I had told them to go ahead, let it out.) Now what I say is, 'Well, when you're through crying, start to sing some of the sadness, some of the loss, some of the appreciation of what you've lost.'

"And there they begin to find a sense of the meaning, the beauty, where the heart was connected with what they've lost. It's a way that humans have of enriching, giving testimony to the enrichment of their lives. Music and song have that ability . . . to give expression to something that may be impossible to express any other way."

A Special Feeling for Special Children

The way singing can tap and release hidden emotions makes it a powerful tool for working with retarded children as well. Paul Nordoff and Clive Robbins, pioneers in singing therapy for handicapped children, describe in their book *Music Therapy in Special Education* (Thomas Y. Crowell, 1971) the effects singing can have on the mentally handicapped:

"Each song has an emotional content that it can impart to the children who sing it; a variety of songs with many different emotional qualities gives them experiences of a spectrum of emotional life. Songs can arouse children to excitement, gladden them with pleasure, calm them to thoughtfulness. Through the feelings of serene warmth that a song can give, the children's consciousness can be deepened and stabilized.

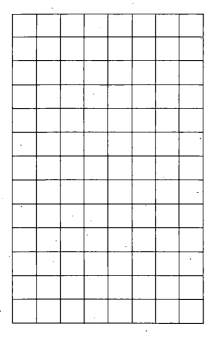

Probably the best thing that could happen to us would be to regain our childhood openness to music and song.

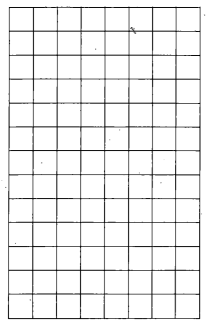

"A handicapped child singing is deeply committed to his singing. The musical instrument he uses is his own body, his voice, and he experiences his singing as a direct extension of himself."

Certainly the physical benefits are enormous. Lawrence Bennett, a tenor in the Western Wind and professor of music at Upsala College, told us, "I don't know how everybody else feels after a voice lesson, but it's one of the most wonderful feelings I've ever had. That physical exercising up and down from the top to bottom of my range, and the concentration involved in it . . ." Words seem to fail him.

"The radiation of that vocal energy really starts right from the feet," Dr. Bellis says. "You can feel it vibrating up and down through your body, when you really are totally into sound."

Music to Soothe Savageness

Music can have therapeutic benefits on violent criminals, too, according to Chuni Roy, M.D., medical director of the Regional Psychiatric Centre in Abbotsford, British Columbia, a 138-bed psychiatric prison hospital. Writing in the *Canadian Medical Association Journal* (November 3, 1979), Dr. Roy, secretary general of the International Council of Prison Medical Services, reports positive, calming effects of classical music on men who have made violence a way of life.

The music program at Abbotsford consists of playing classical music to inmates for one hour every Tuesday afternoon. The program is voluntary and very popular. The inmates, most of whom have been locked up for federal offenses like murder and assault, select the composers and pieces to be played. The program includes a general discussion, led by a school teacher, about the music and about how each listener relates to what he heard.

Dr. Roy's observations confirm that modern society's use of music as a product has forced it to lose a spiritual peacefulness that classical music retains. At one session, he reports: "The group listened to the [classical] music intently without any disruptive behavior. [But] when rock music was played, the group became disruptive, so much so that the [particular] session had to be ended prematurely."

The classical music contained something that was missing from the men's lives; it transported them to a peaceful, introspective place to which they had rarely been. The popular modern music brought them right back to the violent world they hadn't learned to cope with.

To some inmates, classical music even becomes a central focus of their lives. "Of all the composers chosen by the group," Dr. Roy says, "Tchaikovsky seemed to be the most popular, followed by Debussy. A man who had committed a number of murders and had never been exposed to classical music became obsessed with Debussy's music."

Music Speaks a Spiritual Language

William Zukof, countertenor with the Western Wind, told us he sees the group's singing as a way of expressing and preserving our spirituality, a part of our being that is often neglected in modern life. "In addition to the secular repertoire that we sing, we also do a lot of sacred music that was originally intended to be performed within a religious context," he says. "That context either no longer exists or is no longer relevant to an enormous number of people. To many of us the context is no longer relevant, yet the music *is*. The music speaks a spiritual language that is very, very immediate."

Elliot Levine, the Western Wind's baritone and a teacher at the Lighthouse Music School in New York City, discusses a religious context that he has experienced. "I was thinking," he says, "about the tradition of singing which has disappeared a lot from our general culture, but I think it does continue in a lot of different religious settings. I was just in temple. Just conceiving of the immense amount of music that goes on in the High Holy days, the incredible number of tunes and changes and lead-ins . . . everyone *knows those tunes*. There's something really wonderful about that."

Too Many Kids Are Discouraged from Musical Expression

The Western Wind does its best to encourage and extend such communities of song. On its tours the group has conducted singing workshops across the country, and they deplore a tendency in singing instruction in American schools to, as Steven Urkowitz says, "look for polished results very soon. Kids are discouraged from something that is so natural. Instead of having everybody sing, they select a chorus and only the chorus sings." It's "very painful," he says from experience, for the ones who aren't picked. "I remember in this third grade musical, the teacher came along and said, 'Oh, you, just move your lips, Steve.'

"In America, around 1770 to around 1820, professional singers would go around and teach groups of people how to sing, set up singing schools. The children would come and the parents would come at night, and they would teach, from the ground up, the rudiments of singing. A lot of the music we sing was composed specifically for these singing schools. It didn't require tremendous vocal range and was set in the popular poetry of the time.

"We've taken this music back to New England and run the equivalent of modern singing schools, bringing the same music back. When you get a whole hall full of people who've never sung together suddenly making beautiful music together, it's great."

So what are you waiting for? You can't carry a tune? Nonsense. Some killjoy told you to move your lips at the age of eight because you didn't sound like Beverly Sills? You *really* can't carry a tune? Then honk with the other old honkers. There's no excuse not to, really; you've just got to sing – sing in the shower, sing at work, sing at church, sing with your family, sing in bars if you have to, but sing! You were singing songs before you had the slightest idea what the words meant, before you even knew what a word was.

Or, if you still refuse to sing, you can learn to play a musical instrument. According to Jo Delle Waller, assistant professor in the School of Music at the Catholic University of America and head of that school's music therapy program, that's a creative, healthy use of leisure time. She ought to know. She has helped drug addicts become instrumentalists so that they can deal with their emotions in a nondestructive way.

Don't argue that it's too late to teach an old dog new tricks. Just consider how much TV watching or newspaper reading you're about to do in the next 12 months. You could put the same time into letting it all hang out on the piano or guitar. You'd accomplish something, and you'd have an outlet for all those bottled-up emotions and anxieties (caused by TV watching and newspaper reading).

Probably the best thing that could happen to us would be to regain our childhood openness to music and song.

NUTRITION

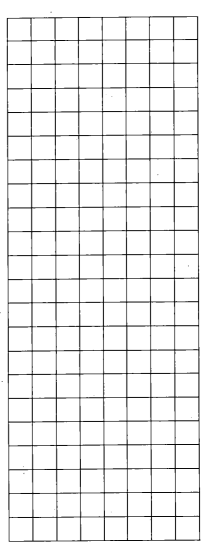

Most of this book is dedicated to explaining exercises and treatments for your body to make it feel better and work better. But we don't expect any raised eyebrows when we point out that the food you eat is also important for your body's well-being. To quote a phrase often used to describe computer operations: garbage in, garbage out. Don't count on good results from a "body-healing" program if you don't take in adequate nourishment.

And getting what's adequate is often a matter of common sense. For instance: eat three good, well-planned meals a day. And eat a large variety of foods to make sure that you're getting a decent supply of all the necessary nutri-ents. But sometimes common sense isn't enough, especially when you're not feeling your best. Then you need to know which specific foods contain the nutrients you need to feel better, and which foods to avoid. If you're feeling dragged out, for example, you may need more *protein.* And you may need it at breakfast.

Don't Overlook Breakfast

Samuel J. Arnold, M.D., from Morristown, New Jersey, sur-veyed his patients who complained of fatigue and fluid reten-tion and found that 88 percent of the women and 67 percent of the men ate a poor breakfast or no breakfast at all. He also found that those symptoms did *not* plague anyone who usually ate a high-protein breakfast, and he advised his tired patients to increase the intake of protein at their morning meal – including eggs, fish, meat, cheese or brewer's yeast – and to reduce their intake of sugar and other refined carbohydrates. All of the men and 95 percent of the women who persisted in their high-protein breakfasting reported substantial improvement. In some instances the reduction in symptoms was "dramatic."

Why did Dr. Arnold's program work? The trick to keep-ing your body perky is to keep up its supply of *blood sugar,* which is the fuel it runs on. Protein breaks down into

If you're feeling dragged out, you may need more protein in your breakfast.

blood sugar slowly, keeping you revved up all day. But sugar and other refined carbohydrates rev you up – and then stall.

Shouldn't sugar keep you revved up, too?

The answer is no, and the reason is that the body is designed to run on a more or less steady, balanced supply of blood sugar. To keep that supply smooth, the body has a regulating system, just as a car has a carburetor to control the burning of gasoline. What would happen to your car if you just dumped a gallon of fuel into the cylinders? It would be flooded and stall. Sugar, too, floods into the bloodstream within minutes after that sugar-coated cereal or that "continental" breakfast of pastry leaves the plate. The body's blood-sugar-regulating system, the pancreas, gets the alarm and tries to lower the blood sugar level by releasing extra amounts of insulin, which causes the blood sugar to be withdrawn from the blood and stored. But the high-sugar, high-refined-carbohydrate meal *continues* to quickly turn into blood sugar and to overstimulate the pancreas until not too long after the sugar and refined carbohydrates are eaten. The blood sugar drops to the point where the body has almost no fuel to burn.

The Right Kind of Carbohydrates

To avoid overstimulating the pancreas, it is necessary not only to eat protein and to avoid sugar and refined carbohydrates, but also to eat the right kind of carbohydrates – the *un*refined kind. Before we talk about them, though, let's define exactly what carbohydrates are.

Carbohydrates, first of all, are not foods; they are molecular compounds in foods. A potato, for example, gets called a carbohydrate, but there is also protein and a little bit of fat in a potato. Breads, crackers, chocolate bars, ice cream, cereals, pastry and fruit are the same way. They are not carbohydrates but are foods rich in carbohydrates. The only foods that are pure carbohydrate, in fact, are table sugar, honey, some jellies and jams, some candies and syrups.

Carbohydrates do not come in just one form. They come in at least 16. The only reason they are all called carbohydrates is that they all consist of varying combinations of carbon, hydrogen and oxygen atoms. Leave it to nature, though, to arrange those three atoms in some miraculously dissimilar ways. The cellulose that goes "crunch" in celery, for example, is a carbohydrate. But then so is the maple syrup you pour all over your pancakes.

Nutritionists have been able to squeeze these 16 major nutritional carbohydrates into two basic categories: simple and complex. The simple carbohydrates are the kind in sugar, fruit, milk and, to some degree, vegetables. They taste sweet, and the reason they're called simple is that, molecularly speaking, that's what they are. That is why they digest so quickly. There are not many chemical bonds to be broken before simple carbohydrates can be absorbed by the bloodstream, so they burn quickly.

Complex carbohydrates, on the other hand, are more . . . complex. They are made up of hundreds of molecules of simple carbohydrates linked together, so they take longer to digest. That's why a baked potato's 100 calories stick with you longer than the 120 or so in a candy bar. They take longer for your body to break down into a usable form. Complex carbohydrates are most prevalent in bread, cereals, beans, root vegetables (such as potatoes and carrots), pasta and rice – foods we commonly call starches.

The Sorrowful Tale of Refinement . . .

If nutrients could sue for damages, carbohydrates would be millionaires. Because there was a time when there was no such thing as a carbohydrate food that was unhealthful. Not until modern-day food processors came along and started taking the protein, vitamins, minerals and fiber out of carbohydrate foods was it possible to get your hands on one that was bad for you. Reach for a carbohydrate food now, though, and it's apt to be regrettably incomplete.

Why are carbohydrate foods refined?

In the case of flour made from grains, it's to make it better for baking. Baked goods made from refined flour are lighter and fluffier. And refined flours, because their natural oils have been removed, can be stored without turning rancid.

In the case of sugar, refinement is simply the most expedient way of getting sugarcane and sugar beets into a form that can be used as an additive. The average American now consumes over 100 pounds of refined sugar a year, two-thirds of which comes to him by way of processed foods.

The Missing Ingredient Is Fiber

The food industry does make efforts to restore some of the nutrients that refinement strips, however; this is a procedure

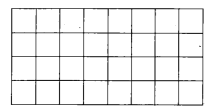

Lack of fiber in the diet has been blamed for increased rates of coronary artery disease and colon cancer as well as obesity, diverticular disease and diabetes.

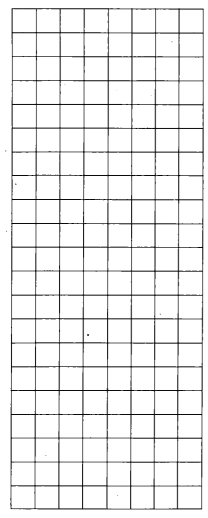

called "enrichment," or "fortification." One nutrient that it doesn't restore, though, is fiber. And fiber is what carbohydrate foods are all about. They are, in fact, our sole source of this all-important material. Without it, we're in trouble.

"The normal human diet has always been high in fiber, and our digestive systems evolved to rely on this common part of food, even though it only passes through our bodies and emerges in a form quite similar to that which it entered," says Sanford Siegal, D.O., M.D., author of *Dr. Siegal's Natural Fiber Permanent Weight Loss Diet* (Dial Press/James Wade, 1975). Indeed, it's been estimated that our prehistoric ancestors consumed about 25 grams of dietary fiber a day. In our modern-day world, we're lucky if we get one-fifth that much.

The results of this fiber shortage? Not good.

- **Increased rates of coronary artery disease** – because fiber has been shown to keep cholesterol out of the blood by inhibiting its absorption in the intestine.
- **Increased rates of cancer of the colon** – fiber's protective effect here is to speed potential carcinogens through the large intestine, thus reducing the chance of their causing damage.
- **Obesity** – fiber is a carbohydrate with no calories, because it doesn't get digested. What's more, it has the ability to take calories out of the foods we eat by inhibiting the absorption of dietary fats.
- **Diverticular disease** – by keeping us regular, fiber can prevent us from "straining at stool," an unpleasantry that can cause ruptures of the walls of the large intestine (a problem for one-third of Americans over the age of 45).
- **Diabetes** – diets high in rapidly digested, fiberless sugars may in time impair the workings of the pancreas, whose job it is to produce enough insulin to see that these sugars get properly utilized.

Fiber, in short, is a very crucial nutrient. And refined carbohydrates just don't have enough of it.

So what does it all mean?

It means fruit instead of candy. Whole wheat bread instead of white. More beans, brown rice, high-fiber cereals and real potatoes. Fewer donuts, lily-white dinner rolls, lighter-than-air pancakes and instant potatoes.

Carbohydrate foods don't have to be unhealthful. They

have the potential, in fact, of being among the most health-ful foods we can eat – low in fat and calories, and high in vitamins, minerals and fiber. Indeed, if there's been a mis-understood nutrient, it's been the carbohydrate. It's time the record is set straight.

But Are They Fattening?

Carbohydrates, regardless of whether they're simple or com-plex, refined or unrefined, contain four calories per gram (the same as protein, and about five calories less than fat). So in terms of calories, you could say that carbohydrates are not fattening. But . . .

Simple carbohydrate foods, particularly refined ones, get digested so fast that they are very unfilling. (We'll include table sugar, jellies, candy and highly sugared pastries in that category.) Even complex carbohydrate foods (starches) that have been refined can get pretty "slippery." (White bread, for example, spends less time in the stomach than whole wheat.) So . . .

In terms of how quickly refined carbohydrate foods get digested, yes, they can be very fattening. You would, for example, be better off satisfying an afternoon hunger pang with 200 calories (about two ounces) of cheese than you would 200 calories of candy, the reason being that the fat and protein in cheese take considerably longer to digest than the refined simple carbohydrates (mainly sucrose) in candy.

How does fructose (fruit sugar) fit into the carbo-hydrate picture?

Like table sugar, fructose is a simple carbohydrate, but it gets absorbed more slowly and more evenly than table sugar. It's also less likely to contribute to the formation of plaque, the bacterial crust that's involved in the develop-ment of cavities. So even though a large apple may contain more total sugar than a candy bar, that sugar, mainly in the form of fructose, is far more healthful. Then, too, the apple is loaded with fiber. The candy bar (unless it has peanuts) contains none.

Complete Protein for Complete Health

As we've already pointed out, protein is a nutrient necessary for good health. Your body, however, doesn't use protein; it uses amino acids, protein's building blocks. Many of these are manufactured right in the body. But nine of them are either not made by the body at all or are produced in too small an amount to do you much good. If one of them is present in your food in a low amount, it "limits" the body's ability to use all of them. Wheat, for example, has low amounts of the amino acid lysine, so all the amino acids in wheat aren't used to the utmost by the body. The way around this problem is to eat a "complete" protein – one with all the amino acids in large quantities.

Meat has a complete protein. So do eggs. Fruits, vegetables and other plant foods don't. But you can combine foods to create a complete protein. For instance, beans are high in amino acid that wheat lacks, and vice versa. Combine them, and the protein is complete. Other combinations include macaroni and cheese, bread and milk, and peas and rice. You should eat a complete protein every day – at every meal, if possible – because the body constantly breaks down and replaces this important nutrient.

When You Need More Protein

The people who need extra protein aren't those you'd expect. The protein myth says that active athletes should gorge themselves with it. Not so, according to Creig Hoyt, M.D., medical writer and editor. The amount of protein that exercising athletes need, he says, "is no more than that which is required in the average sedentary American." What athletes need in extra abundance is food for energy, and this is supplied as efficiently – and more cheaply – by carbohydrates.

In fact, you need more protein if you're flat on your back, recovering from illness, injury or surgery, than if you habitually set the tennis courts on fire. It's easy to understand why, when you consider how protein is used by the body.

Put simply, it's used for building and maintenance. Those parts of you that keep on growing, like hair and nails, are built out of protein. There's protein in your bones, and it's the brick from which muscles are made. Protein is a major component of your heart, lungs and other organs, as well as the blood that flows through and between them, and the enzymes and hormones that keep the whole works in operation.

You need a healthy, constant supply of protein, because

even those parts of your body that seem most stable, like your bones, are always in the midst of tearing down and building up. Old muscle cells are constantly being replaced by new ones. As much as 50 percent of your body protein is in this endless flux of coming and going.

To perform all this construction and reconstruction work, your body breaks down the proteins you eat into amino acids and then combines the amino acids to form its own tissues. The protein from used-up body cells is metabolized and excreted. It's like a weekly budget. If there's as much coming in as going out, you're in "equilibrium," and everything is fine. But if you don't take in enough protein to replace the tissues that are worn out, you're in "negative balance," and that's worse than a pocketful of IOUs. Instead of a spiffy blue-chip stock, you'll feel like a bounced check. A study by Bruce R. Bistrian, M.D., M.P.H., and George Blackburn, M.D., Ph.D., found "a striking prevalence" of protein deficiency in patients hospitalized after injury or surgery at a Boston hospital (*Journal of the American Medical Association*, November 11, 1974). This is reflected by the muscle wastage that turns so many patients into gaunt ghosts of themselves. The worst part of this sudden deficiency is its timing; it can seriously retard recovery and drop the body's guard against infection.

You don't have to be sick to risk protein deficiency, however. You could be healthy – and determined to stay that way – with a low-calorie diet to keep your weight in check. When you cut down on your food intake, your need for protein remains just as high as ever, so it's important to keep this part of your diet intact.

In fact, a reducing program may increase your need for protein. Your body's demand for energy takes precedence over everything else, so when your total intake of calories drops, some of those protein building blocks are liable to end up fuel for the fire.

If your calorie intake drops far enough, some of your own muscle tissue may end up fuel for the fire unless adequate dietary protein is provided.

A High-Protein Menu

What's the most healthful way to get this protein?

You can get it all in one great big daily steak, but you probably shouldn't, because that will also bring you a bonus supply of fats and calories. Instead, put fish and fowl in your diet for more of the good (between 20 and 30 grams of protein in a three-ounce serving) with less of the bad. Have skim milk or yogurt at breakfast (a cup has nearly 9 grams of protein), and when there's a choice to make, choose protein: whole wheat bread and brown rice, for example, instead of their pale refined cousins. For extra protein power in breads, soups and cereals, add brewer's yeast, wheat germ, or soybean or dairy-based powder.

Fat: A Nutritional Villain?

But what about fat? How does that fit into the equation? Many people are afraid of eating too much fat. It seems to be nutrition's version of the mustachioed villain.

Is the fear of fat exaggerated? Not to judge by the research that continues to emanate from laboratories and universities throughout the world. If anything, it implies that the old distinction between "good" polyunsaturated fats and "bad" saturated fats is misleading, and that, to put it bluntly, the only good fat (beyond a bare minimum) may be the fat that has stayed off your table.

At this point, the connection between fat and heart disease should come as a surprise to no one. Atherosclerosis, the buildup of fat on artery walls, is often responsible for the sudden death of heart attack and the lingering disability of stroke. And six decades of evidence, as the *New England Journal of Medicine* (June, 1978) put it, "have provided a considerable degree of certainty" that fat in the diet can promote these fatty deposits in the arteries.

Are Unsaturated Fats Better?

In the case of heart disease, blame does not fall equally on all fats. Chemically, the fats in food come in several varieties. *Saturated* fats (each atom of carbon carries all the hydrogen it can hold; it's saturated with them) are most commonly found in meats. *Polyunsaturated* fats (the carbon atoms have room for more hydrogen) are found more abundantly in vegetables and in fish and fowl.

A large body of research indicates that saturated fats are the ones to watch in keeping guard against heart disease. Where the diet is rich in these animal fats, heart disease is generally a problem. Yet people like Eskimos, whose high-fat diets consist largely of polyunsaturates, suffer very little from heart attacks.

Some studies have found that merely substituting polyunsaturated for saturated fats can lower the level of cholesterol in the blood and presumably the risk of heart disease. In Finland, long-term patients at one mental hospital were given the normal Finnish diet, which is very high in such saturated fat sources as eggs and milk products. In another hospital, much of the saturated fat was replaced with polyunsaturated fat. After six years, the diets were switched.

Researchers found that when patients received the experimental diet, their blood cholesterol levels dropped sharply. In addition, the rate of death from coronary heart disease in the hospital on the experimental diet fell to *half* the rate at the other institution (*Circulation,* January, 1979).

Other studies have suggested that a reduction in saturated fats can raise the level of HDL-cholesterol, the "valuable cholesterol" that apparently resists the buildup of fatty deposits. And that the substitution of polyunsaturated for saturated fats can reduce the tendency of the blood to form thrombi, or tiny blood clots, that may initiate heart attacks and strokes.

The danger here is to see the two kinds of fats, saturated and polyunsaturated, as "bad fat" and "good fat." In fact, the emerging message of much modern nutritional research is the necessity to cut down on *all* fats – animal and vegetable, saturated and polyunsaturated. That may be essential, some investigators say, to reduce the risk of not only heart disease but also cancer.

Some 50 percent of all cancers, they speculate, may be related in part to diet. And fat, according to mounting evidence, is the part of the diet that most bears watching.

The evidence was convincing enough to lead the National Cancer Institute (NCI), in a precedent-setting statement, to recommend that Americans consume less fat (among other dietary modifications) to lessen the danger of cancer. Their directive very definitely includes margarine and corn oil as well as steak and butter.

In fact, some research suggests that polyunsaturated fats may be the more dangerous where cancer is concerned. In a number of studies, animals that were fed polyunsaturated fats developed more tumors than those fed saturated fats. And when researchers at the University of Maryland correlated human diets with cancer rates, they found a strong

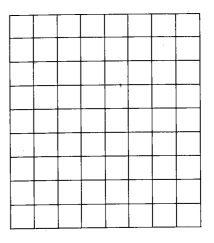

The emerging message of modern nutritional research is the necessity to cut down on all fats.

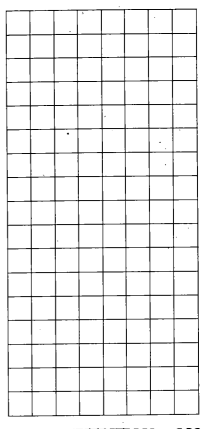

association between cancer and vegetable fats.

Their statistics point to one kind of fat, in particular, as worth being wary about – those containing *trans* fatty acids. *Trans* fatty acids don't occur naturally in vegetables but are produced when polyunsaturated oils are partially hydrogenated – that is, when they are processed with hydrogen to make them more solid or to give them longer shelf life. Many kinds of margarine, salad oil, mayonnaise and snack foods contain significant amounts of these substances.

Quite possibly, researchers speculate, these unnatural *trans* fatty acids alter cell membranes, allowing carcinogens to pass through more easily.

For people who have tried to reduce their risk of heart disease by substituting margarine and corn oil for butter and animal fat, these findings may be particularly unsettling. Is there any diet that will help protect against both heart disease *and* cancer?

What looks best at this point is a diet that markedly cuts down on all fats. For one thing, a very low-fat diet seems quite promising in preventing and treating heart disease. It has been found that vegans, who eat only vegetable foods and consequently consume far less fat than the general population, have significantly lower blood levels of cholesterol and triglycerides. In one study, heart patients who suffered the severe pains of angina showed marked improvement when placed on a vegan diet. A diet that brought fat intake way down to 12 percent of total calories, in another clinical trial, was effective in lowering blood cholesterol levels of patients who had failed to improve with the usual "prudent" 30 percent fat diet.

Cutting down on total fats will also have some very important indirect health benefits. Since fats – animal and vegetable alike – are the most concentrated source of calories (they have twice the calories, gram for gram, of carbohydrates or protein), a reduction of fat intake is essential for keeping weight down. That apparently reduces the risk of both cancer and heart disease. By avoiding overweight, for that matter, you'll help protect yourself against a host of other ills, including diabetes, hypertension, gallbladder problems and liver disease.

Don't Just Trim the Roast

If you want to drop your fat intake down to a significantly

low level, though, you'll have to be aggressive about it. Trimming the fat off the roast is necessary but not sufficient, because most of the fat that finds its way into your body – some 60 percent, according to the U.S. Department of Agriculture – is what they call "invisible fat" and is likely to be overlooked.

Even after the fatty edge is removed from a T-bone steak, for example, the meat itself harbors a considerable amount of fat – some 40 percent of its calories. The same people who keep butter off the table may continue to look at cheese with a fond eye, although *two-thirds* of the calories in some hard cheeses derive from fat.

You may think of sweets as primarily sources of sugar, but their less obvious contributions of fat may be even more significant. Nearly half the calories in ice cream, for example, come from fats, and *more* than half the calories in milk chocolate do. Shortening looks like fat and baked goods don't, but remember that the latter is often full of the former: a croissant, for example, owes half its calories to fat.

Some of the most concentrated sources of fat are to be found in fast-food restaurants. A meal at McDonald's is nearly 40 percent fat, while a serving of Kentucky Fried Chicken has 55 percent fat. Not only do many processed foods harbor a hefty load of fat, but these are often hydrogenated and full of *trans* fatty acids.

Foods that are low in fat, on the other hand, are not hard to find.

There is little fat in fruits and vegetables (with the exception of avocados, nuts and coconuts). Whole grains and beans offer a lot of protein without very much fat, as do chicken and certain kinds of fish.

Making Some Basic Changes

The way to curtail your intake of fats, in other words, is to change the fundamental structure of your diet.

If you follow a few simple guidelines, you'll reduce fats automatically:

- Increase your intake of fruits, vegetables and whole grains.
- Cut down on red meats (beef, pork, lamb and veal), and substitute fowl and fish. When you eat chicken, remove the skin, which contains most of the fat. When

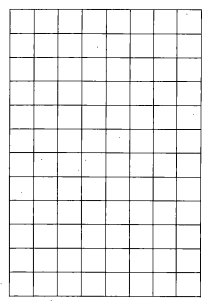

The body needs essential fatty acids to use vitamins A, D and E, to synthesize hormones and to maintain cell membranes. But the amount is only about 2 percent of your calories.

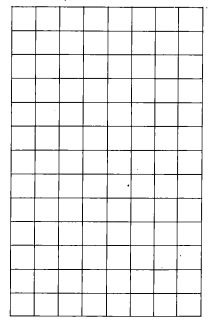

you eat fish, choose less oily varieties, like flounder, sole, haddock and halibut. Buy tuna packed in water, not oil.

- Avoid processed foods. When you prepare your own food, you know exactly what goes into it.
- Read labels and be alert for hydrogenated or partially hardened fats and oils. Natural peanut butter, made from ground peanuts and nothing else, is not hydrogenated; most mass-produced peanut butters are.
- Use low-fat dairy products – cottage cheese, skim or low-fat milk, low-fat yogurt.
- When you eat out, be wary. Fast-food restaurants offer a virtual transfusion of fats. Fried foods in classier eateries aren't any better.
- Don't overindulge in treats like ice cream, pastries and chocolate bars. They are all high in fats.
- Don't eliminate good foods that are high in fat, like nuts and cheeses, but use in moderation.

Is there any danger of getting too little fat in your diet? Not much.

The body needs some essential fatty acids (these are provided by polyunsaturated fats) to utilize vitamins A, D and E, to synthesize hormones and to maintain the membranes that surround each cell. But the amount is quite small, about 2 percent of your calories.

Boost Your Health with Supplements

Even if you're careful about your diet, you may still not get all of the nutrients you need. Michael Colgan, Ph.D., a professor at the University of Auckland in Australia, has found that many foods which nutritionists think contain large amounts of certain vitamins and minerals are actually nutritional washouts.

Dr. Colgan was originally drawn into his investigation of nutrition by "the observation that in the [clinics] which I operated, many of the patients suffering from both mental disorders and physical syndromes of one kind or another manifested what appeared to be signs of malnutrition."

This observation led Dr. Colgan to examine the patients' diets and to analyze the nutritional contents of those diets. He found that "almost all of the [patients] appeared to be on the 'good mixed diet' which is supposed in most nutritional literature to provide necessary vitamins and minerals and other nutritional factors." But when he and his fellow researchers examined the foods that comprised those diets, "we were surprised to find that many of the foods did not contain anything like the amounts of vitamins and minerals given in the nutrition tables. For example, we examined some oranges and found that they contained no vitamin C whatsoever."

When they did blood, urine, hair and tissue analyses of the patients, they found that their bodies' vitamin and mineral levels were as inadequate as the food they were eating.

In order to improve vitamin and mineral intake, Dr. Colgan and his colleagues decided it was necessary to provide vitamin and mineral supplements, since the contents of the food was so unreliable. When they faced the question of how much supplementation was needed for optimum health, they faced a dilemma. The RDAs, or Recommended Dietary Allowances, published by the United States and Great Britain, were inadequate.

"The initial premise on which the RDAs are based is an absence of particular forms of disease," says Dr. Colgan. "Problems with RDAs can best be summed up in the words of Senator William Proxmire in 1974: 'At best the RDAs are only a recommended allowance at antediluvian levels designed to prevent some terrible disease. At worst they are based on conflicts of interest and self-serving views of certain portions of the food industries. Almost never are they provided at levels to provide for optimum health and nutrition.'"

Dr. Colgan and his colleagues studied the medical literature carefully to devise supplementation levels they thought would be adequate. When they proceeded with their research, and compared the health of people who took these supplements of vitamins and minerals with the health of people who took no supplements, they found the supplemented group became substantially healthier. As Dr. Colgan notes, supplementation resulted in "improvements in hair, skin and fingernail condition . . . amelioration of herpes simplex, mouth ulcers, acne, eczema, chronic joint pain, chronic muscle pain, chronic back pain, constipation, pimples, nervous indigestion, headache and sinusitis."

The people who took supplements also showed improvements in blood pressure and blood fat levels, and they had fewer infections and illnesses than the unsupplemented control group.

"We observed," says Dr. Colgan, "that these improvements [in health] were more [pronounced] in older subjects than in younger. . . . We suspect that supplementation [has] a general effect on the health of the subject and might [reduce] some of the degenerative symptoms of aging."

When supplements were given to athletes, the researchers observed notable improvements in performance. Marathoners who received supplementation over a period of six months had an average improvement in race time of around 17 minutes. Supplemented weightlifters showed substantial increase in strength.

Dr. Colgan believes that everyone should supplement his or her diet. "As more and more nutrients are lost during the preparation and processing of convenience foods, which now form a large part of the diet of Western man, it seems likely that the diet will become less and less adequate. In most cases, vitamin and mineral supplementation has proved beneficial in improving physical performance and physical condition of people in apparently normal health."

An important measuring tool you'll discover as you fine-tune your diet and supplement intake is the way your body feels. When you hit the right balance of carbohydrates, protein, fat, vitamins and minerals, you should experience more pep and energy, and you should get sick less often. It's like finding the right blend of fuel for your car. Instead of sputtering, your body engine will hum.

POSTURE

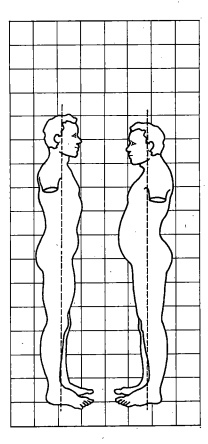

With neither a wrinkle nor a gray hair to mar his youthful appearance, 42-year-old Ted Jonns can nevertheless be spotted from among his group of young trainees – even a mile away. It's his poor posture, that lazy bent-out-of-shape way he carries himself that's the dead giveaway.

How did Mr. Jonns develop such an aged stance? Well, years of improper – or worse, no – exercise helped to accelerate the weakening of those muscles which otherwise hold the bones in alignment.

The Workaday Whirl

Like many executives, Mr. Jonns's workweek revolves around a swivel chair. To make matters worse, the seat of that chair is deeper than the length of his thighs. So, to rest his upper back and shoulders against the back of the chair, Mr. Jonns must bend and tilt his lower back to meet it. This invites a protruding pot and slumped shoulders, to say nothing of the aches of a weakened lower back. At 5 P.M. or thereabouts, Mr. Jonns drags his body from that chair to his car, and home to the sofa. He's also fallen into the American pattern of "eat, drink and be sorry."

Mr. Jonns tries to keep in shape. Unfortunately, all that handball, tennis and, especially, golf does not prevent his slouched entry into the fourth decade of his life. And, even if he had joined a club gymnasium, the dumbbells, bars and rowing machines might have compounded his problem. Exercise equipment that helps to develop certain muscle groups does so at the expense of other equally important muscles.

Correct posture looks good and feels good. But bad posture stresses your body and makes you look sloppy.

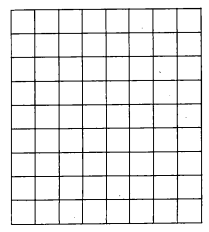

See for Yourself

Whether or not you realize it, you, too, may be falling into a similar stance. To see how you measure up, view yourself nude in front of a full-length mirror.

How's your profile? No cheating – stand the way you normally do. Think of an imaginary plumb line bisecting

(continued on page 335)

329

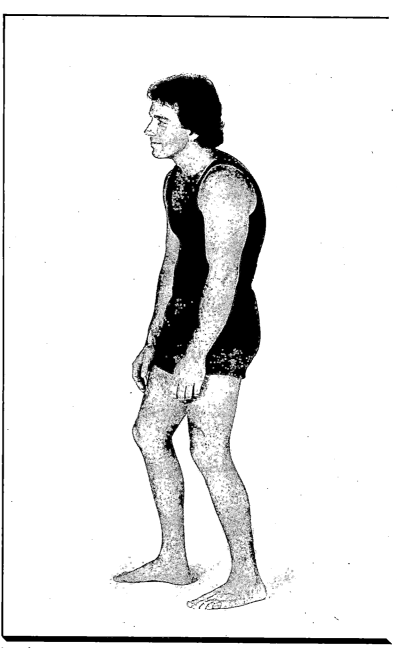

Don't walk with rounded shoulders.

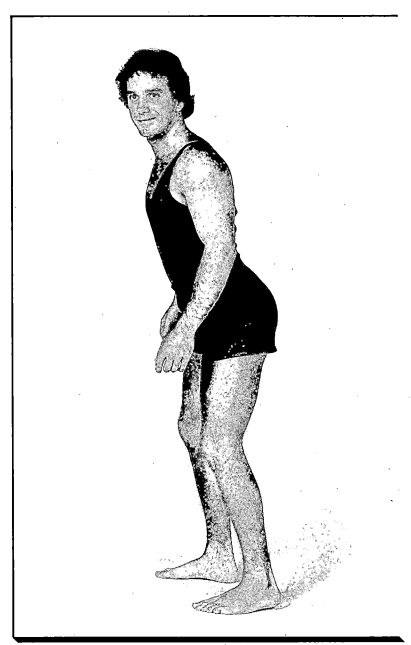

Standing with your back overly curved is stressful.

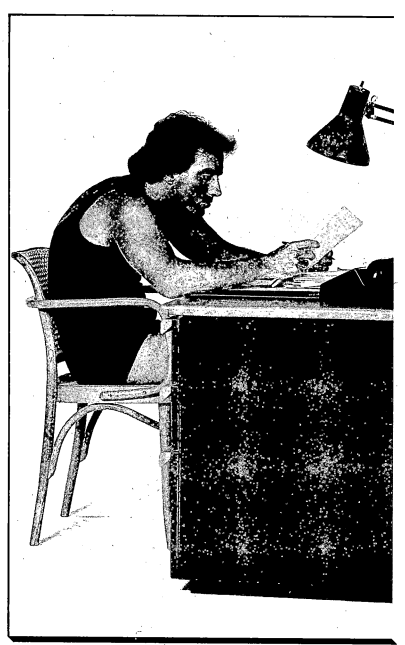

Slouching over a desk strains the back.

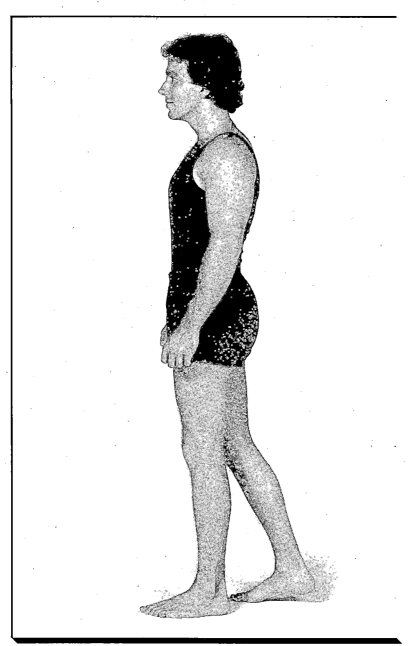

Standing straight makes you feel more alert and graceful.

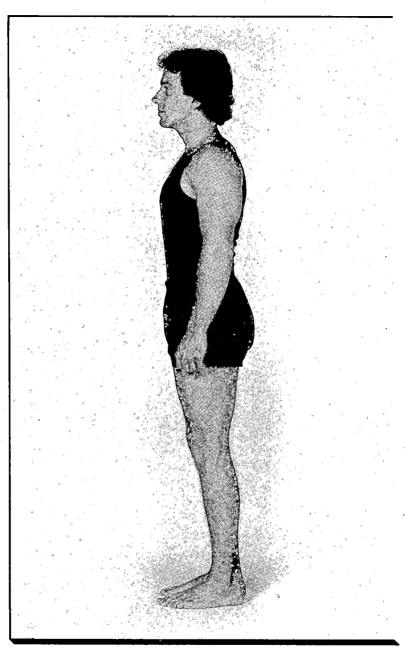

Hold your chest high, and you will breathe easier.

you from the crown of your head through your neck, shoulders and hips to your instep. When the body masses are equally distributed on either side of that line, your weight is efficiently supported without strain on any one muscle group. However, if the head is bent forward, the abdomen thrust out or the back stooped, the body is out of normal balance, and a strain must be placed on various muscles to keep the body from falling.

Here's another test. Stand with your back against a wall, with your head, heels, shoulders and calves touching it. Now, flatten the hollow of your back by pressing your buttocks against the wall. You should just barely be able to stick your hand in the space between the wall and the small of your back. If this space is greater than the thickness of your hand, you definitely have a posture problem.

But before you shrug off those hunched shoulders or that protruding abdomen as something you should have corrected years ago "before it was too late," do yourself a favor and listen to Raymond Harris, M.D., president and director of the Center for the Study of Aging in Albany, New York, and author of *Guide to Fitness After Fifty* (Plenum Press, 1977).

"Bad posture," says Dr. Harris, "can be corrected. And it's never too late to start."

The fact is, it's not easy to face the world with poor posture. When you're slumped forward, it shifts your body weight backward from the vertebrae of the spine to the muscles and ligaments of the lower back, which leads to fatigue, disfiguration such as swayback (the medical term is "lordosis") and pain.

"Swayback is a real problem," explains Benjamin S. Golub, M.D., chief of the back service at the Hospital for Joint Diseases and Medical Center in New York. "The muscles and ligaments of the lower back are just not designed to support our weight."

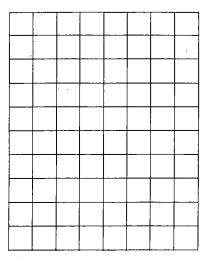

It's not easy to face the world with poor posture. It leads to fatigue, disfiguration and pain.

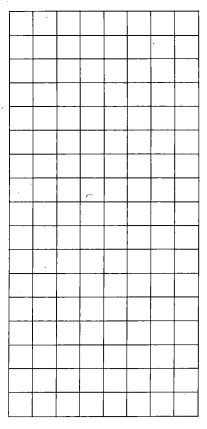

The Foundation of All Activity

According to Dr. Golub, a strong, straight posture is no luxury. "You need good posture for all activities," he told us, "including standing, sitting and bending."

So let's get back to that mirror. This time, you're going to see how you look with the right standing posture – one that will shift your weight back where it belongs, to the spine.

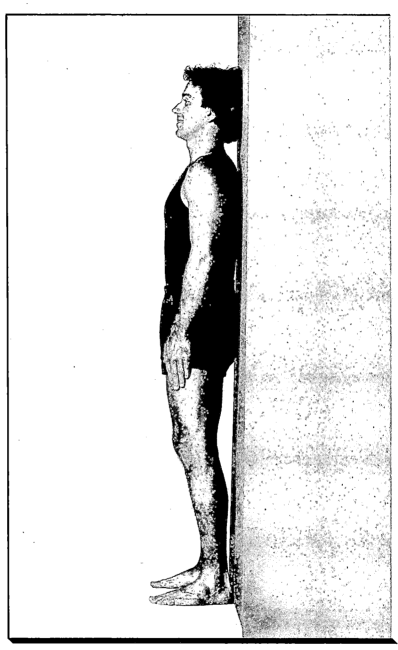

Pressing the back against a wall improves posture.

Stand erect, keeping your body firm, yet flexible.

Relax.

Look straight ahead and distribute your weight evenly on the ball of each foot, not the toes or heel. You should be able to raise your heels without leaning forward.

Slightly tilt your lower pelvis forward and upward. Imagine that you're holding a coin between your buttocks and you'll feel them tightening (don't bend your knees). As you shift into position, your buttocks should tuck in and the small of the back – the lumbar curve – flatten into a slight arc.

"And flattening the lumbar curve," says Dr. Golub, "is the name of the game."

Hold your chest high. As you raise your chest, your shoulders naturally roll back and your stomach pulls in. (A slumping chest or sagging abdomen restricts your ability to breathe efficiently and comfortably.) But don't arch your back and suck in your stomach; this only develops the tense posture of a soldier at attention. "The military style of posture is too rigid," warns Dr. Golub. "Don't be a martinet."

Your goal is good vertical alignment. That is, you should be able to drop an imaginary plumb line from just behind the ear, through the shoulder, the sacrum (the last bone of the spine and part of the pelvis), behind the hip and the knee, and through the ankle.

Three Rules for Good Posture

Although it sounds like quite a goal – connecting all those bones – there are only three maneuvers to remember. Stand erect. Tilt your pelvis. Raise your chest. Everything else takes care of itself and falls naturally into place.

Don't be discouraged if you find yourself twisting like a go-go dancer in front of the mirror while trying to align your body. Chances are your body is accustomed to being "out of line," and at first good posture may seem uncomfortable or unnatural, creating tension in your lower back. But with time – and practice – you will be at ease.

Good posture, then, is a skill, just like playing a musical instrument or riding a bicycle. And, like other skills, it will improve steadily with practice. No matter how bad things look in the mirror, a little determination will go a long way to straighten out your reflection. Once you make up your mind to put in the effort, in fact, you may be surprised at how easy it is to improve your posture.

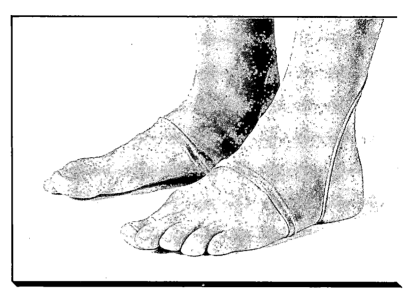

Your weight should be on the balls of your feet when you stand.

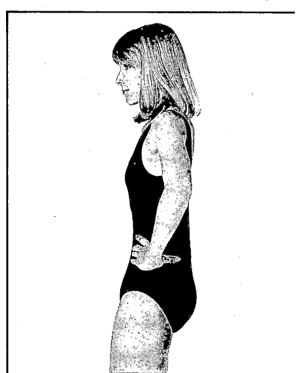

Tucking in the pelvis straightens the back.

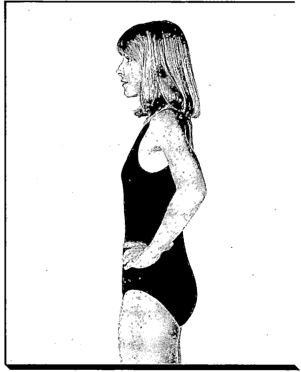

The back curves when the pelvis is untucked.

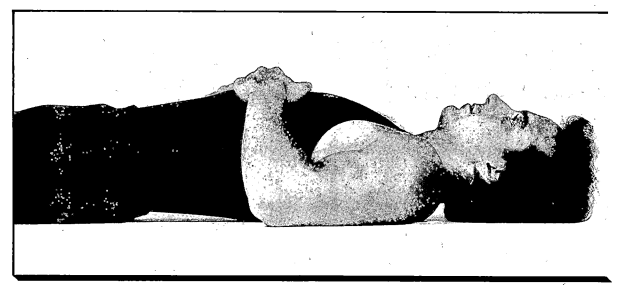

Relax on your back before doing this pelvic tilt.

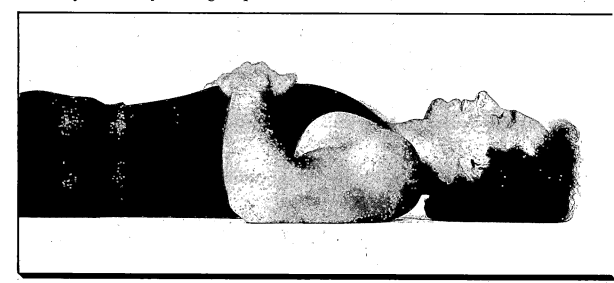

Then push the lower back down against the floor.

Three More Steps to Straightness

According to Dr. Harris, there are three basic parts to the process.

First, he says, be aware of your posture. Monitor your posture in mirrors and store windows instead of combing your hair or straightening your clothes.

"The idea," explains Dr. Harris, "is to mobilize your thought processes. The best way I know to do this is to walk as though you are wearing a crown."

Second, consciously place yourself in the proper positions. Dr. Harris suggests that you practice lying flat on the floor or on a slantboard (a piece of wood built on a slant so that you can rest with your feet higher than your head) or on a wide, strong ironing board with the small end propped up about six to ten inches. In this position your spine will straighten and your back will flatten. Muscles are relaxed and at ease. Small pillows can be placed behind the neck and the knees to ease any strain on the spine.

The final component of the good posture process is stretching, massaging and exercising your muscles.

"Gentle massage is especially helpful for those over 50," says Dr. Harris. For some, he also recommends hanging from a chinning bar: "It stretches muscles gently and gets them working properly . . . it brings the back into proper alignment and relieves pressure on the nerves and discs."

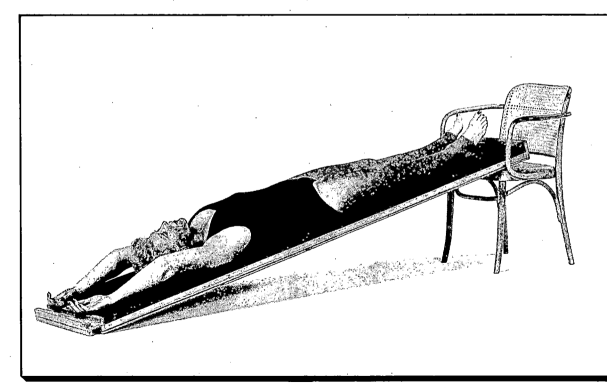

Lying on a slantboard with your feet higher than your head is supremely relaxing.

Even rolling around on a padded or carpeted floor is beneficial. Dr. Harris claims it restores joint mobility by improving muscle tone and helps the muscles hold the body in proper posture.

When you think about posture, don't overlook the impor-

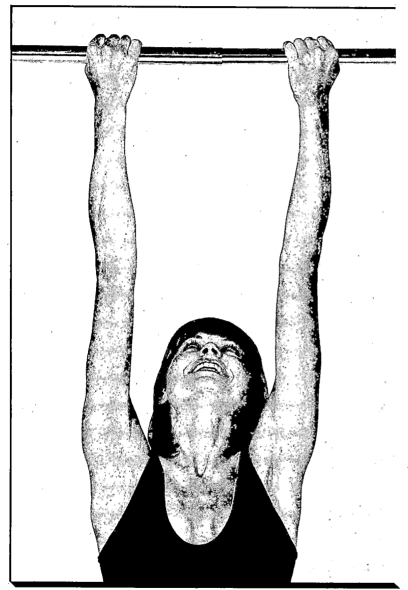

Hanging from a chinning bar helps straighten your back.

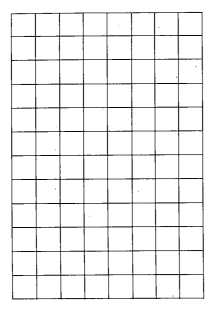

The best exercises for improving posture are those which strengthen the stomach muscles.

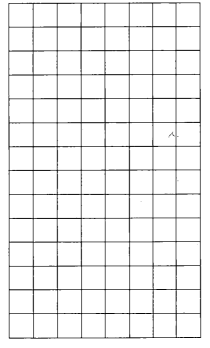

tance of proper breathing, he adds. Diaphragmatic – or belly – breathing is the basis for really good health.

Let's take a moment and try it.

Place your hand between your navel and ribs and take a deep breath. Your hand goes out as your diaphragm drops. Exhale, and your hand goes inward as the diaphragm rises. Again, practice makes perfect.

Good Posture Eases Back Pain

If you suffer from back pains, improving your posture is especially important, according to orthopedist Golub. While good posture won't correct osteoporosis, fractures, disc degeneration or other back problems, it can help reduce the effects of back disease. "And bad posture superimposed on other back disorders only compounds your problems."

The best exercises for improving posture, he says, are those designed to strengthen the stomach muscles. "The stomach muscles are the key to the back. When tight and strong, they automatically tilt the pelvis and diminish the lumbar curve."

Whatever exercises you use to improve your posture, the important thing is to do them regularly. So says Hyman Jampol, director of the Beverly Palm Rehabilitation Hospital in Los Angeles and author of *The Weekend Athlete's Way to a Pain-Free Monday* (J. P. Tarcher, 1978).

"You can't exercise only when you feel like it. You need to have a program, just like you have one for brushing your teeth or your hair or for going to the beauty parlor," he says.

"You should strengthen your stomach muscles and stretch your back muscles for about ten minutes the first thing each day. Soon this will snowball. The more you do, the better you feel, and the more you want to do."

Back Exercises

The best exercises for improving posture are those which strengthen the stomach muscles. The following routines designed by Dr. Golub do just that. Start in the position shown – lying on your back, hips and knees bent, feet flat on the floor – then proceed as follows:

1. In basic position, with arms folded across chest, tighten lower abdominal muscles. Hold five seconds, then rest. Repeat five times.
2. Move elbows to floor, then use them to push lower back against floor. Hold five seconds, then rest. Repeat ten times.

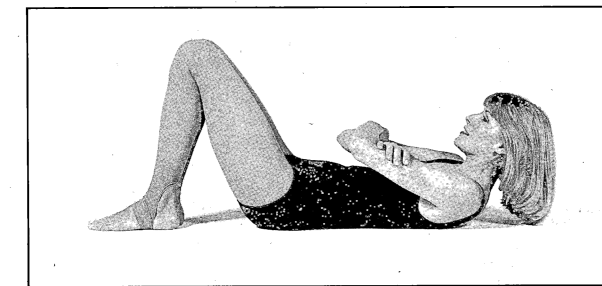

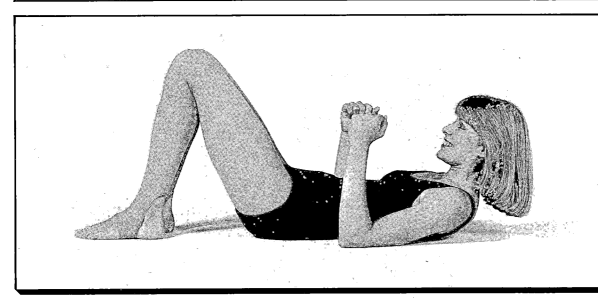

1. Start this posture exercise with your arms folded. 2. Put your elbows on the floor.

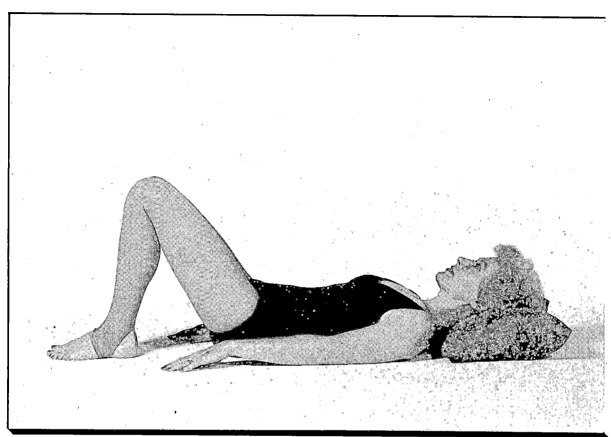

1. Put a pillow behind your head.

1. With a small pillow under your neck, inhale and exhale fully and slowly while contracting abdominal muscles. Rest. Repeat ten times.
2. Put hands behind your head. Inhale deeply, elevating chest. Exhale by contracting abdominal muscles and pulling abdomen upward. Hold five seconds, then rest. Repeat five times.
3. You can end your routine with partial sit-ups. With hands behind your neck, elevate shoulders and upper back two inches off the floor. Hold five seconds, then rest. Repeat five times.

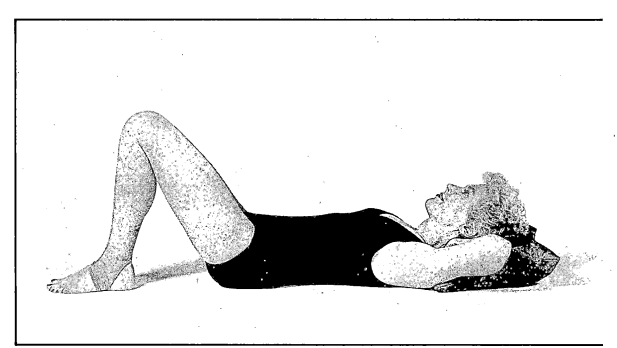

2. Place your arms behind your head.

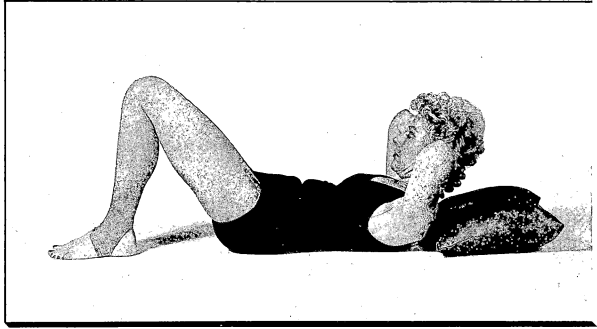

3. Lift your head off the floor.

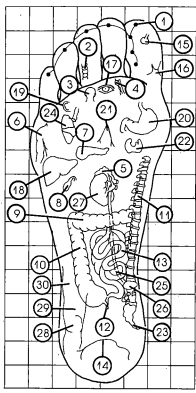

1	Sinuses	15	Pituitary
2	Bronchial Tube	16	Neck
3	Back of the	17	Eyes
	Head	18	Liver
4	Throat and Tonsils	19	Ear
5	Adrenal Gland	20	Stomach
6	Shoulder and	21	Solar Plexus
	Arm Joints	22	Thyroid
7	Pancreas	23	Coccyx
8	Gallbladder	24	Lung
9	Transverse Colon	25	Ureter Tubes
10	Ascending Colon	26	Bladder
11	Spinal Vertebrae	27	Kidney
12	Ileocecal Valve	28	Knee
13	Small Intestine	29	Thigh
14	Sciatic Nerve	30	Hip Joint

A massage map for your foot.

346

REFLEXOLOGY

You're lying on your back in a dimly lighted room. Your shoes, socks, billfold, watch and belt have been set aside. There's a rolled-up towel tucked under your knees, and the bare soles of your feet lie even with the end of the table. You relax; you take a few deep, slow breaths.

Two hands, moistened with hand lotion, grasp your left foot and begin kneading it, prying at the toes, loosening the foot's 26 bones, 56 ligaments and 38 muscles. You relax more, and close your eyes.

After the left foot, the right foot. Then back to the left. This time a thumb methodically probes along the sole, between the toes, digging in painfully at points. Sometimes there's a crackling feeling, like mashing Grape Nuts with the back of a spoon. Then the right foot again, the sole, the toes, around the ankle. Then both feet at once, energetically at first and then gently, and more gently.

You open your eyes. An hour has passed. You're so relaxed that you can hardly sit up. You've just experienced a foot reflexology treatment.

For most of the last 40 years, ever since a woman named Eunice D. Ingham published a thin how-to book called *Stories the Feet Can Tell* (1938), foot reflexology has remained on the occult fringe of medicine. Only in the last few years has this cousin of acupuncture begun to attract serious attention from outside a circle of initiates.

Both reflexology and a more refined technique called "reflex balance" are based on the theory that distinct points on the feet and on the palms correspond to specific organs inside the body. Massaging these points, reflexologists say, promotes better circulation to these organs, stimulates them to function and eliminate waste efficiently, and drains tension from the body as a whole. "Reflex balance does not heal," says one textbook on the subject. "Reflex balance helps your body's self-healing mechanism do its job more efficiently."

The National Institute of Reflexology, located in St. Petersburg, Florida, estimates that 12,000 people have taken its courses. The American Medical Association has no official position on reflexology, and few doctors are using it.

Gurney's Inn, a well-known resort and spa at Montauk Point, Long Island, New York, furnishes a reflexologist for its guests. People who receive these treatments regularly describe it as "absolutely marvelous."

Laura Norman is a certified reflexologist who also holds a master's degree in the treatment of emotionally disturbed children. She lives in New York City, and for about the last ten years she has been treating the feet of housewives, businessmen, elderly people, handicapped children, dancers and athletes in Manhattan, Boston, Long Island, New Jersey and Connecticut. "Laura," says one client who's been seeing her for five years, "has got a great pair of hands."

She Begins with Your Medical History

Her treatments generally begin with a brief sketch of your medical history: any major illnesses or surgery you've had, or where you experience the most tension. That alerts her to potentially tender areas on the feet. The treatments are, as a rule, received on an empty stomach. You remove your shoes and socks and lie on a folding examination table.

"You're going to do this for an *hour?*" a first-time visitor asks.

"Maybe a little longer. Beginners need more time," she says.

As you lie down, she instructs you not to talk and not to cross your arms. She feels that crossing the arms would short-circuit the current that runs through patient and therapist.

The session begins. At first, it feels like nothing more than a massage. Then you begin to relax. She rolls her thumb along the heel, and there's that feeling of mashed Grape Nuts. "Feel that?" she says. "Those are the crystals."

The "crystals," reflexologists say, are waste deposits that build up in the nerve endings and the capillaries of the feet and hinder the free circulation of the blood. The treatment supposedly breaks up the crystals so they can be flushed out of the body.

The treatment lasts for a little more than an hour. It seems like 20 minutes. You sit up, and if your movements are jerky at first, that's tension being released. "Most illness is caused by tension," Ms. Norman says, as she offers a glass of water and advises that liquids help carry off any waste stirred up by the treatment. She tells you not to lift anything heavy at first, and she asks if your thoughts are noticeably clearer. The treatment "gets rid of mental chatter," she says.

Guide to Self-Treatment

Ms. Norman's technique of weekly, one-hour sessions is based on Eunice D. Ingham's books. There are other schools of thought. Another New Yorker, Michael Andron, calls his method "reflex balance" and has published a manual entitled *Reflex Balance: A Foot and Handbook for Health* (1980), which demonstrates how people can learn to massage their own hands and feet. Where Ms. Norman's massage proposes to flush out crystals, Mr. Andron's massage supposedly balances and corrects an "electromagnetic field" that surrounds the body. (He feels he has confirmed his theory by producing measurable changes in the electrical current within the body.) Most of the massage techniques and the results of the two systems are similar. The advantages of this method, Mr. Andron says, are that it requires people to "take responsibility for their own health" and that it costs nothing.

Rub Away Aches and Pains

A businesswoman in Oceanside, Long Island, New York, has received weekly foot treatments for five years. For about 15 years prior to that, she suffered from chronic, serious back trouble. She'd been in traction three or four times, and each time she left the hospital in a body cast. Describing herself as a "walking testimonial," she says her back pain responded immediately to foot massage. And she says that a pain in her hip, for instance, meant that the hip's reflex point on her foot would be unbearably sensitive. "The feet don't lie, I found," she says.

Two more reflexology enthusiasts are brothers who own a chemical plant in Bayonne, New Jersey. The younger, who is 70, receives a weekly treatment nine months out of the year. His older brother, who is 74, gives the massage to himself and his wife. "The treatment works," the elder brother says. He feels that reflexology helped him recover from a stroke in 1971 and that it cured his wife's heart problems. His brother says, "It makes me feel like a new man. My ankles and legs used to swell. Now, no matter how hot it gets or how far I walk, my ankles don't swell. It gives me such a boost."

"I didn't believe it myself at the beginning," says Julie Etra of Lawrence, Long Island, New York, who works with diabetics at Mount Sinai Hospital in New York City. She's received foot treatments for three years. "It makes you feel marvelous, like a shot in the arm," she says.

Ken Miller was director of the residential center at the Maimonides Institute, a private school for handicapped and disturbed children in Queens, where Ms. Norman worked as a special education teacher from 1974 to 1979. By giving foot treatments, she was able to calm down and increase the attention spans of hyperactive children, he says. He calls her results "quite exceptional" and adds that she relieved a back problem he had.

Reflex balance has been used in New York City by at least one physician, a resident in pediatrics at Mount Sinai Hospital, who learned reflex balance techniques from Michael Andron in August, 1979, and since then has used it on about 20 of her patients.

In one particular case, she used reflex balance to help save the life of an infant girl born four weeks premature by emergency cesarean section.

One hour after the child was delivered, she developed a pulse rate of 250 and was taking 150 breaths per minute. These high rates were the infant's attempts to compensate for an as yet underdeveloped heart and lung system, but both rates were dangerously high.

On the second day of the baby's life, the doctor began applying pressure to the point on the child's foot that corresponded to the heart and lung. According to reflex balance charts, that would be the ball or pad of the foot. Using either her pinkie or the eraser end of a pencil, she tested how much pressure the child could tolerate before she began to cry or withdraw her foot.

"When [pressure] was applied to the heart-lung border and held steady for 60 to 90 seconds," says the case report, "respiratory rate dropped to 60 to 80 per minute. . . . If [pressure] was held for over two minutes, respirations dropped to 40 per minute and rose to 80 to 90 per minute within 30 seconds after relief of pressure. This event was consistently reproducible." She noted that the pressure had no effect when it was applied to any other part of the foot.

Even though other standard medical procedures, such as an oxygen tent, were used in treating the infant, the doctor still feels that reflex balance may have played an important role. "I was impressed," she says. Asked if she would use reflex balance again, she says, "Definitely."

Like Mr. Andron, the Mount Sinai physician thinks that people should be taught how to apply the massage to their own feet. She has shown the technique to some of her teenage patients, but few of them stayed with it.

Do-It-Yourself Foot Rubs

In the final analysis, reflexology may or may not be all that it claims to be. The soles of the feet may or may not be a way of gaining access to the body's internal organs. Explorations of tender points on the foot may or may not be an accurate diagnostic tool.

But even without these reputed benefits, the foot therapy is a deeply relaxing experience, something more than just an ordinary rubdown. It may very well stimulate better circulation in the outermost extremities of the body, as it promises. At the least, the treatment feels very, very good.

The best part is that reflexology is a drugless, surgery-free therapy that anyone can learn for next to nothing. You can pay a specialist, but you don't have to.

And with the smallest of precautions (such as not doing it too hard or too often), there's no way it can hurt you.

To experiment with foot reflexology, all you need are a pair of willing hands and a pair of willing feet.

The person receiving the treatment should lie on a couch, table or bed. The masseur should sit on a low chair or stool, facing the soles of the subject's feet.

The amount of time you spend on each foot can vary from 5 to 45 minutes. Some people like to warm up the feet with a general rubdown, while others like to start working on the reflex points right away.

According to traditional reflexology technique, the thumb should be bent at the joint, and the tip of the thumb should then dig with a rotary motion into the reflex points. The pressure should be firm but gentle at first, then gradually increased to as much as the subject can tolerate without pain. Thumbnails should be cut short for this, and you should keep an eye on the subject's face to see if he or she is wincing in pain.

One young woman who received a 20-minute treatment from a local, inexperienced masseur said the massage made her feel "warm all over." She described it as a "pleasant state of suspension." She said she felt a relaxation as deep as that attained through meditation.

Masseur and subject can switch places after the treatment. But they don't have to. Some people claim that it's just as relaxing and rewarding to give a foot massage as it is to receive one.

ROLFING®

by Jason Mixter, Certified Rolfer

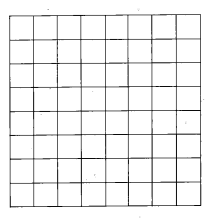

The term "Rolfing" now refers to a system of body education and physical manipulation originally called "structural integration." It is the product of 50 years of study and practice by Ida P. Rolf, Ph.D., and, since her death in 1979, the many people she trained to carry on her work. Fundamentally, Rolfing consists of some simple ideas about human structure: (1) most human beings are significantly out of alignment with gravity; (2) we function better when we are lined up with the gravitational field of the earth; and (3) the human body is so plastic that its alignment can be brought into harmony with gravity at practically any time of life.

Rolfers insist that the human body is so plastic that its alignment can be brought into harmony with gravity at practically any time of life.

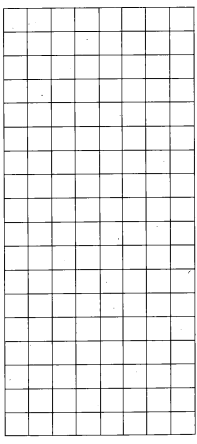

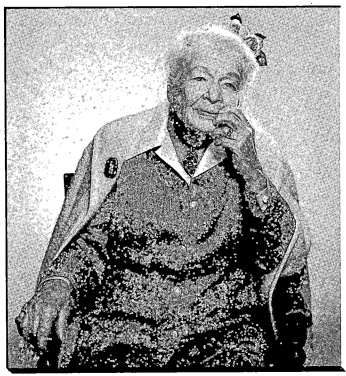

Ida Rolf, founder of Rolfing.

Ida Rolf's Discoveries

Ida Rolf earned a Ph.D. in biochemistry from Columbia University in 1916. Somewhere in her scientific research, she made a fundamental discovery about the body: *the same network of connective tissue which contains and links the muscle system when it's healthy can be used to reshape it when it's been pulled out of proper order.* Each muscle (and each muscle fiber) is enveloped in a connective tissue called *fascia.* Toward the end of each muscle, this fascia thickens into straps we call tendons or ligaments, which work to bind muscle to muscle and muscle to bone. In fact, this strange stuff we term connective tissue might better be called the *prima materia,* the basic stuff of the body. Part of it evolves into bone, and the muscles actually develop as tissue tendrils growing out through the fascial network in the embryo.

Dr. Rolf's discovery of the importance of the fascial system revolutionized thinking about the body. Instead of muscles, her followers emphasize their covering, much as if, when looking at an orange, one emphasized the rind rather than the meat. The enwrapping fascia supports the muscles and holds muscle and bone combinations in place. But it has one troublesome property: it can support *whatever* patterns of movement and posture the body adopts. The fascia can aid normal balanced posture. Or, when muscles are overloaded by the constant strain of off-balance movement, these connective tissues may take over some of the load by shortening and giving up their elasticity. In this way the body actually changes shape to reflect how it's being used. Fortunately, the fascia can be restored to health by returning muscles and bones to their proper alignments and inducing proper movement.

Dr. Rolf's discovery of the importance of the fascia was based upon another insight. She recognized that gravity is the basic shaper of the body. We have to balance our bodies, somehow, against the pull of gravity. From birth to death, gravity is always working on us. Because it is, deviations in the muscle-bone system are never merely local. Gravity's influence spreads them throughout the body. If the natural balance of the body is disturbed – if it doesn't follow the best geometry of the skeleton – then the *whole body* will gradually change form to adapt to the deviation. For example, a child falls from a bicycle and injures a knee. To avoid pain, he or she tightens the muscles around that knee. Since the body must work against the tug of gravity, the entire muscle and fascial system gradually shifts to compensate for the first change. Movement through the pelvis is influenced, as is the pattern of breathing and the set of the head. Because muscles alone cannot carry the additional tension, the fasciae shorten to support the new movement, and, in time, the shape and function of the whole body alters with them.

The human body is like a house. It's structured so that each part has its proper place, and each piece interlocks to balance the load of the others. As in the well-built house whose every post and beam is in place, the well-used (more than well-built) body functions efficiently. Because gravity pulls down on everything, out-of-place body parts – beams out of alignment and unsupported by a post – are pulled into painfully unnatural positions. What the Rolfer seeks is a return of the construction to its original blueprint specifications. This is often compared to, first, grabbing the client by the hair and lifting him or her straight up until he or she is hanging in a perfectly vertical position and, then, setting the client going again. Putting one out-of-whack piece back into place is usually not enough. *Everything* should be right before a house can stand or a body can work smoothly. *This* kind of arrangement, in turn, produces what Dr. Rolf called "the gospel of Rolfing: when the body is working properly, the force of gravity can flow through it. Then, spontaneously, the body heals itself."

The Body's Geometry

Dr. Rolf's view of the role of the fascia in posture led to still another major discovery. It might be called the theory of *body geometry.* When an elbow, knee or any other joint is properly balanced, the individual experiences an internal sense of rightness. The body senses that it is aligned along the true *planes* of movement. The hinges of the legs (hips, knees, ankles, even toes) all work within a single plane. The paths of the legs have parallel courses. The head and spine feel a clear sense of "up." The elbows move naturally through their angle in a smooth course. Compared with this new organization, the previous functioning of the body appears random, even chaotic. In contrast, the new geometry, this new orientation in space, feels much more secure. The goal of the Rolfer is to bring the body close to its

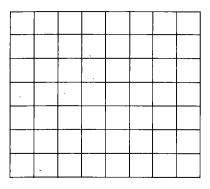

The human body is like a house. It's structured so that each part has its proper place and each piece interlocks to balance the load of the others.

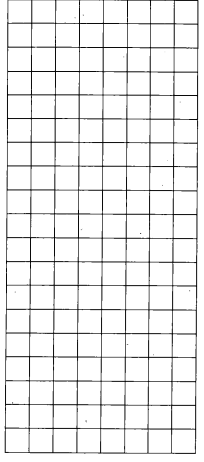

center line of gravity so that fewer muscles are required for basic standing and sitting. "Posture" is no longer an immobile holding action but a floating balance and ease. It is this attention to the proper body geometry that distinguishes Rolfing from those forms of body work that simply seek deep tissue massage and relaxation.

Naturally, each person has his or her own version of this ideal geometry, which depends on the person's height, the length of his or her limbs, and other similar factors. But Rolfers consider five basic points when planning individual goals for a client. In order for the human body to function properly and maintain an upright position, these five landmarks must be in alignment: the ear, the shoulder, the hip, the knee and the ankle. The head, neck and shoulders tell the story of the structure below them. The body should glide along, rather than look as if it has to do extremely hard work with every step. The head and neck must be centered over the middle of the body, and the spine that supports the structure must be at the back of the pelvic section. The spine must then curve in conjunction with the natural back curvature until it enters the base of the skull in a central direction. Any damage or constant pressure will disturb the balance of the upper torso.

In quite a few words, that's Rolfing, but the definition may make no sense to you because you've never seen or felt Rolfing. To remedy that, let's follow a client through her first session and then get into a little routine that will give you a few of the feelings that a Rolfing client has in that initial encounter.

A Visit to a Rolfer

Marcia had known about Rolfing for maybe ten years. She knew that the technique was developed by a biochemist and that it was designed to improve posture and flexibility. She had also heard that it was sometimes painful, although people she knew who had been Rolfed did not emphasize this aspect as much as people who had not been Rolfed. She decided to try it.

After answering a health questionnaire and discussing what she hoped to gain from the sessions with her Rolfer, Marcia was asked to undress down to her underwear and pose for some "Before Session One" photos. Then she stood in front of the full-length mirror and was introduced to her body through a Rolfer's eyes. She began to see that her body was far from organized: not only were her shoulders a different height, but they were also rotated distinctly to the right, while her pelvis was turned to the left. She noticed that she could breathe either from her upper chest or from her abdomen, but not both. From the side, she saw that her midsection protruded out in front because her upper back slumped ahead of her pelvis and abdomen. Following her shoulders, her neck and head also came forward. The Rolfer helped her to see that if her head were balanced properly on her spine, the muscles in her back would not have to support its 12-pound weight.

Finally, she was asked to lie down on the cushioned table, and the Rolfer began to work on her ribs. She felt a brief burning sensation as he did, as if the skin was being stretched and kneaded. He worked around her left armpit and asked her to perform an arm movement as he did. The discomfort was different here – sharper, more precise. His hands seemed to know just where to find tightness and tension. First in front, then along her side, back under her shoulder blade, down under the line of her rib cage. Soon she was feeling light and airy. She was breathing more deeply and with less effort. Her left arm was moving easily, almost by itself. But when she moved the right one, it seemed blocked. She had never noticed a problem there before, but the difference between her arms was very noticeable.

As the session continued, Marcia felt more at ease. The Rolfer worked on her hips and then on the back of her thighs. He explained that years in high heels had caused her knees to hyperextend, or "lock" backward. This had cut off circulation in her lower legs and left her with a tendency toward cold feet. He also connected the locked knees to the forward jut of her upper body. As he continued to work, the back of her thighs had that same burning sensation for a moment, but it was soon replaced with a new sensation of "length" and freedom.

When she stood up, she felt straighter, even though she had not previously thought her posture was especially crooked. As she walked around the room, her legs seemed to glide under her; her knees did not lock as before. Looking in the mirror, she saw that her upper back was pulling back, but it did look better. Her body felt alive and tingling. The Rolfer gave her a mental image to think about: her motion should come from deep inside her body. She felt more expansive, taller. When she sat, she sat straighter and liked it. When she slouched, the position was uncomfortable!

Intrigued? Try this self-help routine.

Feel What Marcia Felt

One of the major distinctions made by Rolfers is the difference between *holding* and *supporting*. As children, most of us are told to "sit up straight." The well-meaning relatives who usually make this command are trying to teach us good posture, and by good posture they generally mean some variation of "chest out and shoulders back!" Try this posture right now as you read. Notice that when your shoulders are pulled back, they cannot be SUPPORTED by the rib cage, that, instead, your trunk is lifted up off the pelvis and HELD in an uncomfortable imitation of good posture.

While sitting, most of us droop forward and let our bodies hang off our spines in various forms of collapse. When we do remember to "sit up straight," we often reverse everything and hold our chests up and keep the shoulders high and aloft. Some people even become locked in this position. Although they look good to the untrained, most trained observers agree that the body structure is not supported from below in this posture; it is uncomfortably held from above. In either case, with the held posture or the collapsed one, energy is being expended, which might be conserved with proper structural support and balance.

To see how much better efficient posture can make you feel, first sit down. Then, let your chest fall so that your spine curves to the front. Now sit up so that your spine arches to the back. Do you feel relaxed, or is it an effort to hold your body in this second position? Return to the collapsed position, and put a hand on each hip bone. Push your hips forward until you feel the bottom of your pelvis (the two "sit bones") touch the chair seat. As you do, notice that your chest floats up as the pelvis rolls forward. Now *rest* on the forward part of your "sit bones." Notice that you can sit and maintain a feeling of support without either collapsing or holding your body up.

Learned body patterns become so much a part of us that, at first, you may not be able to sit in this new, supported fashion for very long. You may also need to "play" with it until you can feel your body learning to support itself. But most people eventually find that they do not feel quite "right" unless they are using this supportive posture in place of the old holding patterns.

What, Exactly, Is Rolfing?

Rolfing is normally taught or applied in ten sessions of variable length. Each segment of the process is both a continuation of the previous one and an introduction to the next. The body is systematically and physically manipulated during this initial series of ten sessions, each of which lasts about an hour and may be scheduled as often as twice a week. Some people choose to schedule their sessions once a week, others once a month. The cost of each session varies from $50 to $75, according to local economic conditions and the experience of the Rolfer.

Rolfing's ten-session series is designed to uncover a structural ease and kinetic balance that is unique to each client. Rolfing cannot accurately be described as therapy or as a returning of the body to a "natural" state from which it has deteriorated. Rather, it is a process of education in which a Rolfer seeks to help a client discover the most efficient way of using his or her body, given the limitations, liabilities *and* virtues of that body. In effect, the plan of each group of ten lessons must be created anew for the needs of the particular person seeking help. However, there *are* certain guidelines and landmarks which every Rolfer follows in each program of sessions, and it is to these basic tenets that we must turn to complete our description of the treatment process.

The First Session

The intent of the first Rolfing session is considered superficial by most Rolfers, but they have a very special meaning for "superficial." The session's goal is to systematically release the body's "stocking," or the fascial sheath that lies just below the skin's surface. Some lengthening of the trunk up and out of the pelvis is also anticipated, as well as a relaxation of the legs below the hip joint. Most people appear to be jammed into the pelvic structure from both above and below. After the initial session, clients usually feel longer and experience freer movement in the pelvis.

The breathing pattern of the client is also affected by

this session. Most of us employ only the upper rib cage when we breathe instead of using the bottom of the cage and the diaphragm. By skillfully working with the superficial fascia as it spans the ribs, shoulder joint and costal arch, a Rolfer can help fashion a breathing pattern which uses the diaphragm and the front, sides and back of the rib cage to create one smooth, bellowslike motion. As breathing becomes deeper and easier as the sessions go on, more oxygen is available for metabolic and catabolic activities, and the client feels an increase of energy.

The end of the first session often involves some freeing of the fascial planes around the neck and shoulders, a lengthening of the structures on either side of the spine and those covering the lower back. Finally, the client is asked to walk and describe what changes he or she feels. Reports of a "lightness" and ease, and the strange sensation that one is taking up more space are common. Some kind of "homework" is usually assigned in order to reinforce the session's results. The Rolfer might suggest that the client imagine a string hanging from a helium-filled balloon and tugging on the top of his or her head as he or she walks. Or the client might be told to allow his or her breaths to press against the sides of the ribs or to both rise toward the head and drop to the navel.

The Second Session

The second Rolfing session centers around the legs and, especially, the feet. Most people carry their weight on the outside edge of each foot, even though the inside appears better able to support the stresses of body weight. In addition, most people walk by allowing the legs to pull the upper body along after them. This habit puts too much pressure on the heels and can reduce flexibility in the toes and metatarsals. If, on the other hand, the upper body initiates a step by "falling" lightly forward, the legs can easily swing forward in response, the body's weight "caught" on the whole foot. To teach this behavior, the second session begins with the feet.

After one leg has been worked with, clients are asked to walk and compare the action of the two legs. Invariably, they report that the leg which has been Rolfed feels stronger, more secure. Often they notice that the weight travels on the inside of the Rolfed foot and that there seems to be less pressure on the heel. The other leg will then be Rolfed and some work done on the back and neck to complete the session.

The Third Session

The third Rolfing session is an integrating one. It attempts to tie the first two sessions together into a complex whole. It is the last of the "superficial" sessions and a crucial point for both Rolfer and client. If, for any reason, either one wishes to delay the series, it is advantageous to do so before the fourth Rolfing session, which begins to deal with the deep structures of the pelvis.

Fundamentally, the third Rolfing session deals with what's called the "lateral line" from the head of the humerus, or upper arm, to the greater trochanter of the femur, or thigh bone. The client lies on his or her side as the Rolf practitioner works to arrange the shoulder, ribs and pelvis into an even stack. He tries to differentiate the rib cage from the shoulder girdle on top and the pelvis underneath. The Rolfer's goal is to set each in its own space without crowding from its neighbors. The result will eventually be freer breathing and less painful crowding of the structures.

Typical homework after the third session might be to imagine that the pelvis is hanging from the rib cage like a swing hanging from a tree limb.

The Fourth Session

The fourth Rolfing session represents a change in the therapist's intention and commitment. His or her focus is no longer on the superficial fascial planes and is now concentrated upon what's called the body's "active core." Rolfers define "core" structures as those that lie close to the spine and the body's midline; they are differentiated from the "sleeve," consisting of the shoulder and pelvic girdles, and the "lateral" structures of the legs.

The agenda for the fourth session is deceptively simple, and the session may actually take less time than those which come before. The inside of the legs, from the ankles to the pelvic floor, is treated, followed by work on the hamstring muscles and some "organizing" of the back and neck. The goal of the session is to establish improved support for the structures that make up the pelvic floor. Although most of

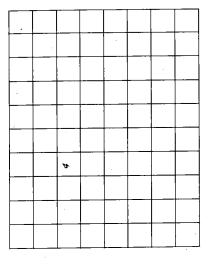

A typical Rolfing mental exercise is to imagine that the pelvis is hanging from the rib cage like a swing hanging from a tree limb.

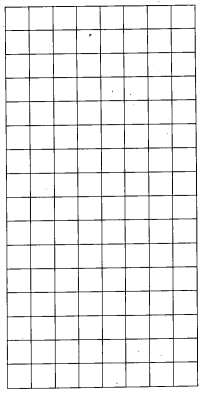

the work is on the legs, a client will also often feel a "lift" throughout the torso. The fourth Rolfing session seeks to establish an inner pillar from which the limbs can be hung. That is, the Rolfer wants to hang the body's "sleeve" from the supportive "core."

The Fifth Session

The fifth Rolfing session is a continuation of the fourth. It is recommended that not more than two or three weeks separate these sessions. Its province is the relationship of the superficial abdominal muscle (the Rectus abdominis) to the deep-seated hip flexor (the iliopsoas). Most people wrongly use the wide band of external stomach muscles to do the work of stronger, deeper-lying muscles. During this session the Rolfer slowly lengthens and separates the outer structures to allow room for the inner structures to reassert themselves.

Sometimes clients become anxious about this particular session, especially when they know a bit about anatomy. They fear manipulation deep in the body and in the area of crucial organs. However, Dr. Rolf discovered an ingenious and remarkably safe method of examining these deep structures with a minimum of discomfort. Only a properly trained Rolfer should attempt this method, but with the right education and experience, the fifth Rolfing session often becomes more enjoyable and produces less discomfort than those preceding it.

The deep stomach muscles have certain properties that make them unique in the body. They are the only muscles that extend from the legs to the trunk. All other muscles of the leg or trunk attach directly to some part of the pelvic girdle. As a result, the proper training and toning of these leg *and* stomach muscles are usually better for bad backs than traditional sit-ups.

In fact, sit-ups are likely to exaggerate back problems by shortening the front of the body from the collarbone to the hip joint. But the balancing exercises of Rolf movement work are designed to bring health and vitality to the under-used deep structures, and they can do much more than the surface muscles to cure weak backs.

A healthy, active psoas muscle also helps other conditions. The nerve fibers located near the psoas become stimulated as the muscles respond to new movement. Menstrual cramping, constipation and excessive gas are often lessened as a result. A satisfying feeling of the leg-trunk connection of these muscles often emerges as the client learns to move his or her legs from the lumbar spine rather than from the hip joint. The holistic nature of the body becomes physical reality rather than an intellectual idea. The "pelvic tilt" is sometimes taught during this session to give the client a way to practice moving with the psoas at home.

The Sixth Session

In the Rolfing series, each session focuses on some aspect of the pelvis. Even in the second session, work on the legs and feet is designed to establish support for the pelvic basin. However, the sixth session is very specific in its approach to the pelvis. The muscle structures that are the keys here are the deep rotating muscles under the buttocks. If the client's legs are unable to function smoothly while walking, balancing the "rotators" deep in the buttocks will usually even out the operation.

By this time in the sequence, both the Rolfer and his client have become aware of the balancing of the pelvic structure. As the body becomes more symmetrical and organized around a vertical line, disparities between the right and left sides become less apparent. In the sixth session, this symmetry is enhanced and extended above and below the pelvic girdle.

The incorrect use of the term "posture" to describe the results of Rolfing can now be better understood. The Latin root of posture is "positus," meaning "to place, to put." Consequently, "good posture" usually implies the "placing" of the body into a position that is considered appropriate and balanced. The goal of the Rolf process in its sixth session, on the other hand, is to create a *structure* which *rests* on a well-supported vertical core and demands a minimum effort to maintain while the person is standing. Rolfing, therefore, is concerned with the *integration of human structures* and not with notions about posture.

The results of the sixth Rolfing session are generally dramatic and welcomed by clients. A sense of "bigness" and space are reported, as well as an ability to breathe through to the spine; that is, the spine appears to undulate during respiration in a wavelike motion. People who have decreased or eliminated chronic back pain through Rolfing usually point

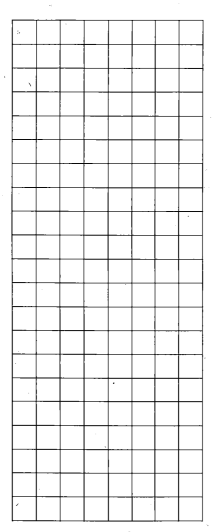

to the sixth session as pivotal in their progress. Others, who come suffering from anxiety, may also claim a great easing of emotional distress after this session.

The Seventh Session

Referring to the seventh Rolfing session, Dr. Rolf often remarked: "The seventh session is the last chance to 'horizontal' the pelvis," but in fact, the work of the seventh session is directed entirely toward balancing the neck and head on the spine. During a seventh session, the Rolfer works on the fascia of the neck, opens the connective tissues around the skull and face and helps to improve breathing further by opening constricted nasal passages.

The Eighth, Ninth and Tenth Sessions

In each of the first seven sessions of Rolfing, the practitioner focuses on one area of the body. The goals of a particular session center around placing its part in the vertical balance of the whole body. With the eighth session, a broader and more comprehensive approach to the problem of integrating the entire structure becomes necessary. These last three sessions are called the "integrative hours," and in them the client prepares to end his Rolfing series.

The dictionary defines "integration" as "a combination and coordination of separate and diverse elements or units into a more complete and harmonious whole." This is the job of the client and Rolfer in these final sessions. "It is easy to take a body apart," Dr. Rolf would declare, "but it takes skill and understanding to put it back together."

In the last three Rolfings, the practitioner tries for a body that is poised on a narrow base and can move in any direction with equal ease. Large fascial sheaths are related one to the other, and a "silky" quality in the muscle tissue is sought. Several times during these sessions, the client will be asked to stand up and walk about in order to assess the result of the manipulations. Much work will be done with the client sitting or standing, because the relationship of a particular body part to gravity is the most important goal in these hours.

In these sessions, it is time to get the client ready to leave Rolfing, and it is suggested that he avoid more deep structural work for six months to a year after the initial

After being Rolfed, you're encouraged to look within your own body for new ways to use the changes that Rolfing creates.

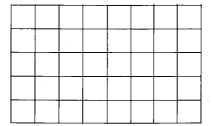

series, because the change that is initiated by the first sessions will continue for months, even years, after the series is completed. During this fallow time, however, many clients see Rolf movement teachers who are trained to teach them ways of using their "new" bodies to maximum benefit. The Rolfed individual is encouraged not to lean on the Rolfer for further changes by his or her body but to look to the intelligence within it for new ways of using the initial changes.

Advanced Rolfing

Six months to a year after completing an initial series, many clients need a refresher session, or "tune-up." Many Rolfers also recommend one or two sessions per year after the first ones to maintain the benefits of the original ten. But it is possible to have too much Rolfing, and most practitioners recommend that clients use what they've already learned rather than seek more and more material.

Somewhere between one and five years after an initial series, most clients return for the shorter (four to six sessions) "advanced" series, which is conducted by Rolfers who have completed the "Advanced Rolfing Training" program. This sequence concentrates on ways of balanced *movement* in gravity using the organization established by the original ten sessions. Often areas that were painful and frozen even during the first sessions are found to be pliable and free during the advanced work. As one client described her advanced sessions:

> On going back . . . there was so little pain in my body, I accused my Rolfer of getting soft. The intense emotional experiences weren't there after the later sessions either, but what joy I felt walking on the beach afterward. The pure and simple joy of being ecstatic in my body!

Training and Certification

Certified Rolfers and movement teachers undergo a training program which is considered "postgraduate" in nature. Many aspirants to either of the training programs must spend up to three years meeting the Rolf Institute's prerequisites and preparing their applications for admission.

Persons seeking admission to Rolfing training are required to have an extensive background in the biological and behavioral sciences, training and professional experience in body manipulation, and a facility in working with people. A written application is submitted to the Rolf Institute, and the candidate is interviewed by the Institute's admissions committee to determine the person's qualifications for the work.

Having been admitted to Rolfing training, the student attends a series of classes at the Rolf Institute over a period of about a year. Throughout the training program, each student's progress and readiness for continued training is evaluated by the instructor and his or her assistant. Classes are kept small in order to give students personal attention.

Rolfing students are committed in writing to a program of continuing professional education and must gain advanced training within five years of their initial certification. Certified Rolfers are governed by a Code of Ethics and Standards of Practice. In order to practice Rolfing and to identify themselves as "Rolfers," they must be members in good standing of the Rolf Institute. Rolfing training is available only through the Rolf Institute, the sole certifying agency for Rolfers. A directory of certified Rolfers is published by the Rolf Institute and is free to requesters. Rolfing movement teachers receive an additional year of training and must participate in an apprenticeship. Movement teachers also agree to a program of continuing professional education.

To obtain information about Rolfing and Rolfing movement integration or a list of certified Rolfers and their addresses, contact The Rolf Institute, P.O. Box 1868, Boulder, CO 80302.

ROPE SKIPPING

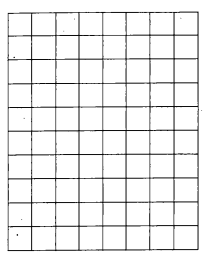

When the cold winter of the North Pacific would close in on our ship, many of us would retreat below decks for our exercise. Unsailorly as it might sound, we often gave our sea legs to rope jumping. Although the yaw and tug of the ship often made rope jumping a rollicking dance, we did quite a lot of it at sea, both above and below decks.

Anyone who has the notion that skipping rope is intended only for bored sailors or Sally next door is very wrong. It is a remarkably complete, exhilarating routine destined to make muscles and lungs sing. It is also an exercise that can take an adult to the end of his rope, as any boxer knows.

According to Dr. Rodahl, skipping rope trains the heart, strengthens the legs and arms, and improves posture and coordination.

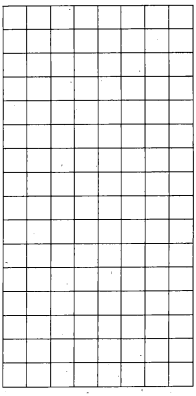

Boxers traditionally have the reputation of making the rope whir beneath their ring legs. Although I had seen enough film clips of Sugar Ray Robinson and Floyd Patterson talking to the rope, I was curious as to why boxers spend so much time with this simple exercise.

To answer my question I visited Ring 23, a boxing clinic for young men not far from my home in Pennsylvania, where, sure enough, the men were bending the rope. I asked one of the trainers why so much time is spent jumping rope. He replied, "I've always believed that time with the rope was as good as time on the road. Skipping rope builds up your wind, your legs, arms and chest. It's good for you all over."

If champion boxers have learned a valuable exercise routine from the children, there is no reason why we shouldn't take it up, too. Our fitness is no less important than a fighter's. And it makes sense to start an exercise that we can be confident about sticking to.

A discouraging dropout rate is associated with many exercises taken up to combat flab and fatigue. The advantages of a rope skipping program in this regard are readily apparent. The health benefits of this exercise are good, the time required is minimal, and the equipment is inexpensive and easily acquired. The rope jumper's season never stops. He or she can change his or her exercise space from the sidewalk to the cellar with no fuss. He or she can skip anytime during the day or night. If the rope skipper is going to travel, he or she can take along a rope. The rope jumper can skip in hotel and motel. Rain or snow is never a factor for a man or woman with a rope.

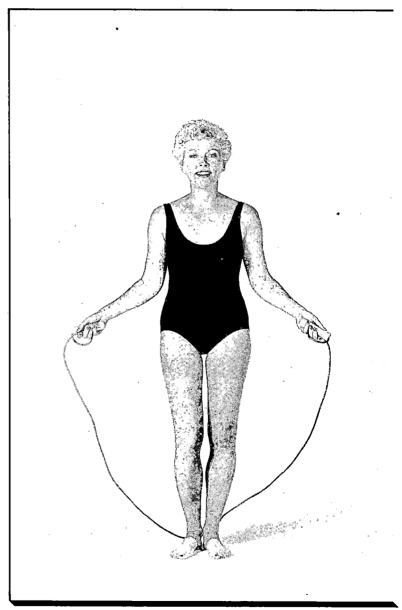

Jumping rope improves coordination.

Simple and Efficient

But can something as mundane as skipping rope really make a dent in our "unwellness?" One doctor who thinks so is Kaare Rodahl, M.D., a man who has probably done more than anyone else in Europe and America to promote rope skipping. Dr. Rodahl, in his *Be Fit for Life* (George Allen and Unwin Ltd., 1968), has built an entire fitness program around the humble art of jumping rope. "Of all the different exercises we have investigated," he writes, "we find that nothing surpasses the simple skip rope in producing the greatest fitness in the least amount of time. Five minutes of rope skipping a day, five days a week, improved the physical work capacity of a group of our young laboratory technicians by 25 percent in one month.

"We have also found that rope skipping is superior to many of the complicated and time-consuming physical education programs. If a couple of very simple physical conditioning exercises that will strengthen the arms, legs, back and abdominal muscles (push-ups, sit-ups, knee bends) are added to the rope skipping program, one may achieve a maximum of benefits from a simple 10- to 15-minutes-a-day program.

"The advantage of the skip rope is that it not only trains the heart, resulting in improved physical endurance, but also increases the muscle strength of legs and arms in addition to improving coordination and posture." Dr. Rodahl advises that "the individual skip rope should be about eight and a half feet or longer, according to the person's height. The thickness should be about three-eights of an inch or more, depending on the weight of the rope. The lighter the rope, the thicker it should be. A very satisfactory skip rope can be made from sash cord of half-inch diameter. The cord comes in varying lengths and can be purchased in most hardware stores. The ends of the rope should be tied in a knot to prevent fraying. There are also fancier ropes available, of course, ropes made of nylon with handles supplied with ball bearings for smooth operation."

A lot of people have trouble in determining the size of the rope they should use. A rule of thumb says that the rope should be long enough to reach from armpit to armpit while passing under both feet. The professional skip rope with ball bearings in the handles is easier and smoother to use.

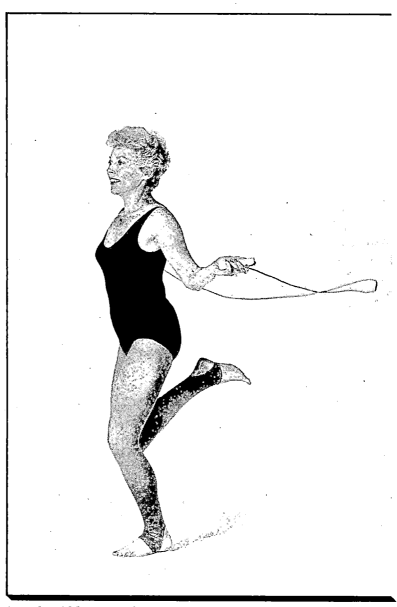

You should keep good posture when jumping.

Contrary to what a lot of people think, jumping rope punishes the foot almost as much as running. Accordingly, a soft surface is better to skip on than a hard one. Curtis Mitchell in *The Perfect Exercise* (Simon and Schuster, 1976) recommends skipping "on a rug or mat, or wearing shoes with a thick rubber sole. Old football knees are sometimes a problem. But treat your joints with care for the first two weeks of your program, and they will return the favor with interest."

How to Jump

Jumping rope can be compared to swimming or riding a bike; once you learn it, you will never forget. If you've never learned it, start practicing without the rope. First, stand with your forearms down and out at a 45-degree angle and hands about eight inches out from the hips, with the upper arms near the ribs.

Then, suggests Lenore Zohman, M.D., in *Exercise Your Way to Fitness and Heart Health* (CPC International, 1974), "start bouncing one inch off the floor with a slight bend at ankles, knees and hips. Do about 25 bounces to get the rhythm. Then make a forward circle of the hands by moving the wrists as you bounce off the floor.

"When you have mastered this coordinated movement, try it with the rope. Place the loop behind the heels with the arms slightly to the front. The rope is swung over the head and under both feet. The jump should be just high enough for the rope to pass under the feet – sometimes only an inch off the floor. Try only one jump [per revolution] and try to work up to 25 [revolutions], which will be very similar to the 25 bounces plus hand rotation you mastered previously.

"You can also learn with the rope. Hold both ends of the rope or both handles in one hand. Try coordinating your bounce off the floor with the swing of the rope. Try to arrange the sequence of events so that the rope slaps the floor when your bounce has taken you into the air. This is the type of coordination needed for the rope to pass under your feet when you hold it in both hands. When you have mastered this technique, place the loop behind your heels and jump as explained above, only one jump at first, later up to 25 in a row."

Among sedentary, elderly or cardiac patients using rope skipping for fitness, Dr. Zohman reports, "stepping over the rope one foot at a time, rather than bouncing over it with both feet, has been found to be easier and to prevent rapid increases in heart rate. It also avoids ankle and foot discomfort which is common in new jumpers who are not conditioned to landing on both feet. The step-over method is very similar to the foot motions used in jogging."

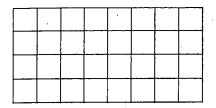

Jumping rope is like swimming or riding a bike. Once you learn how, you never forget.

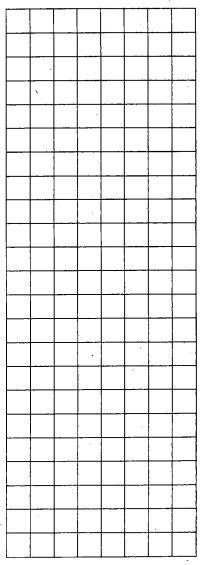

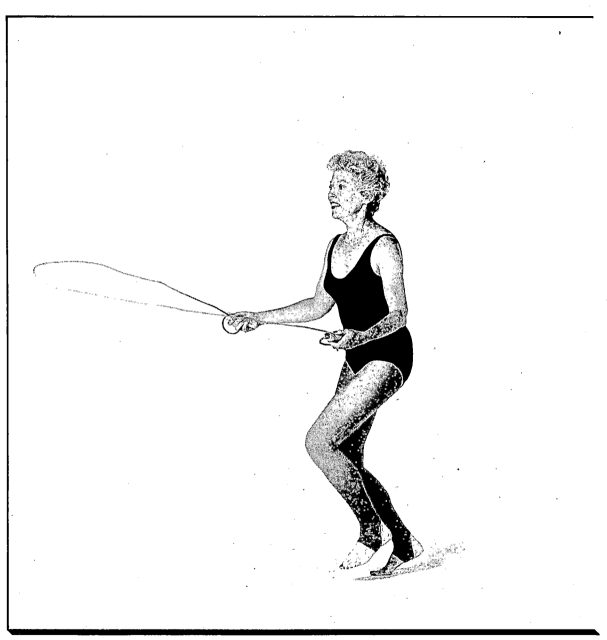

Try to land on the balls of your feet.

An Easy Plan for Action

Although your enthusiasm to reap the benefits of a rope jumping exercise program may be overwhelming you, don't rush to get your rope until you've taken some common-sense precautions. If you have any heart problems, high blood pressure, asthma, arthritis or any other health problems, including being more than 20 pounds overweight, check with your physician before starting. If, however, you are under 40 years of age, have been exercising fairly regularly and feel pretty healthy, you probably could forgo the medical checkup. If you notice that after exercising you feel dizzy, have chest pains or abnormal heart rhythm, stop exercising and see a physician.

Once you begin jumping rope, remember not to rush. The quickest way to lose interest in exercising of any kind is to work yourself to exhaustion. Take it easy.

Planning a Skipping Routine

You might begin with a few warm-up hops without the rope, then jump rope a few times, rest for a few minutes, then jump a few more. Gradually increase the jumps, a few each day at a comfortable speed, until you are able to jump for ten minutes at a time without exhausting yourself. After a skipping workout, warm down by walking around.

You can work any number of variations into your skipping routine. Teach yourself to jump high enough to allow the rope to pass under you twice before you come down to earth. You might even get yourself a copy of a book like *Jump Rope!* (Workman, 1974) by Peter L. Skolnik. It contains much of the information presented here, plus hundreds of traditional jump rope rhymes and games, skipping routines from all over the world that allow you to vary the speed and make-up of your exercises effortlessly.

Skippers should remember to come down on the balls of their feet in a "soft" landing. Relax while you skip so that each landing is on ankles, knees and hips that are slightly bent. Make yourself comfortable. Wear loose-fitting clothing. Skip to your favorite music if you can.

Above all, remember that the music you make with the rope will make your body sing.

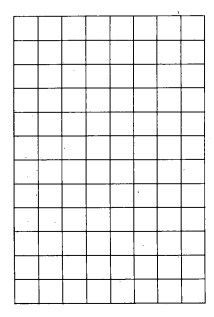

For getting rid of depression, running is much better than taking medication. And it's cheaper than psychotherapy.

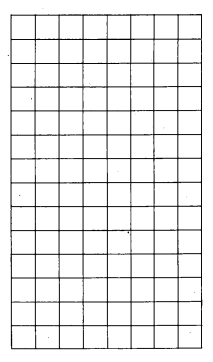

RUNNING

Many runners begin running for health reasons. Some want to lose weight. Or do something good for their hearts. Today 20 to 30 million Americans run. A recent survey by *Runner's World* magazine (December, 1980) showed that 82 percent of all runners planned to keep on running for the rest of their lives. Now, even a casual observer of the United States scene could tell you that 20 million Americans would not continue to do something over and over again simply because it was good for them. There's got to be more to it than that. And there is.

Those people out there pounding the roads in their multicolored running shoes are not only changing the shape of their bodies; they're also doing things to their minds. Good things. Medical folks haven't yet figured out the chemistry of how running massages your mind with good feelings, but there's no doubt about the reality of its effects. Just listen to Thaddeus Kostrubala, M.D., a California doctor who has had great success prescribing running for his depressed patients.

"For getting rid of garden-variety depression, which seems to afflict an awful lot of people, running is much better than antidepressive medication. And it's cheaper than psychotherapy.

"All you've got to do is be sure it's safe for you to start. Your anxiety will burn off right away.

"If you run longer than a half hour, you begin to notice a change come over you. The running is no longer as much a chore as it was. You feel like you're doing something extremely good. You might even feel a kind of euphoria. Once or twice a year, that euphoria can be really intense. A lot of runners have told me about their experience of this moment of aesthetic 'arrest.' In all cases it seems to be a profound experience in which they become aware of things they were never aware of before. Symbols suddenly have meaning. Things fit together like never before. Now, you get a little of this quite often, if you run long enough and regularly enough. And it sticks with you throughout your life.

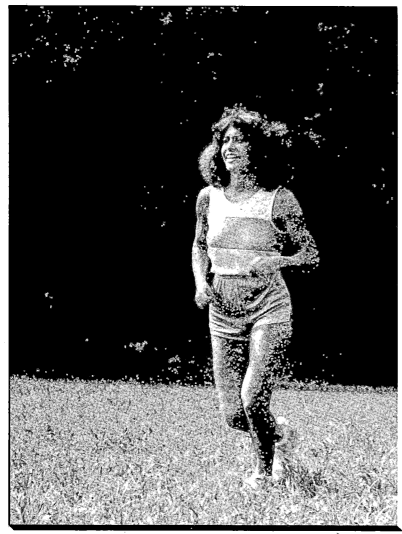

Running in the country soothes the body and the mind.

A Natural High

" 'Runner's high' isn't just our imagination, either," says Dr. Kostrubala. "There are hormones involved. Running stimulates adrenal hormones, which are antidepressants. And the stimulation is enough to cause runners to sometimes mimic the behavior of people who are 'high' on a drug. The runner can get so high that he or she can fail to recognize that everyone else doesn't appreciate the euphoria. People who are standing by – or not taking the drug – are in a different world, so to speak.

"I started running when my doctor 'prescribed' that I join a group of men who were getting into running as rehabilitation, after their heart attacks. I hadn't had a coronary, but I was a high-risk normal. I was actually the fattest of the group, and I was terrorized by their stories. There they were, living more or less normally, and then, the next thing they knew they were in the hospital with a 50-50 chance of surviving! I had never really associated with that pathos, that pain and terror. But I wasn't there as a doctor, I was there as a patient, so I had to associate with it now.

"Of course, these fellows were depressed. I was depressed, too. But the first thing that happened was they said they had a sense of increased energy at the end of a run. Now that makes no sense. Any study of energy expenditure would lead to the opposite conclusion. But as anyone who exercises this way knows, you do feel better. Energy is increased, not decreased. This is a very important clue, because if something is violating what you think is supposed to happen, that is exactly the spot where you should look. Either something is out of kilter, or you've struck pay dirt.

"The second significant thing these men reported was that their depression was less. Even their wives reported it. And that 'shouldn't' happen, either. So immediately I lit up. It was happening to me, too. I said, 'Aha! Something is happening here!' "

Dr. Kostrubala began using running as a treatment.

"I started using running as a therapy for my patients, and they've mostly done quite well. One of that first group was a schizophrenic. But as long as he keeps up his running, there's no trace of his disease visible in any kind of examination. But his symptoms come back very clearly if he stops running. He has an absolute choice available to him. He can choose to be schizophrenic or well. There were two women in that first group of my patients. One was a drug abuser, the other suffered from anorexia nervosa. They're now both symptom-free.

From the Playground to the Marathon

"We had a temporary school project in which we demonstrated that running outside the classroom can change the kids' behavior inside. At a local grammar school, we had kids from grades one to eight running for an hour three days a week after school. The parents were informed, for their approval. We encouraged the kids and their coaches to do whatever they wanted to do. Four weeks after we started we held a 20-kilometer run and about 30 kids finished it. Six of those kids went on to run a marathon, and continued running marathons. And the parents started running, too. And I've seen other clinical examples of kids responding to running. I've seen hyperactive kids whose parents have gotten into running, and after they start running with their parents, they don't need the medication anymore.

"As a preventive tool, it's great. Naturally, besides helping you avoid depression, running will help keep you out of the coronary care unit. Your cardiovascular system will grow stronger and healthier. Heaven knows what other wonderful things running probably does for us, in terms of psychological health. If it can affect the minds of severely ill people, bring about positive changes, imagine what the effect can be on people who aren't ill."

Body Chemistry

There are many theories about why running does good things for your brain. One idea is that it stimulates the body to produce endorphins. Endorphins are powerful antidotes to depression. They lift spirits the way that express elevators pop tourists' ears on the way to the top of the Empire State Building.

Another theory links running to increased production of norepinephrine. Norepinephrine is a hormone released by the adrenal glands. Its presence in the blood is associated with euphoric emotions. Right now no one knows if norepinephrine causes euphoria. We only know that it seems to arrive in the blood at the same time and that running can triple its concentration in the blood.

But aside from any internal chemical effect, running gives many people a sense of self-fulfillment. When they run, they do something outside of the mediocre, normal range of behavior. Running makes them extend themselves, giving them a chance to see what their mind and body can do. When you get yourself in shape, and you can run longer and longer distances without exhaustion, you become a member of an elite group. If you can run four miles continuously at a nine-minute-per-mile pace, then you are able to perform a task that most people can't.

As you push yourself beyond the normal limits that modern society requires, you begin to see yourself differently. You acquire more self-respect and introspection as well as a different view of those around you. The process puts you more in touch with yourself. Dr. Kostrubala says:

"You have to reevaluate your relationship to pain. One of the biggest things in our culture is that people are afraid of pain. Anything that smacks of pain is to be avoided; it's considered abnormal. If it's got pain, it's no good. But you don't want to deny or ignore the pain, you don't want to lose it artificially. You want to own up to it. Say something like this to yourself: 'This pain is my own, it's nobody else's. It's maybe the only thing in the world I can own. It's mine. It's precious. It really lets me know I'm here.' If you acknowledge the struggle, you're much more likely to appreciate it."

"We're *Supposed* to Run"

In our own informal survey of runners, we found that the beginning of a running program often coincides with a change in people's lives. Relationships may break up. New ones begin. Jobs are lost. Careers launched. Several people reported that they began running during a time of stress, and the running helped them get through it. All continued running after the period of stress ended. One person says that he originally used running to relieve the anxiety of a mentally demanding job but continued running because it had made him a calmer person. One woman said that running made her feel more self-reliant. When questioned closely, almost all the runners said that running, once begun, often felt like something they *had* to be doing. Dr. Kostrubala's observations confirm this:

"Of course, you have to keep in mind that running may not be what you might call a 'supplementary' health-producing activity: we're *supposed* to run. If you don't use an organ system for the purpose for which it was designed, it will deteriorate. By running, you're not only using a tool to reach optimum health, you're going after what the body was designed for. I believe that we evolved into conscious beings through running and hunting. We're designed to run. Our 'machine' is a running machine. We're built to be long-distance runners. Slow runners, but long-distance over periods of time. Our whole physical structure supports long-distance running, right down to the way we deposit fat. So if you start using the 'machine' properly, for the right purpose, it will run better and longer."

The Human Machine

Running is powerfully good medicine for the human machine. And runners feel better about themselves simply because they are healthier. Running fine-tunes the circulatory system. It lowers blood pressure. It strengthens your heart, protecting you from heart attack. If you do have a heart attack and you are a runner, you'll have a better chance of surviving. A Paris study showed that exercising regularly drops your chance of heart attack by 40 percent (*New England Journal of Medicine,* October 9, 1980).

Running helps you lose weight through the alteration of your body chemistry. Running raises your metabolic rate, the rate at which you burn off those calories that might otherwise go into the production of body fat. The exercise not only raises your rate while you run, but the rate stays elevated even after you've finished, taken a hot shower and stretched out to relax. So even while you're sitting or lying down, you're still burning off more calories than you would have if you didn't run.

If you run at least three times a week, you can expect to lower your body fat percentage, drop your weight and raise your HDL level. (HDLs are high-density lipoproteins, substances that help prevent cholesterol and fat accumulation within artery walls.) All of these things occur as physiological results of running and also because running leads to a healthier lifestyle. Dr. Kostrubala feels that "as a runner you start doing other things that bring you closer to optimum health. Sometimes you can't help it. A lot of people, including myself, at one time or another run in order to be able to eat a lot but not put on weight. But the system tricks you. Something changed inside of me. I didn't *want* to eat a lot more. Your sensitivity to food increases. You get away from junkfood. And you gravitate more toward a vegetarian diet. Other things change, too. You start to do what feels right for you. Some people develop peculiar sleep patterns when they become runners. At one time I used to run between 2 and 3 in the morning. That's when it felt right. I'd be out there in the dark running around with a flash-

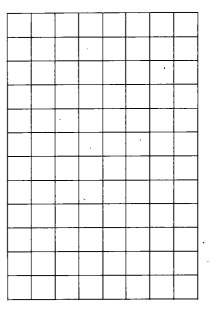

Running is powerfully good medicine for the human machine.

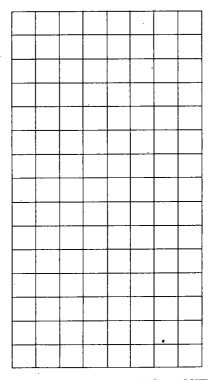

light, scared to death. But it felt right. A lot of changes can take place. You may have to change your diet, your lifestyle, even your job.

Putting One Foot in Front of the Other

"The best way to begin running is to just do it. Take it easy at first, feeling out what your body can do, but get out there on the road or track and move," says Dr. Kostrubala.

"There's nothing you can do as expeditiously and easily as running. The first step has nothing to do with anything physical, nothing to do with getting an exam or buying the right shoes or anything. The very first thing you should do is simply determine that you're going to do it. It's a principle borrowed from Zen.

"When a Zen archer aims at his target, he actually visualizes the entire process in his mind, including the flight of the arrow into the target. If you can do that mental imagery, in a sense send the signals to the muscles to prepare them for what is going to occur, you can achieve some remarkable things. So the first step is to say, 'I'm going to do it.' No equivocation, no hedging, no qualification. It's a leap of faith. And I think that's necessary in order to gird yourself for the first few months, which can be pretty hard if you're in as bad shape as I was."

If you do have a serious question about your health and your ability to run, you may want to see a doctor first. In talking to runners, however, we have found that most, when they began, were in average health and felt no need to consult a physician. If you do wish to consult a physician, it is important that you talk to one who is knowledgeable about exercise and that you understand the kind of tests you may undergo. Otherwise, there is a strong possibility that you will get incorrect advice. (According to George Sheehan, an MD/philosopher in Red Bank, New Jersey, "The worst enemies of runners are drivers, dogs and doctors.")

As you overcome your initial resistance to running, using what Dr. Kostrubala refers to as a "leap of faith," you'll want to develop proper running technique.

Contrary to what many people would like to believe, proper running form is not a natural ability that can be mastered without practice. Most runners run incorrectly. They run inefficiently, wasting energy in extraneous motions that slow them down, and they run stressfully, bouncing and overusing certain muscles. That inefficiency and stress can lead to injuries that would be avoidable by using proper running technique.

Leroy Perry, D.C., a chiropractor at the Chiropractic Corporation in Pasadena, California, who is an expert at treating athletes, uses the term "jogging" to describe what most people do when they think that they are "running." According to Dr. Perry's terminology, "Jogging is one of the worst things you can do to your body. It is done by people who strike on their heels with a vertical or backward lean to their bodies as their arms twist in a rotary motion around them. By corkscrewing their arms around themselves as they jog, they are literally screwing themselves into the ground. They also concentrate tension in their upper back by keeping their shoulders tight while either sticking out their heads or pulling their ears into their shoulders.

"The bouncing motion of jogging sends stress right up the body from the foot, through the ankle, tibia, knee and thigh into the lower back through the spine to the base of the skull, eventually causing injury. I've even seen patients with headaches resulting from stress that started in the foot!

"In proper running technique, there is a forward lean to the body. The faster you run, the more forward lean you should use. A long-distance runner should lean forward about 15 to 20 degrees. This means a 5-degree lean from the ankle to the knee, a 5-degree lean from the knee to the hip, another 5 degrees from the hip to the shoulder and about 5 degrees from the shoulder to the head.

"The forward plant of your foot should land about one-half to three-quarters of an inch in front of your heel and, in a fluid motion as you move, you should roll through the length of the foot and push off between your first and second toes. Proper running means pushing off with your back foot, not pulling with the front one! Too many people never use their toes.

"Your arms should move in an easy pendulum type of motion, a free arm swing forward and backward, each arm coordinated with the opposite foot. On their forward swing the arms should come up to about the level of your chest. Your shoulders should be level and you should always look straight out in front of you. Don't look at the ground.

"Proper running, like proper walking, is related to proper posture. A common problem is that many people, when they stand, walk and run, stick out their buttocks, which leads to stress on the lower back. During running, and all

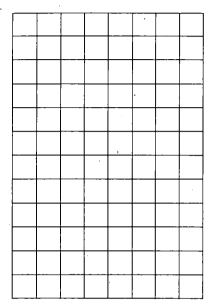

According to Dr. Kostrubala, the best way to begin running is just to do it. Take it easy at first, feeling out what your body can do, but get out there on the road or track and move.

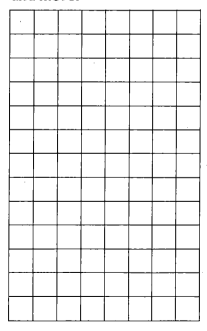

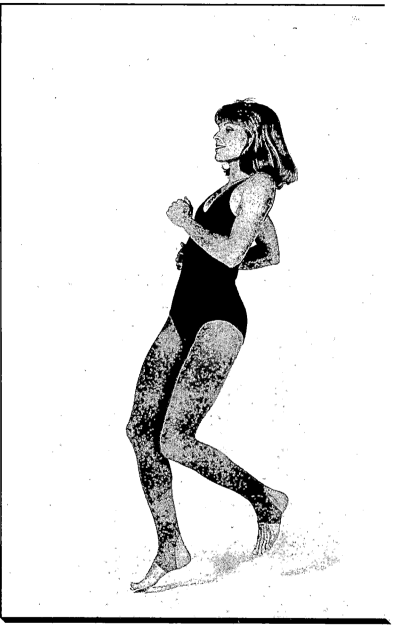

The wrong way to run – leaning backward.

body movement, your pubic bone should be tilted upward toward your belly button. This reduces the stress on the lower back muscles.

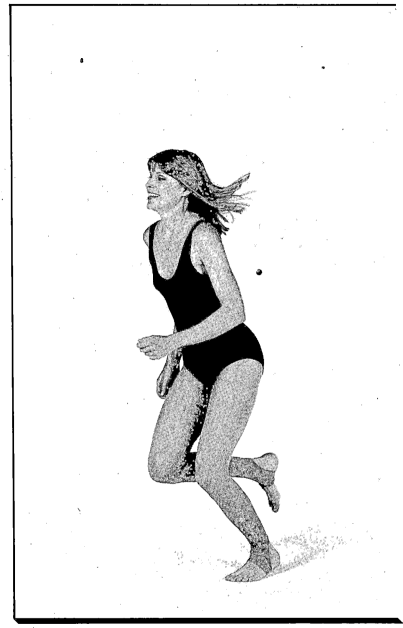

Lean forward slightly when you run.

"One of the main differences between jogging and running is how you deal with stress. Proper running motion dissipates the stress behind you, not through you. In running, both feet leave the ground after you push off with the back foot. After the front foot lands, a full rolling motion takes place, enabling you to come up onto your toes quickly, so that to an onlooker it almost looks as if you are running on your toes.

"When I teach people how to run, or to perform any sport, I try to give them mental images they can use to keep their bodies in the right position. I tell runners to imagine that they have a helium balloon attached by string to each breast and another attached to the top of their head. As they run, they can imagine that a gust of wind comes from behind, pushing the balloons forward and up. If you can picture these make-believe balloons pulling your chest and head forward and upward, it will help you retain the proper running posture."

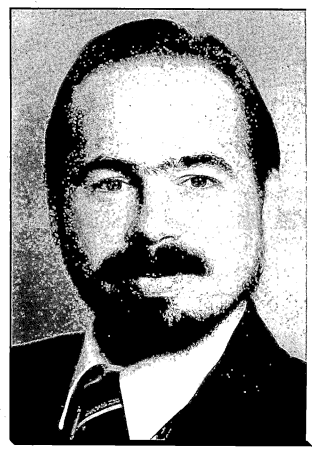

Dr. Leroy Perry, expert on running.

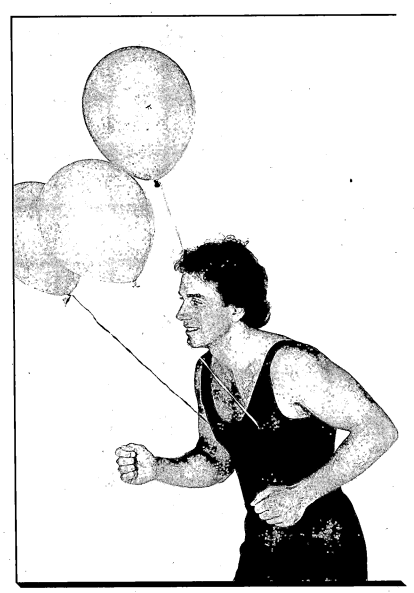

Imagine balloons lifting up your chest, and your running posture will improve.

Running Uses Your Whole Body—Not Just the Feet

"Running," according to Dr. Perry, "is as much an upper body exercise as it is a lower body activity. Developing upper body strength is just as important as developing the lower

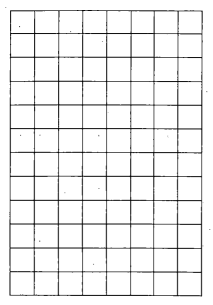

Dr. Perry says that running is as much an upper body exercise as it is a lower body activity. Developing upper body strength is just as important as developing your legs.

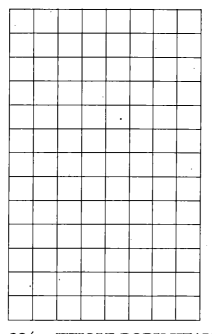

body. An exercise I recommend to develop upper body muscles and which aids vital lung capacity is 'reverse windmills.' This exercise also helps posture and body alignment.

"From a standing position, push your arms out to the side as straight and hard as you can. Bring your hands up at a 90-degree angle to your arm and push out as hard as you can, like you are Samson spreading the walls apart. Now rotate your arms backward – only backward.

"Reverse windmills bring your upper body back, and they bring the head back between the shoulders so that you don't stick your head out like a pelican. In treating my patients I recommend doing reverse windmills 50 times per minute for three minutes, twice a day, as long as they don't have a structural problem.

"We had a lady patient 68 years old who had been a secretary since she was 17 years old. She was suffering with osteoarthritis. Her spine was bent forward quite a bit, and we brought it back six inches in nine months mainly by using this exercise. Much of her problem was caused by bending over her desk every day for 51 years.

"Another important exercise for runners is the 'pelvic tilt.' To do this, lean forward against a wall at a 45-degree angle, your arms extended so your hands are resting against the wall. Using the stomach muscles, pull your pubic bone in to your belly button and then relax. Do 50 repetitions of this per minute for two minutes, twice a day. This will strengthen your stomach muscles and help keep your lower back in proper alignment, with the pubic bone tilted in (rather than your buttocks sticking out).

"A good exercise for further strengthening the stomach muscles is the '30-degree abdominal trunk curl.' To do this exercise, lie on your back on the floor, your knees bent and your heels resting on the ground. Your arms are crossed across your chest. Using only your stomach muscles, lift your head while curling your trunk forward off the ground until the angle of your spine is 30 degrees from the floor, then lower yourself back to the ground.

"Doing exercises to develop the stomach muscles is particularly important to combat fatigue and pain of the lower back muscles. These lower back problems are usually caused by a muscle imbalance; the back muscles are much stronger than the stomach muscles and overpower them. The resulting constant use of the back muscles causes stress. The traditional method of doing sit-ups only adds to the imbalance problem. Regular sit-ups (where you sit all the way up

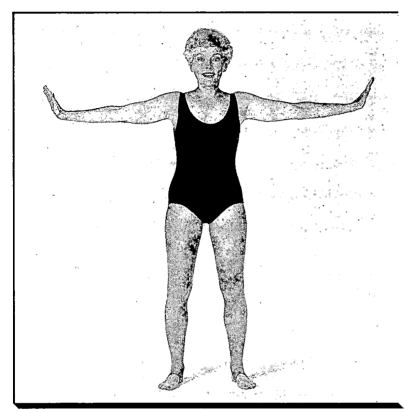

The reverse windmill develops upper body strength.

touching your knees or your toes) actually exercise the back muscles more than they do the stomach muscles, and the imbalance of strength actually becomes more pronounced rather than being relieved.

"For general muscle development and prevention of injuries, I also recommend that all runners have a swimming program. Running tends to create short, tight muscles, which are prone to pulls and tears. Swimming elongates the muscles and aids in creating muscle balance. A good minimum swimming program for runners includes 30 minutes in a pool three times a week. Fifteen minutes are spent doing the crawl while wearing a water ski belt (the belt helps lift the back, decreasing the sway and emphasizing proper muscle balance). The leg kick should be performed from the hips without bending the knees. The other 15 minutes should be spent doing the backstroke. The flotation belt should not be worn while doing this stroke."

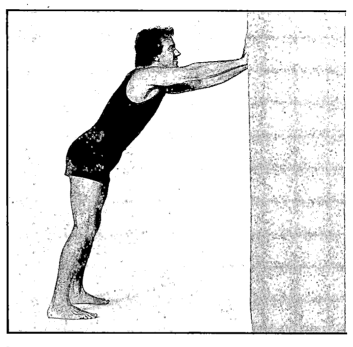

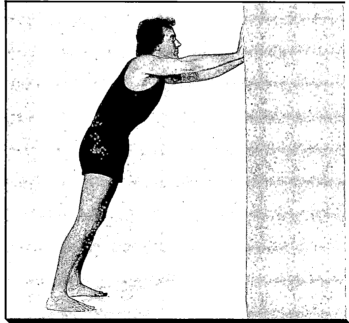

1. This version of the pelvic tilt starts with lower back curved. 2. Then tuck the pelvis and straighten the back.

Preparing to Run

One of the best ways to destroy your running career is to jump out of bed first thing in the morning, get dressed in your running gear, open the front door, step outside and begin running immediately. Using that kind of approach to running, you'd be lucky to last a month. Before doing any running, in the morning or later in the day, but especially in the morning, it's important to prepare your body. This preparation consists of warming up and stretching. If you run with cold, tight muscles, you increase your chance of injury. Several studies have shown that an unusually large number of running injuries occur in the morning. This is probably due to people trying to run without proper preparation on muscles that have just spent eight hours in bed.

While doing your prerunning stretching, remember to do it with a slow, relaxed motion. Never bounce for any reason. Bouncing may seem to help you stretch farther, but it actually makes your muscles tighter instead of more relaxed, by triggering the "splinting" reflex. When you do a stretching motion, reach only until the movement starts to be uncomfortable and then hold that position. Don't reach far enough to cause intense pain. If you stretch daily, over a period of time your body should become somewhat more limber, and you will be able to stretch farther. You must have patience and wait for that to happen without trying to rush its development.

The first stretching exercise to try is the "wall push-up." This is not related to a regular push-up (which exercises the arms) but is, instead, intended to stretch the calf muscles. Standing at least three feet away from a wall, and keeping your knees locked and your heels flat on the floor, lean into the wall, supporting yourself with your hands on its surface. Lean forward until you feel a dull, aching, pulling sensation. Hold for ten seconds. For the "modified wall push-up," keep your toes pointed toward the wall and slide your right foot back, bending the left knee. Then bend the right knee until you feel a different set of calf muscles stretching. Hold the bent-knee position for five seconds. After stretching the right leg, repeat the procedure on the left leg. Murray F. Weisenfeld, D.P.M., a podiatrist who is a consultant at the New York College of Podiatric Medicine, recommends in his book *The Runners' Repair Manual* (St.

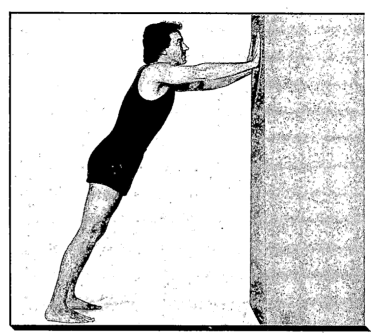

The wall push-up.

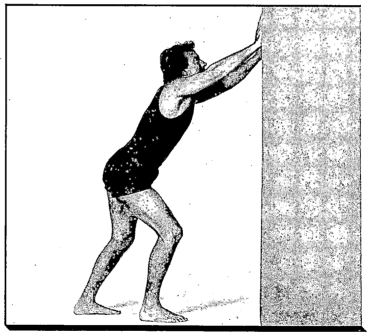

Modified wall push-up.

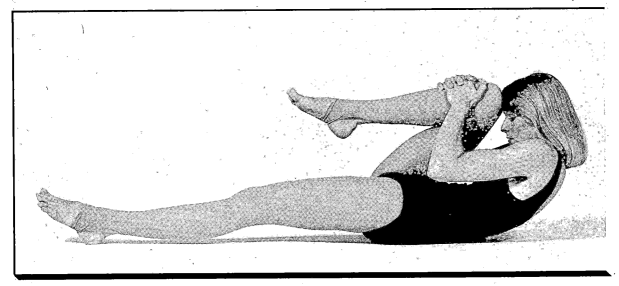

The knee and head press.

Martin's Press, 1980) that this stretch be used on each leg five times, alternating legs, before running.

Another important stretch to do before running is the "knee and head press." This will stretch the neck and shoulder muscles as well as the hamstrings and lower back. Lie down on your back. Pull your right knee up to your chest by grasping your hands around it and pulling it toward you (the left leg stays on the ground). At the same time you pull up your knee, lift your head off the ground and try to touch your forehead to the knee. Hold this position for ten seconds. Do each leg five times, alternating sides.

Next, you should do a "hamstring stretch." With both legs straight and your knees locked, put one foot up on a chair or table in front of you. (The height of the surface depends on how limber you are. Beginners should probably use a chair.) While bringing your face toward the knee of the extended leg, reach out with one hand and try to grasp the foot on the table. Stop when you feel extreme tightness, and hold your body there for ten seconds. Then, relaxing the arm you just used, reach for the same foot with your other hand, again pressing your face toward your knee. Hold this position for ten seconds also. Do the same motions with the other leg up on the chair or table, and do each leg five times.

Isometric exercises, recommended by Dr. Weisenfeld for strengthening the leg muscles, should round out your prerunning stretching. The first is the "foot press." This exercise strengthens the quadriceps, or thigh muscles. To do this isometric exercise, sit on the floor or on a chair. With the legs straight in front of you, put one foot on top of the other. Pull your lower foot toward your torso while you push down with your upper foot. Press the feet together for ten seconds, then switch feet and repeat. Press down on each foot five times, alternating feet.

The last exercise is called "inner and outer thighs." It is also done sitting on a chair or on the floor with your legs straight out. Point your toes toward your knees, tighten your thigh muscles, and then point your toes in toward each other, pigeon-toed style, as far as you can. Hold them there for ten seconds, then turn them out and hold for ten seconds. You should keep your thigh muscles tight the entire time. For best results, alternate between pointing your toes in and out and do each position five times.

According to Dr. Perry, an exercise you should avoid, which some books recommend, is the "backover." During

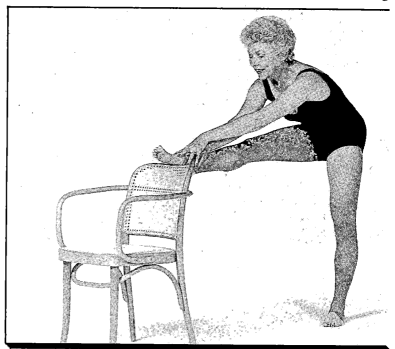

Hamstring stretch.

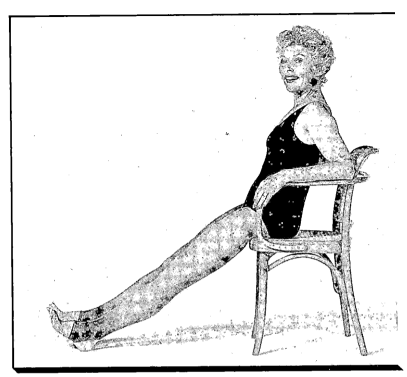

The foot press.

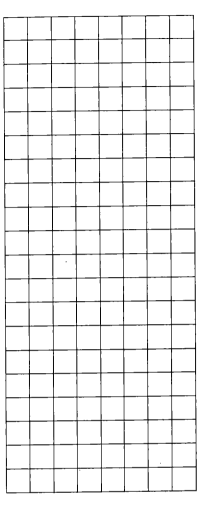

this exercise you lie on the ground on your back and throw your feet up over your head, trying to touch the ground behind your head with your toes. The exercise puts too much strain on the neck and upper back muscles, says Dr. Perry, which subjects them to a great deal of pressure. If you have neck or upper back problems, this exercise will make them worse. If you don't have those problems, the backover may help create them.

Doing stretching before and after running will help prevent injury by counteracting some of the tightening forces that come into play when you run. You should do a minimum of ten minutes of stretching before you start and after you finish. In addition, walk before and after running. Suddenly running after sitting at a desk all day or after a night's sleep taxes the heart as it strains to supply more blood to the working muscles. A five-minute walk before running increases the heart's pumping action and brings it closer to the rate at which it will have to work during running. Walking after running helps clear lactic acid out of

It is always better to run a little less and hold yourself back than it is to strain by running too much.

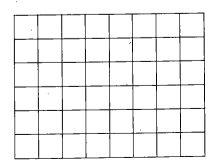

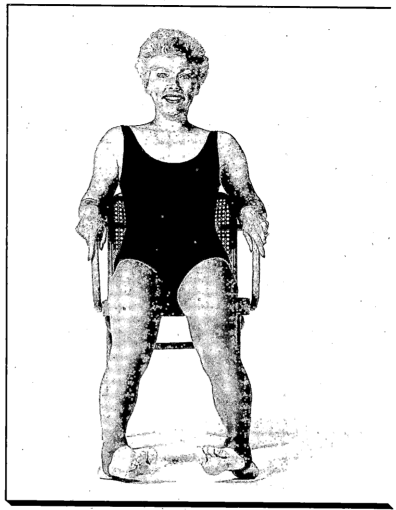

The inner thigh press.

the muscles, reducing fatigue. Lactic acid, one of the waste products created by working muscles, builds up in your legs during running (and can cause cramps if you are trying to run too fast). Walking after your run will shorten your recovery time by helping to break up the lactic acid accumulation in your legs.

How Far and Fast Do You Want to Run?

Having done your warm-up stretches and walking, you are finally ready to run. Now you have to decide how far and at

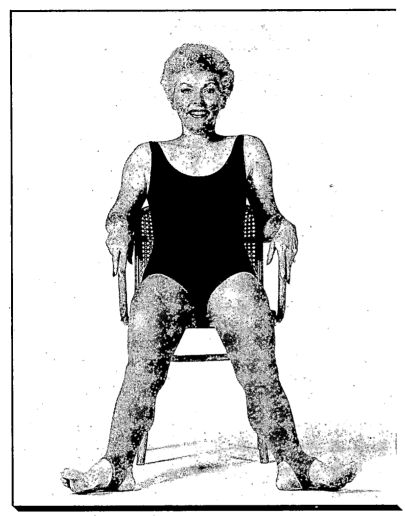

The outer thigh exercise.

what pace you want to run. Remember that it is always better to hold back a little too much than it is to strain by pushing yourself too hard. A good beginner's pace is to alternate intervals of running a quarter of a mile with walking a quarter of a mile. As you run, you should not be so winded that you are unable to speak. If you are so out of breath that you are unable to carry on a conversation as you run, then you are going too fast. The idea is to do aerobic exercise, and that means exercising moderately enough to avoid oxygen debt yet vigorously enough to produce a training effect. You are coaxing your lungs, heart and muscles to work a little bit harder than they are used to but not so hard that they rebel in the form of wheezing lungs, cramping legs and pounding pulse. (For more details on aerobics, see the chapter on aerobic exercise and dance.)

Your running sessions should last at least 20 minutes each and be done at least three times a week. Your exact speed and distance are unimportant as long as you spend enough time working toward your goal of fitness. Let the way your body feels be your guide to how fast you accelerate your program. If you get very serious about running, you will probably run every day. That's the best way, once you start to develop endurance, to improve your staying power as a runner. But the best way to remain satisfactorily fit and limit the chance of injury is to run every other day. The day off in between runs allows the body to recover from the stress of pounding the roads.

Injured? Relax—It Happens to Everyone

Talk to any experienced runner and you'll find out that at some time in their running career they've been injured. This includes everyone from those runners in the back of the pack (like one of the authors of this book, Carl Lowe, who as he writes this is suffering from shin splints) to champions like Alberto Salazar, who has won the New York City Marathon several times.

Mr. Salazar was injured during his training in the months before one of the marathons and was forced to take time off and do alternative exercises like swimming to maintain his level of cardiovascular fitness. Despite his injuries, he was still able to run the marathon in the second fastest time ever run by an American.

Given enough rest, relaxation and encouragement, the body will usually heal itself. Along with rest, the best remedies for injuries are corrective exercises, practicing a correct running style and running on a soft surface. Sometimes changing your style of running shoes will help.

The best surfaces for running are dirt paths and flat asphalt roads. Grass can be deceptively dangerous, with hidden holes and depressions waiting to catch your foot and twist an unwary ankle. The hardest running surface is concrete. Stay off it when you run! It's just too hard on the feet.

RUNNING INJURIES

If you run correctly, using the methods we outline in the chapter on running, you will lower your chance of injury. You won't eliminate it, however. Running is not a riskless sport. You can get a lot out of running, including physical fitness and the mental satisfaction of accomplishment, but you don't get something for nothing. Both your mind and body have to put out. It's an effort that most people won't give. That's one reason why not everyone is a runner. If you talk to people opposed to running, they'll usually tell you all about the dangers involved, the stress of 800 pounding steps each mile, the horror stories about people who ran even though injured and limped for the rest of their days, and the running addicts who let running take over their lives the way alcoholics let booze wipe out theirs. Let's face it – disaster can happen, but the chances that running will destroy your life are pretty remote if you use your head as well as your feet.

How far and how fast you run is going to have an effect on your risk of injury. If you are running every day, it's important that you don't do two rough training sessions back to back. Alternate hard and easy days. If you run fast and far on Monday, you'd better lay back on Tuesday. That gives your body a chance to recover from running's rigors. Getting physically fit is a gradual process. You can't do it all in one day, one week or one month. Trying to do it too fast is like blowing too much air into a balloon – it will blow up in your face. Pushing your body too hard will make it rebel in the form of pain and injury.

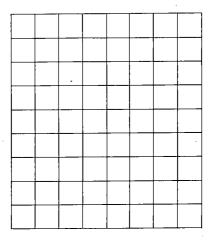

Training too ambitiously is like blowing too much air into a balloon—it will blow up in your face. Pushing your body too hard causes injury.

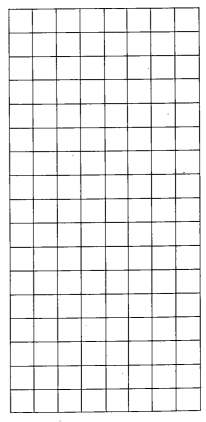

The Side Stitch—It's Not Serious, but It Hurts!

The side stitch is a pain. Literally. And since no one is sure exactly what it represents, if you get one you'll know as much about it as anyone – it hurts. Some people describe it as a cramp, a sharp ache or a burning sensation. It can start anywhere on your torso, but most often it's on the side of your chest or stomach. Some runners seem to get side stitches at random. Others report getting them running

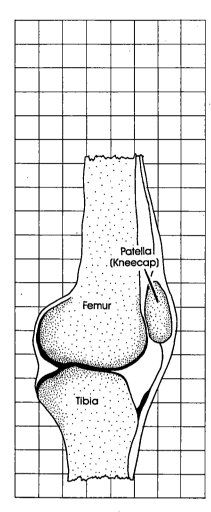

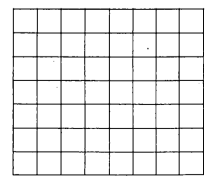

The kneecap rides on a layer of fat over the joint where the upper and lower leg meet.

uphill or downhill or at the end of a long run. They may be symptomatic of an abdominal weakness, and some athletes combat side stitches by doing the 30-degree abdominal trunk curls we described in the previous chapter.

Side stitches can be "run through" without risking serious injury, as long as you can stand the pain. One runner we talked to, Tom Dybdahl, who has been running for eight years and who has completed several marathons in close to three hours, says, "If a side stitch comes on slowly, I can control it by belly breathing. I usually get them after a long run or after going downhill. I had one last year during the New York Marathon, but it went away after I belly-breathed for a while – luckily it wasn't too bad. If a stitch comes on suddenly, without any warning, it hurts worse and is harder to get rid of. I do find that I get more stitches nowadays than I used to, and I think it's because I've been neglecting my stomach exercises."

The belly breathing Mr. Dybdahl describes is an exaggerated motion of your stomach muscles while you run. As you inhale you stick your stomach out more than usual, and as you exhale you tuck it in. Saying something as you exhale, like "Ah!" or "Oh!" also sometimes helps break up side stitches.

Knee Pain—It Hurts to Slip Out of the Groove

The knee is an up and down joint. In running, its job is to connect your thigh to your lower leg while they propel you forward. As you move, the thigh and lower leg move at different speeds and constantly change angles relative to each other, forcing the kneecap, their point of connection, to slide up and down on the patellar groove. As long as the kneecap stays in this groove, located on the thighbone, things run smoothly and painlessly. But the groove is like a railroad track through the Rocky Mountains – slide off it, and you get a bumpy ride that grinds to a quick halt. And there are probably as many ways to slip out of the groove as there are runners. That's why runner's knee is the most common injury among runners. Any imperfection in motion as your foot strikes the ground and takes off puts "sideways tension" on the knee, edging it out of its groove, grinding it against the condyle, a knob on the thighbone. This uneven motion damages the cushioning cartilage around the knee and causes the pain.

What can you do for runner's knee? The most important thing to remember is that you can't run through knee pain as you can a mild side stitch. Trying to run with knee pain will only make it worse because, untreated, you're grinding your cartilage into "dust." The first place to look for the source of your pain is your feet. Your problem may originate with pronation. Pronation means that your ankles are rolling in when your feet hit the ground, and your feet are literally sagging inward as you run. This motion pulls your whole leg to the inside as your weight presses down, forcing your knee out of its groove. If this is the cause of your trouble, then arch supports will relieve the problem. The supports, which you insert in your running shoes, act as bridges, holding up your arches and keeping them in alignment. With this support, they don't sag and tug at your knee.

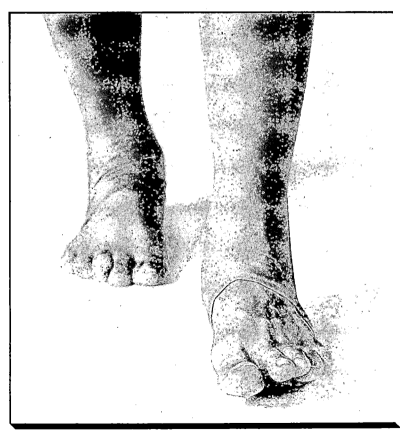

There should be even weight distribution on the feet.

It's possible that a problem with runner's knee might involve other foot structural problems or a severe pronation problem that cannot be helped by "over-the-counter" arch supports. In that case, you should consult a podiatrist who is familiar with runners' ailments. A good podiatrist should be able to analyze your problem and devise customized orthotics for your shoes. Orthotics are shoe inserts that compensate for your foot irregularities and weaknesses by modifying the inside surface of your shoes.

Besides toying with shoe inserts, a good way to fight runner's knee is through the use of exercises that strengthen your thighs and increase flexibility in your calves and hamstrings. Do the knee press isometric exercise and the inner and outer thighs stretch that we describe in the previous chapter on running. The thigh muscles developed by these exercises help to hold your knee in the proper position

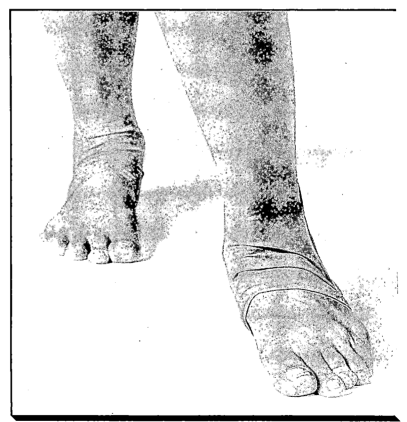

Overpronation means the ankle rolls in too far.

while you run. Likewise, from the same chapter, do the wall push-ups and the knee and head press; these are flexibility stretches. Doing these exercises will cut down on the stiffness that tends to pull your knee out of place on every running step.

Injury on the Rocks

All the treatments we've described so far for knee pain will help get your knee back in the "groove," but they won't kill the pain very quickly. The best way to help your knee (or knees) feel better right away is to ice them immediately after running and then use heat on them later in the day. This follows a general cold/hot method of treating injuries. The cold you apply right after activity reduces the swelling and inflammation caused by running. The heat at night enhances healing by encouraging the flow of blood to the injured area.

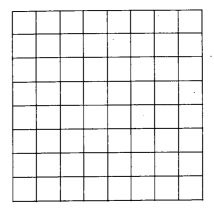

When in doubt, rest is the best treatment for any pain, big or small.

When you apply heat or ice to your knees, do it in moderation. Keep the ice on for about 15 minutes; any longer and you may hurt yourself by making your leg too cold. To keep the ice on your knee, all you need is a plastic bag of ice cubes from the freezer. This bag can be used over and over again. As the cubes melt on your leg and then refreeze back in the freezer, the bag will take on the shape of your knee, making it easier to apply next time. Another way to cool off your knee is to soak a towel in water, then stick it in the freezer. The cold towel can then be wrapped around your leg after you run. This method can be messy, however – the towel will drip as the water thaws.

A heating pad or hot water bottle can be used to heat your knee at night. If you use an electric heating pad, keep the heat on low. Even on low, with some heating pads you may have to move it off your leg periodically to keep your knee from getting too hot. Use the heat for about half an hour. Probably the best place to use it is in bed; there you can relax and put your feet up. But don't fall asleep with the pad on your knee, or you might end up overheating it.

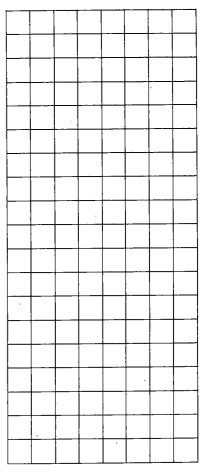

Shin Splints—Too Far, Too Fast, Too Soon

A runner friend of ours decided he wanted to increase his speed and endurance in a hurry. He started doing intensive interval workouts at the local high school track. That meant that he would run quarter-mile intervals as fast as he could, giving himself two minutes to rest between each sprint. At the end of each workout, after he got too tired to do quarter-miles, he'd do a few 100-yard dashes and then run home. He started doing these workouts every other day. Two weeks into this new training schedule he was invited to dinner at a friend's house almost exactly ten miles from where he lived. "Aha!" the runner thought. "A perfect chance to do a ten-mile workout and impress everyone by running there instead of driving!"

Running to his friend's house, he discovered that the wind was against him all the way, making the run more difficult than he had anticipated. Heavy auto traffic forced him to do most of his running on sidewalks, and he constantly had to go up and down curbs. Toward the end of

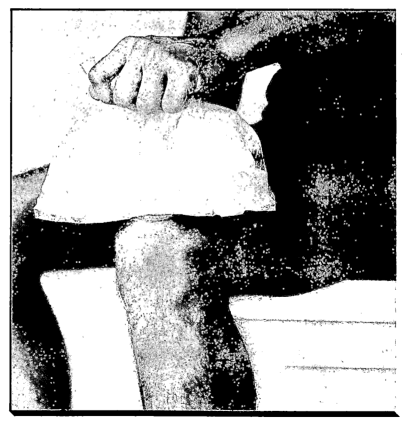

Ice is good for injuries – it relieves pain and swelling.

this trek, the longest distance he had ever run, he began to get pain in the outside front part of his left leg. With a mile left to go, a car cut him off at an intersection just as he was leaving the sidewalk and stepping onto the road. As he changed direction, his foot came down with a twisting motion, toes on the road, heel jammed into the side of the curb. This made the pain worse. Too proud to telephone for a ride, he finished the run despite the pain. That night, and for the next few days, his lower leg hurt when he walked, and running was impossible. He had a classic case of shin splints.

Many people call shin splints an "overuse" injury. The word "overuse" is a catchall term describing an injury that occurs when a part of the body has been used too much. The injured muscles that cause shin splints, on the front outside part of the leg, work as shock absorbers for the feet. Each time your foot hits the ground, these muscles fight the stress of contact and hold the foot together. Without these muscles, your feet would flatten out like blobs of jelly every time you took a running step, and your legs would fall apart. When the shock of hitting the ground becomes too much for these muscles to handle, they tighten up in spasms of pain. That's what happened to the runner in our story when he tried to run ten miles on concrete.

One of the main causes of shin splints is too large an increase in training speed and distance. Muscles that can easily handle a five-mile run on a dirt path at an easy pace freeze in agony when pounded during a long run on hard concrete sidewalks or a series of quick sprints around a high school track. When you run for miles on sidewalks and go up and down curbs as you cross the intervening streets, it's just like driving your car over miles of nasty potholes. In both cases, the underside of your vehicle gets pounded to smithereens. With your car, you'll end up in a service station, your auto on a lift, looking up at bent and twisted metal. With your legs, you'll be looking down to find the source of pain – overworked muscle.

The first treatment for shin splints is rest and ice. Get a bag of ice cubes from the freezer, sit down, put your feet up and put the ice where it hurts – the outside front part of the leg. Ice the shin splints the same way we told you to ice your knees in the section on runner's knee – for 15 minutes after running. This will bring down any inflammation. Inflammation and swelling can be a serious problem in shin splints. The muscles involved expand from the heat of exertion, but because they are boxed up in a small, narrow compartment along the outside of the leg, they have nowhere to go. Because of this tight fit, they can hurt a lot when they swell.

The second treatment for shin splints is a cutback in running. If you have been doing extra speed work or hill running, take it easy for a while. If necessary, don't run at all for a week. To maintain your fitness while you lay off running, try another aerobic exercise (for a wide range of suggestions, see the chapter on aerobic exercise and dance). Two possible substitutes are swimming and bicycling. Both of these activities are good for cardiovascular fitness but do not put a strain on your lower leg muscles.

Weak Muscles Are the Ones That Get Hurt

You may be getting shin splints because the muscles on the back of your calf are overpowering the sore muscles on the front of the leg, and you can treat the pain by strengthening the muscles that are hurting. A good way to do this is an isometric exercise that flexes the foot without moving the rest of your leg. While sitting, tuck your toes under any large, heavy object like a desk, couch or table. Pull your toes upward, trying to move the object with your toes. Murray F. Weisenfeld, D.P.M., in *The Runners' Repair Manual* (St. Martin's Press, 1980), recommends doing this ten times a day, pushing for ten seconds each time.

Also, don't forget to do the wall push-ups that we explain in the previous chapter. Increasing the flexibility of your calves should help to relieve some of the pressure on those front leg muscles. Other things to try when you have shin splints include changing your running shoes for a pair with better cushioning or adding a foam heel support to your present pair.

Achilles Tendinitis—Don't Ignore That Pain in the Back of Your Leg

A story from *The Physician and Sportsmedicine* (February, 1979) demonstrates the danger of trying to run through intense, untreated pain. William P. Morgan, professor of physical education at the University of Wisconsin in Madison, tells of a college professor who ran for a year, five miles a day, even though the pain in his legs was close to unbearable. As a matter of fact, his legs were in such bad shape that he could only walk down a flight of stairs backward. Walking down the right way made the pain excruciating. After 12 months of pain, he awoke one morning and discovered that he couldn't walk downstairs using any method at all. The professor had to undergo surgery, is now unable to run and walks with a limp.

That kind of story leads some people to think that running is a crazy thing to do. Well, it is crazy to keep running when the pain of injury won't even let you walk down the stairs! That's why we say you have to use your head as well as your feet. When you do, then running is just about the best overall exercise there is.

Apparently, the professor in the story systematically destroyed his Achilles tendon, a cord that joins the heel to the calf muscle. When the back of the lower leg starts hurting, it usually signals an attack of Achilles tendinitis. Running strengthens the calf muscles and makes them short and bunchy. As they shorten, they pull more and more on the connecting tendon. It's when the pull becomes more than the tendon can comfortably accommodate that the pain begins.

The Achilles tendon, with its surrounding fluid and cover, resembles a taut rubber band surrounded by gelatin, shrink-wrapped in crinkly plastic. The body's reaction to excessive pulling on this structure is to increase the amount of fluid inside the wrapper. But it's a tight fit. Try to get more fluid inside a real shrink wrapper, and the plastic will crackle as it resists. Likewise, your body will send crackling messages of pain to your brain when your Achilles tendon becomes irritated, and the fluid builds up around your tendon.

The best thing to do for Achilles tendinitis is to get a shoe with good heel lift or insert a sponge-rubber heel lift into the shoes you are using now. The higher heel reduces the distance that the tendon has to stretch in order to keep the heel attached to the calf muscles.

You can treat Achilles problems with ice and heat, in the same way you treat shin splints and runner's knee. Use the ice after running, to hold down the swelling, and the heat in the evening to speed healing. And don't forget to cut back on hill work when you're having any kind of problem with your legs. The extra stress involved in going uphill will irritate your injury.

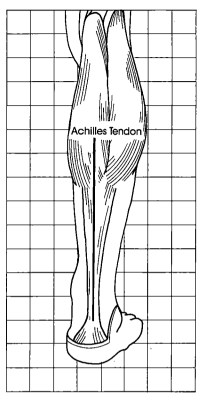

Achilles Tendon

The Achilles tendon—high-heeled shoes make it shorter and less mobile.

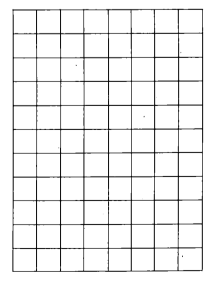

Pain Is the Body's Way of Getting Your Attention

One of the great things about running is that it puts you in touch with your body. As you run, you're opening up the lines of communication. You meditate on how you feel, on who you are, on what your body is and what it is able to do. These things can't be done as effectively by someone who is always sedentary. There is knowledge in movement. Your body will tell you about itself if you can listen. Running clears out your internal ears.

No two human beings have bodies that are identical. That's why, if you get hurt from running, your injury may respond to a cure that wouldn't help someone else. And vice versa. So you have to listen for the pain that signals an injury as well as for the indications that something is relieving the pain. No one can do it for you, because after you've been running for a while, no one will know your body as well as you do.

If something hurts, don't be afraid to try different cures. Your body will tell you if they are working or not. Just don't keep pushing your body onward if the pain persists or increases. Back down. It's better to miss a day of running now than it is to provoke a small injury into a big one. When in doubt, rest is the best cure for any pain, big or small.

SEX AND EXERCISE

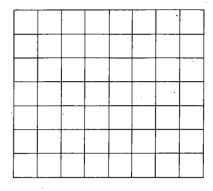

Ever wonder why ads for almost every product – from avocados to new cars with zebra-striped interiors – have a sexy lad or lass in them? Probably not. You know, as do the people who think up the ads, that sex is a basic drive. To attract, to love, to enjoy the sensations and intimacy of physical pleasure is one of the most desired of human experiences.

But how sexy we are – interested and interesting – depends on how healthy we are. A bad heart is likely to be lonely; a worn-out body uses the bed to sleep. But if poor health is a turn-off, good health is an aphrodisiac. And exercise fills you with the glow and energy of health.

Exercise whets our sexual appetite. It also whittles away the fat and torpor that block sexual fulfillment. And that's not just our opinion. When scientists turned their attention to the facts of life, they found that exercise was one of them.

Exercise is a potent medicine, one that riles up your hormones and rejuvenates your body—and your desires. But it may have some unexpected side effects.

Get Your Sex Drive into High Gear

John R. Sutton at McMaster University in Ontario, Canada, has found that blood levels of the male sex hormone testosterone tend to rise during periods of physical exertion. He studied highly conditioned Olympic oarsmen and swimmers as well as lesser-trained medical students. With the Olympians, sessions of extreme exertion produced more testosterone than workouts that were easy. And with the students, levels of the hormone reached a peak after 20 minutes of pedaling a stationary bicycle. In other words, production of testosterone seemed to vary according to each subject's particular degree of fitness, but in all cases it was "work" that triggered the goods.

Muscles store energy in the form of glycogen, and glycogen, studies have shown, keeps best in the company of testosterone. Scientists say the hormone may also help muscles to metabolize carbohydrates. Either way, a body that's active asks for more testosterone than one that is not. And it's testosterone that fuels the sex drive.

Studies show, too, that secretions of testosterone depend

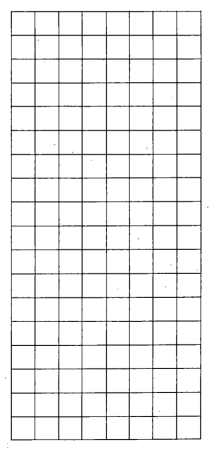

on the amount of blood that flows around the testes. Because the hormone is secreted directly through the testes walls, it needs good circulation to move it around. No blood, no testosterone. Like commuters waiting to board the 8:05 train, testosterone molecules get backed up, and it isn't long before the testes stop producing passengers. Exercise, by increasing blood flow, gives testosterone the lift it needs.

Fewer studies have been done with women, though one study done by researchers on women who were dieting showed that while female hormone levels dropped in those who ate less only, standards held constant in those who supplemented their reduced food intake with exercise.

Exercise Is Perfect for Two

Exercise is a potent medicine, one that riles up your hor-

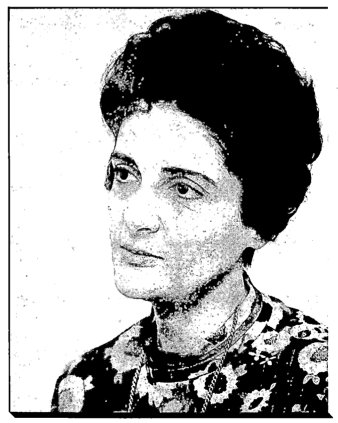

Dr. Domeena Renshaw, sex therapist.

mones and rejuvenates your body – and your desires. But that medicine may have some unexpected side effects.

For instance, if you start an exercise program, it's a good idea to urge your spouse to start one, too. Otherwise, you may set yourself up for sexual *problems.*

Domeena Renshaw, M.D., professor of psychiatry and director of the Sexual Dysfunction Clinic at Loyola University in Illinois, told us about a sexual disaster when a wife, but not a husband, started to jog.

"She reported that she felt invigorated and more interested in sex. But her renewed enthusiasm scared her husband off." The husband, says Dr. Renshaw, felt he couldn't keep up with his wife's newfound energy, so rather than risking failure and humiliation by not being able to perform as well as he thought his wife expected, he didn't (or couldn't) perform at all.

But husbands could scare off their wives, too. "Suppose a husband starts exercising and losing weight, looking better, and his wife does not," Dr. Renshaw explains. "The wife may find her husband's new, attractive, Don Juan image scary, and that will cause problems."

And once you've started your exercise program, you should keep it reasonable. As Dr. Renshaw points out, "Not tonight, dear, I have a headache," can easily be replaced by "Not tonight, dear, I'm tired from jogging."

"A lot of this depends on people's expectations, personalities and self-image. One partner starting a jogging program can be similar to one partner giving up smoking. The message is, 'Look at me – I'm good and you're bad.' It can turn into a threatening situation."

But the optimal situation is for *both* partners to exercise. That way, no one feels left out.

"We know of excellent situations where both husband and wife have started jogging together," Dr. Renshaw says. "They say that it makes them feel better and brings them closer together."

And being closer, in every way, is what sex is all about.

SHIATSU

The word *shiatsu* means "finger pressure" in Japanese. It is an effective Oriental therapy, similar to acupressure, that treats bodily ailments by using the palms and thumbs to press on the skin.

How effective is it? Shiatsu is effective enough to have converted Jerry Teplitz from a straightlaced lawyer into a shiatsu therapist who travels the country giving lectures and demonstrations of this traditional Japanese treatment. Mr. Teplitz started out as a doubter who soon found himself drawn to shiatsu as a way of life. And he finds that his lecture audiences are also strongly influenced by shiatsu's healing potential.

The toughest audience Mr. Teplitz has ever had to work with was inside a prison. "The prisoners didn't know who I was or why I was there or what on earth I was going to do," recalls Mr. Teplitz. "They were basically told they could either work or see my program, so they obviously chose me over work."

Later, there were moments on stage when he wished they hadn't. Usually, five minutes into his program, he would have nearly 100 percent audience participation as he instructed people how to use various techniques to relax or to energize their bodies. But the prison audience was problematic – restless, talkative, smoking, shuffling around and indifferent to his presence.

To make matters worse, in order to demonstrate shiatsu, Mr. Teplitz usually chooses someone from the audience who has a headache. Unknowingly, he picked a prison ringleader from the fidgety crowd.

"He sat down on stage, and I demonstrated the headache relief technique on him. When I got done, he said his headache was worse," laughs Mr. Teplitz, who still remembers the misery of the moment and his own discomfort. "I talked to him a little more and discovered he was having a migraine headache, which he gets all the time. So I did the shiatsu treatment for migraine on him, and his pain completely disappeared."

When Mr. Teplitz arrived at the meditation part of his program, he led the prisoners through a meditation exercise and lectured on the merits of meditating twice a day.

"I told them they needed to get up 20 minutes earlier in the morning to meditate. Then all of a sudden I began wondering – do they get woken up by bell? Are they allowed alarm clocks? Do they have 20 minutes?"

Positive Feedback

Before the prison performance, Mr. Teplitz always had been astonished by the success of his program. Whether he faced a crowd of college students, business executives or older adults, his program seemed to have something for everyone. Maybe an audience full of convicts was stretching his luck just a little too far. Then the prisoners' performance evaluation forms were turned over to him. To his surprise, the prisoners had written that they believed shiatsu and meditation would help them in their lives.

Subsequent feedback from prison staff members further boosted his spirits. "The monetary system of the prisoners is cigarettes," relates Mr. Teplitz. "A staff member told me that one prisoner earned two packs of cigarettes by doing shiatsu for another one's headache. And the toughest guy in the prison is a Muslim who carries a file folder with all of his prayers in it. Tucked within that folder is the shiatsu headache diagram I left with them," he says. "It was the toughest audience I ever went through, but there, too, it worked."

In Mr. Teplitz's program, audiences learn by doing different techniques used to relieve headaches, migraines, sore throats, sinus colds, eyestrain and neck fatigue. "It's a seed-planting profession," he says. "I'm planting the seed for people that they can heal themselves in a whole variety of ways. They've got more power and potential than they probably ever thought they had."

Mr. Teplitz admits he faces a roomful of skeptics at the beginning of every performance. He promises to pay $4 to anybody who comes to the demonstration and does not leave feeling more relaxed. "I've done the program now for about 100,000 people, and I've had only 3 people ask me for the $4," he adds.

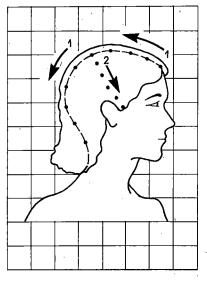

To relieve headaches, press points along arrow number 1. Then massage points along arrow number 2, pressing both sides of the head simultaneously.

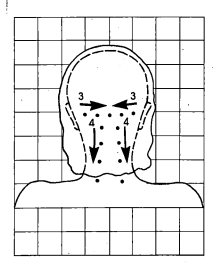

More headache relief can be had by pressing points along the number 3 direction and then pressing along the spine (number 4).

Ex-Lawyer, Ex-Skeptic

Actually, Mr. Teplitz admits he isn't anyone to quibble over skepticism, since he was the biggest skeptic of all when first introduced to what he does now.

"If you had asked me in law school if I could see myself doing this five years after I graduated, I would have thought you were crazy," he quips. "As a lawyer you are trained in skepticism and to tear things apart. I tried to tear these things apart. They wouldn't tear. The more I tried, the more I experienced, and the more excited I got."

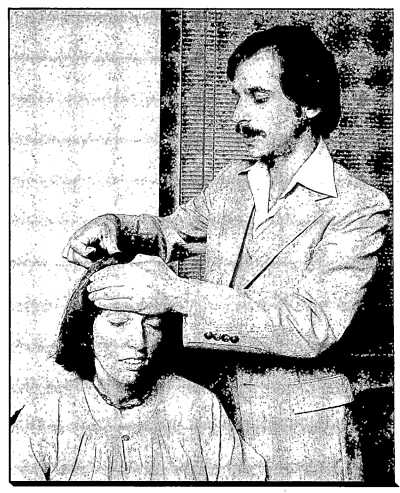

Jerry Teplitz pressing shiatsu points on the head.

Mr. Teplitz has written a book with Shelly Kellman entitled *How to Relax and Enjoy* (Japan Publications, 1977), which describes some shiatsu methods, hatha yoga exercises, general relaxation and meditation techniques and discusses proper nutrition. With several other books in the planning stages, he continues to lecture to groups around the United States and Canada. He claims that in as little as two hours he can teach people relaxation and energizing techniques that they will be able to use for the rest of their lives.

"You can use shiatsu on yourself as well as on other people," he explains. "My goal is to make people self-

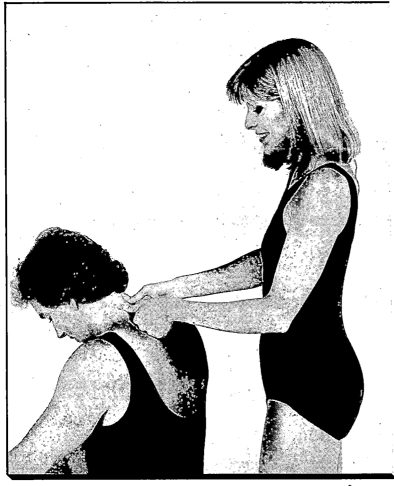

Shiatsu technique employs the thumbs.

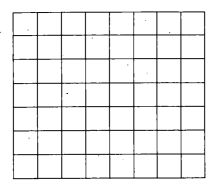

Mr. Teplitz reports that shiatsu can vanquish headaches and hangovers in as little as a minute and a half.

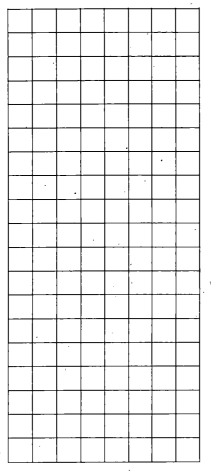

sufficient. My real purpose in doing a lot of this actually is to put me out of business. That will mean everybody is running around healthy because they know how to do these things. They will be practicing shiatsu, meditation and good nutrition and will be feeling a lot better as a result."

Shiatsu is an ancient therapy that is older than Japan's recorded history. Practitioners wanting to relieve a headache use the fleshy part of their thumbs to bear down on a series of pressure points along the skull and the back of the neck. Mr. Teplitz reports that headaches and hangovers can be relieved in as little as a minute and a half. In some cases, a third treatment is necessary to alleviate all pain. "Of course, if anyone has an ongoing problem, I recommend seeing a doctor," he adds. "The individual should look at what is going on in his or her environment. Something is really pretty intense either physiologically or externally that needs treating."

But for ordinary ailments, shiatsu is quite effective, says Mr. Teplitz, although no one really knows why. "There are several theories," he continues. The hard pressure exerted by the thumbs may cause extra blood to circulate through the painful area. The blood acts as the natural cleanser of the body, bringing antibodies and oxygen to the area and removing waste products and carbon dioxide, he says. A second possibility is that shiatsu may act like acupuncture, stimulating certain nerve meridians and motivating the body to heal itself. Others suggest that when pressure is put on the head, natural substances called endorphins are released in the brain. Endorphins act as pain inhibitors, which block the pain signal throughout the body. Another theory is based on the physics concept that every action has an equal and opposite reaction. "With a hangover a person has restricted blood vessels," adds Jerry. "The shiatsu pressure may cause the blood vessels to expand and relieve the pain."

Whatever the scientific explanation may be, Mr. Teplitz says that shiatsu often works as long as people follow directions. "When people work on the neck area, we tell them they must not press directly on the spine. Instead, the pressure is placed on both sides of the spinal column. Also, the practitioner instructs the person to say 'ouch' whenever pain is felt during a treatment. At that point, the practitioner leaves that area and continues with the treatment," he explains. When the practitioner returns to the pain point, he presses gently at first and then gradually presses harder. "You'll either be able to get more pressure on before they say 'ouch' again, or in many cases, the pain has just disappeared completely."

Shiatsu practitioners are told to press no more than three seconds when working in areas of the neck and above. They press no more than seven seconds on each area below the neck, says Mr. Teplitz.

Although he has worked with the therapy for several years now, Mr. Teplitz still is surprised at times by its effectiveness. He relates the story of a friend with wisdom teeth problems who called him long distance for help. He was in intense pain, but his dentist could not see him for

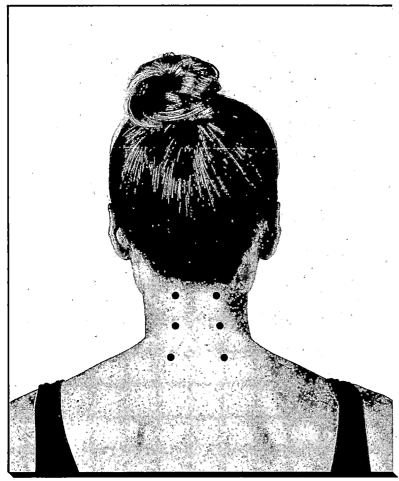

Press these shiatsu points for headache relief.

several weeks, says Mr. Teplitz, so "I proceeded to give him instructions for the shiatsu treatment for toothache over the phone. I saw him a few months later, and he said not only did it work, but after several treatments the pain completely vanished. He still had to go to the dentist, but he was totally painless to the point of going."

In the case of toothache, shiatsu may provide three or four hours of pain relief. When the pain returns, all the person may need to do is to repeat the shiatsu treatment. "Shiatsu is a good alternative to aspirin and to the negative effects of any chemical on the body," Mr. Teplitz asserts.

Dressed in a blue three-piece suit, Mr. Teplitz may still look like an attorney on his way to court, but "Exhibit A" for his presentation is a diagram of a shiatsu technique. Conducting a small workshop in Washington, D.C., he illustrated for us how companies can help their employees to help themselves. He demonstrated shiatsu on a woman in the group who had complained of having a severe headache before the program began. "I thought, am I going to make it to this meeting or not?" she mused. After getting relief through Mr. Teplitz's therapy, she announced with amazement, "I really feel great. It's gone! It was really making me sick."

What people like this woman also find is that shiatsu, when shared among family and friends, brings people closer together. It's a nonthreatening way of touching those close to you while making them feel better at the same time.

SLEEP

Ever turn off your car only to find that it *won't* turn off? It coughs, sputters, shakes, rattles and rolls, and won't stop. That reaction is known as dieseling, and it's caused by bad gasoline and/or a bad tune-up job on your engine. Leftover fuel in the cylinders keeps igniting, making your car chug like an old jalopy.

Your body can do the same thing. You get into bed, turn off the light, close your eyes . . . but sleep won't come. The events of the day run through your mind. You toss and turn and feel aggravated. Your body just won't turn off. And the more you try to sleep, the further away sleep recedes.

Well, the answer to your body's dieseling problem may be similar to your car's – better fuel and a better tune-up. In your body's case, this translates into the right kind of food and relaxation. First, let's take a look at the food you've been pumping into your body's engine.

Asleep at the Meal

Alice Kuhn Schwartz, Ph.D., is a former insomniac – and also a sleep therapist, a type of psychologist who helps other people overcome insomnia. Part of her therapeutic program involves putting into practice the results of current laboratory research on how what we eat can change what happens inside our brain and, in turn, our sleep.

Dr. Schwartz has identified five different types of insomnia; they include short sleep; very light sleep; dream-troubled sleep; and waking up and not being able to fall back to sleep. "But," she says, "by far the most common type of insomnia is what I call 'initardia,' which is simply difficulty in falling asleep in the first place. If you suffer from initardia, eating the proper foods can be quite important. But it's not only that. You also have to eat the right foods at the right time."

What might the right foods be? "Basically," says Dr. Schwartz, "there are two different kinds. First, foods that are high in the essential amino acid tryptophan. As you know, amino acids are the basic building blocks of protein.

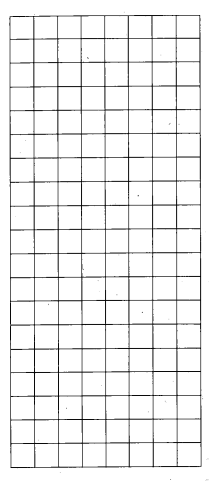

What we eat can change what's going on inside our brain and affect our sleep.

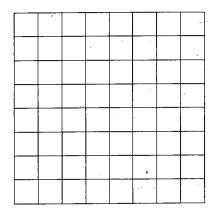

415

Eggs, almost any meat, certain fish such as salmon or bluefish, and dairy products, especially cottage cheese – all of those protein-rich foods have a hefty amount of tryptophan, and tryptophan has been shown in the lab to increase drowsiness and help bring on sleep.

"But," says Dr. Schwartz, "there is a second type of food you should eat as well. You see, in addition to tryptophan, there are many other amino acids. Once these different amino acids get into the bloodstream, they compete with each other for entry to the brain. For someone who wants to get to sleep, the trick is to give tryptophan a competitive edge."

Rather like fixing a horse race, we mused. And how do we give tryptophan the edge? "It's really quite simple," she says. "Animal studies have shown that eating carbohydrate foods – those that are starchy or sweet – liberates tryptophan and gives it greater access to the brain. In fact, the tryptophan in food is hardly used at all by the brain unless a carbohydrate is also eaten, or, interestingly, a food with a carbohydrate-fat combination.

"The implications of this are fascinating," she explains. "If you've been eating high-protein, high-tryptophan foods during the day, and you want to fall asleep at night, then it may help to eat some bread, have a banana, drink some grape or apple juice, have some figs or dates – all of those high-carbohydrate foods and many others will help activate tryptophan."

Dr. Schwartz explains further that it's important to eat your carbohydrate food two to four hours before bedtime so that the food will reach its peak effect when you are ready to retire. On the other hand, if your problem is frequent awakenings during the night – quite a common complaint after the age of 40 – or short sleep periods, or light sleep, you should eat your carbohydrate immediately before "lights out." Since falling asleep in the first place is not your problem, you will want your carbohydrates to operate at top efficiency after you have been asleep for a few hours.

"In any case," concludes Dr. Schwartz, "if you tend to fall asleep during the day or early evening, you must try to eliminate carbohydrates during the day. If you usually eat dessert after your evening meal, you should defer your dessert until the time appropriate to your particular sleep problem."

We could not resist asking Dr. Schwartz one final, burning question: if you wake up in the middle of the night, is it too late to eat your granola cookies? "Indeed, it is," replied

Dr. Schwartz. "There is a small child in all of us, and if that child gets used to waking up every night expecting to be 'rewarded' with cookies or something sweet, it will become a habit. If you wake up in the night and cannot get back to sleep in a half hour, I recommend getting out of bed and performing some boring, routine task until you feel sleepy."

Rewiring Your Nervous System

Now let's turn away from an examination of the fuel in your gas tank and take a look under your hood. Since your body's engine ignites after you try to turn it off, the problem might be in the ignition's wiring – otherwise known as your nervous system.

A good way to check that is to measure the "voltage," or amount of activity, in your autonomic nervous system, the part of you that controls involuntary functions like heartbeat and breathing. Well, when scientists measure the nervous systems of insomniacs, they usually find enough voltage to light up the Christmas tree on the White House lawn.

"Many poor sleepers are more aroused than good sleepers," writes Northwestern University sleep specialist Richard R. Bootzin, Ph.D., in a recent survey of sleep research. "Poor sleepers [have] higher rectal temperatures, higher skin resistance, more vasoconstrictions [narrowing of blood vessels] per minute and more body movements per hour than good sleepers," says Dr. Bootzin in *Progress in Behavior Modification* (vol. 6, Academic Press, 1978). All of those symptoms mean that the insomniac's autonomic nervous system is preparing him perfectly for dodging rush-hour traffic – but not for sleep. If he can put his autonomic nervous system to sleep, the theory goes, the rest of him should follow, according to Dr. Bootzin.

And one way to calm down the autonomic nervous system is "progressive relaxation." Originated in the early 1900s by physiologist Edmund Jacobson, progressive relaxation or variations of it are still widely taught. One of these variations has been evaluated by Thomas D. Borkovec, Ph.D., a psychologist at Penn State University.

"We have the person start with the muscles of one hand, making a fist, holding it for seven seconds, and then relaxing it," says Dr. Borkovec, who teaches four-week and nine-week courses in relaxation.

"We ask the individual to learn to identify what both

tension and relaxation feel like so that he will be able to detect tension when trying to fall asleep. After sufficient practice, most people are able to deeply relax themselves within five minutes."

His students gradually learn to relax 16 of the body's muscle groups, Dr. Borkovec says. They also inhale when they tense their muscles, then exhale and relax very slowly (for about 45 seconds). That is good therapy for people whose main problem is falling asleep, and its effect improves with practice, Dr. Borkovec says.

Proper breathing, just by itself, is another way to reassure the autonomic nervous system that it can tone down for the night. In one experiment in 1976, volunteers were asked to "focus passively on the physical sensations associated with their breathing and to repeat the mantra [a word or image to fix the mind on] 'in' and 'out' silently." Results indicated that this technique is as effective as progressive relaxation.

"Breathe through Your Fingertips"

Other fine points of breathing to relax are described by psychologist Beata Jencks Ph.D., in her book *Your Body: Biofeedback at Its Best* (Nelson-Hall, 1977).

"Imagine inhaling through your fingertips," Dr. Jencks writes, "up the arms into the shoulders, and then exhaling down the trunk into the abdomen and legs, and leisurely out at the toes. Repeat, and feel how this slow, deep breathing affects the whole body, the abdomen, the flanks and the chest. Do not move the shoulders while you breathe.

To inhale deeply, Dr. Jencks advises, pretend to inhale the fragrance of the first flower in spring, or imagine that your breathing rises and falls like ocean waves, or that the surface area of your lungs – if laid out flat – would cover a tennis court. That's how much air you should feel yourself taking in, she says.

Sleep-inducing imagery can accompany breathing exercises, and your choice of images doesn't have to be limited to the traditional sheep leaping over a split-rail fence. Any image that you personally associate with feelings of peace or contentment will work well.

One sleep researcher, Quentin Regestein, M.D., director of the sleep clinic at Brigham and Women's Hospital in Boston, says that one of his patients imagines a huge sculpture of the numeral 1, hewn out of marble, with ivy growing over it, surrounded by a pleasant rural landscape. Then she goes on to the numeral 2 and adds further embellishment, such as cherubs hovering above the numeral. "She tells me that she usually falls asleep before she reaches 50," Dr. Regestein says.

"Insomniacs come here from all over the world," he continues, "and ask me to prescribe a sleep cure for them. They are sometimes surprised to find that careful scientific investigation substantiates that commonsense remedies really work."

Heaviness and Warmth

Autogenic training is another natural and potent sleep aid. This technique acts on the premise that your mind can compel your body to relax by concentrating on feelings of heaviness and warmth. Through mental suggestion, the "heavy" muscles actually do relax, and the "warm" flesh receives better circulation, resulting in "a state of low physiological arousal," says Dr. Bootzin.

In an experiment in 1968, researchers taught 16 college-student insomniacs to focus their attention on warmth and heaviness. At the end of the experiment, the students had cut their average time needed to fall asleep down from 52 to 22 minutes. These results matched the findings made by Dr. Bootzin in the Chicago area in 1974: "Daily practice of either progressive relaxation or autogenic training produced 50 percent improvement in time needed to fall asleep by the end of the one-month treatment period."

A Raggedy Ann doll, says Dr. Jencks, is one image that can facilitate autogenic training. To feel heavy, she says, "make yourself comfortable and allow your eyes to close. Then lift one arm a little and let it drop. Let it drop heavily, as if it were the arm of one of those floppy dolls or animals. Choose one in your imagination. Choose a doll, an old, beloved, soft teddy bear." Once the mind fixes on the doll's image, Dr. Jencks says, lifting and dropping the arm in your imagination works as well as really letting it drop.

To invoke feelings of warmth, Dr. Jencks adds, "imagine that you put your rag doll into the sun. Let it be warmed by the sun. . . . You are the giant rag doll, and you are lying in the sun; all your limbs are nice and warm, but your head is lying in the shade and is comfortably cool."

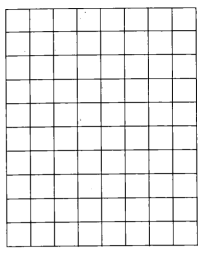

Autogenic training is a natural and potent sleep aid. It teaches your mind to relax your body through feelings of heaviness and warmth.

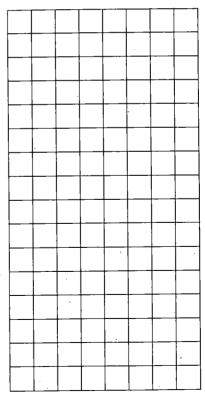

A Good Suggestion

Rituals also play a role in falling asleep. Dr. Regestein told us that when dogs go to sleep, they always sniff around for a warm and comfortable spot, circle it and finally coil up in their favorite sleeping position. People are a bit like this, he says. They fall asleep most easily when they proceed through a nightly ritual – flossing their teeth, for example, and then curling into their favorite sleeping position. In support of that theory, researchers in 1930 found that children who assumed a particular posture when going to bed fell asleep faster.

The last but not the least effective route to immediate relaxation is sexual activity. Dr. Schwartz says that sex "alleviates tension. It is a powerful soporific. And what is more, it's fun. . . . The road to sleep branches into other byways. Explore all of them."

Finally, if none of the above techniques seem to work for you, there are several changes in daily habits that can, with practice, help you to fall asleep a lot faster in the future. Here are some hints that many sleep researchers recommend:

- Go to sleep and wake up at regular hours.
- Go to bed only when sleepy.
- Don't nap during the day.
- Use your bed only for sleeping and sex; don't read, eat or watch TV in bed.
- Keep your bedroom fairly cool.

If the inability to fall asleep becomes a chronic problem, the researchers suggest that you inspect other aspects of your life and behavior. Anything that can raise your blood pressure will keep you up. A constant state of tension over finances can do that; so can the habit of bottling up all kinds of emotions.

Two studies conducted by a team of researchers at the Penn State University Sleep Research and Treatment Center in Hershey, Pennsylvania, suggest that cigarette smoking is associated with insomnia and that quitting improves sleep within days after the last pack is thrown away (*Science,* February, 1980).

If, however, your lifestyle doesn't include any violations of those rules, then any serious attempt to relax – by tensing and releasing the muscles, by deep breathing, by imagining yourself on a tropical isle, by self-hypnosis or by any mixture of the above – ought to soothe your autonomic nervous system and help you slip into restful sleep.

Tucker Yourself Out and Tuck Yourself In

There's one last tip we can give you to help you fall asleep – get tired! Seem a little too simple to be helpful? It's not – the right kind of wear-yourself-out exercise done at the right time can make you fall asleep faster. But there's a catch. The wrong kind of exercise at the wrong time will probably keep you awake.

Remember, there are basically two different kinds of exercise – dynamic and static. Dynamic is the kind that gets you moving, like running, bicycling or swimming. Static exercise is the weightlifting kind, where you move something heavy or do isometric types of muscle contractions. You expend a lot of effort but don't get too much movement.

If you run ten miles just before bedtime, you'll get tired, but chances are you won't fall asleep easily. Although you're fatigued, a dynamic exercise like running has a *mental* arousal effect that'll keep you up.

So if you want to do exercise just before bed, try the static variety. Do some barbell curls or isometrics; the sandman should show up soon.

As for dynamic exercise, try that in the afternoon. The time between the exercise and your bedtime lets the mental arousal dissipate while the fatigue from the exertion settles in.

Sweet dreams!

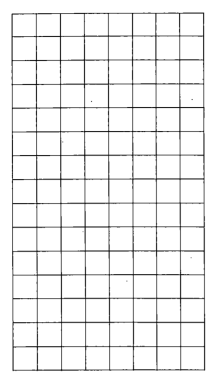

Sometimes the natural healing process needs a boost. Then there's need for an outside healing force, or at least advice on how to speed the natural healing process.

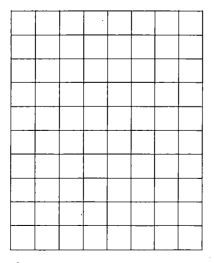

SPINAL MANIPULATION

by Robert Rodale

If you are like me, there are times when your body won't carry you as far as you'd like to go – at least not without complaining more than you think it should. In my case, these hurts usually spring from overexertion. I love to walk, ride a bike, dig, saw wood and do other outdoor work. In moderation, such activity is totally beneficial. But every once in a while I find myself caught up beyond all logic in the good feeling of being active and end up with a persistent ache or pain.

Most of these "pain events" are very slight irritations, and as the doctors say, they are self-limiting. That means they go away by themselves, without the use of any medication or treatment, especially if the afflicted part is allowed to rest. The body has tremendous recuperative powers. Sometimes, though, the natural healing process needs a boost. Some injuries and strains to the body's framework are too serious to be left just to time. There is need for a healing force applied from outside, or at the very least informed guidance on the best ways to help speed the natural healing process.

Manipulation: The Healing Force

Manipulation is one excellent answer to many of these painful problems. A medical book on manipulation calls the therapy a "passive movement with therapeutic purpose using the hands." That definition refers mainly to the kind of manipulation of the spine and joints done by chiropractors, osteopaths and those few MDs and physical therapists who have been trained in pressing and pulling the body back into shape. I would go further and call any kind of pressure and reconstructive force manipulation; that is, such things as traction (pulling), certain kinds of bandaging, the use of braces and arch supports, deep friction massage and even the application of heat and cold. The prescribing of pain-killing drugs and muscle relaxants is an approach entirely opposite to that of manipulation. A major purpose of this hands-on technique against pain is to avoid drugs which can have serious side effects. Drugs also seldom get to the root of the problem. The whole idea of manipulation is to find a spot in the body which has become misaligned (or cramped), reach it physically in therapeutic ways, and thereby allow normal activity to resume as quickly as possible.

The spine is the most frequently manipulated part of the body, and for good reason. The backbone is central to many aspects of health and well-being, and it is made up of many small bones (vertebrae) that can slip out of position. It also has numerous discs between these bones that can become compressed or even herniated. Whenever heavy work is done, the spine bears much of the stress and pressure. The many large muscles of the back that connect to the spinal area are also an important part of the picture, as are nerves, ligaments and other kinds of connective tissue.

I'd like to talk to you specifically about medical manipulation, which is somewhat different from that done by chiropractors and osteopaths. While the chiropractor usually manipulates to align the vertebrae properly, the orthopedic manipulator tries to stretch the supporting tissue of the joints. MDs actually use traction much more than strict manipulation. Sometimes the pull applied – during a neck manipulation, for instance – is well over 200 pounds.

Obviously, this technique is not something you can always do for or to yourself. You need a doctor's diagnosis and care – and sometimes also the skill of a physical therapist. But there is at least one kind of manipulation that you can continue at home once it's prescribed by a physician and you're given the proper instruction. Let me describe it through my own experience with the technique.

One Tree Too Many

"You ought to write something about woodcutters' injuries."

My friend Tom Dickson, an orthopedic surgeon, said that to me last winter. The wood-burning season was in full swing, and a parade of walking wounded was passing through his office.

"I'm seeing some pretty bad cases," he continued. "One man had a piece of steel from a broken splitting wedge in his leg. It was the size of a .38 slug. A woman broke two fingers trying to hold onto an ax that twisted when it hit a tree. It's an epidemic."

I was thinking of those unfortunate people a few days later when I went out into my small woodlot to cut down 25 pine trees that were crowding each other. No splitting wedges for me, though. And no axes to twist in my hands, either. Just a Scandinavian bow saw, which I thought was as safe as safe could be.

What wasn't safe, though, was the large number of trees. After felling about ten, I realized that I was tackling too much and quit. But the damage had been done. That night I experienced a type of pain that was entirely new to me. When I turned on my side, after having slept flat on my back for several hours, a sharp pain flashed under my right shoulder blade, not far from the center of my back. That was it – just the one burst. The rest of the night I felt okay. But the next day, the pain came back.

"It will go away," I said to myself. All other pains I ever got from working too hard had passed. This one would, too. But it didn't. In fact, it got progressively worse. After about six weeks of waiting it out, my right arm hurt so much that I couldn't do much more than turn the pages of a book.

There was nothing to do but to see Dr. Dickson and tell him that I had acquired my own personal woodcutters' injury. "You may have bursitis," he said first off. But then he felt around my shoulder and could find no tender spots. "There's a possibility the problem is in your neck. I'll need an X-ray to find out for sure."

Now, Dr. Dickson knows that I like X-rays as much as I would enjoy living next to a nuclear power plant. So, he promised that only one exposure would be needed to see whether something happening in my neck could be causing the persistent shoulder and arm pain. I finally said okay, reasoning that in cases where there might be a specific injury, the use of X-rays in moderation made sense.

"Here could be your trouble," he said a few minutes later, pointing to the X-ray of my neck. "There should be space between the vertebrae, but *these* two are too close." What Dr. Dickson was showing me was a classic case of a compressed cervical disc. The word "cervical" refers to the neck area. Discs are soft-tissue bodies that provide padding between the vertebrae. When healthy and full-sized, they space out the bones properly, cushioning the nerves, blood vessels and muscle tissue that service the spine. When there is too much spinal stress or pressure, one or more discs can become compressed. That puts pressure on the nerves extending from the spinal cord to other parts of the body. Pain can result in the area to which these pinched nerves extend.

"How did that happen?" I asked. What puzzled me was the connection between a squeezed disc in my neck and a sore shoulder caused by sawing too much wood too fast. Maybe, I thought, the two weren't related at all.

"A compressed disc in the neck can be caused by many different kinds of injuries, or blows to the head or neck," Tom said. "Whiplash from a car accident can do it. I see it in rugby players, who push each other with their heads. Maybe it comes from sleeping with too thick a pillow or sleeping on your stomach. Both are bad."

Bending the head forward, Dr. Dickson continued, naturally puts more pressure on that area of the disc, which is the part usually squeezed. Any posture which causes the head to hang forward for long periods also may put too much pressure on those discs. One doctor has said that secretaries often get cervical disc problems, because they work all day long looking down at their typewriters. A fall forward, stopped by your hands, causes your head to snap to the front. That could do it, some doctors believe. I have a large head, which could make me more vulnerable to disc strain than someone with a small hat size.

"Seeing a compressed disc like this on an X-ray isn't proof that it's causing a problem," Dr. Dickson explained to me. "Sometimes we X-ray the neck of a person who has been in an auto accident and find several old degenerated discs. Yet they say they never had any pain before the accident."

All the time these facts about discs were being explained to me, I was doing some low-key worrying about the treatment that would be suggested.

"I used to operate on cases like yours," Dr. Dickson told me.

Those words "used to" were comforting.

"Then I found out about what could be done with home traction. In fact, in the seven years I've been prescribing traction at home, I haven't done a single cervical disc operation."

Stand Up (or Sit Down) to Neck Pain

The home traction apparatus Dr. Dickson prescribed cost me $19 and was simple to use. It consists of a pulley arrangement that fits over a door, a length of rope, a plastic bag, and a harness that fits under the chin and around the back of the head. When everything is put together and water placed in the bag, enough upward pull is exerted on the head to stretch the cervical spine and relieve the pressure on the disc.

"Put 10 to 15 pounds of water in the bag at first," Dr. Dickson told me. "Give yourself 20 minutes of traction twice a day, morning and evening. You can read to make the time go faster. And every week add two more pounds of weight, until you feel it's enough."

"How much do you think will be enough?" I asked. I had visions of turning into something like one of those native African ladies with a neck a foot long.

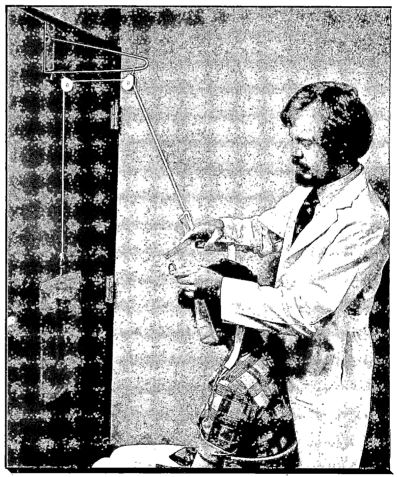

Dr. Dickson's home traction apparatus.

"One patient of mine, a rugby player, went up to 35 pounds," Dr. Dickson said.

As it turned out, 25 pounds was enough to do the job for me. Since I started at 10, and added 15 more, the course of treatment lasted seven weeks. I found that traction was not exactly fun but not unpleasant, either. The harness does irritate your chin somewhat, but the pulling sensation is vaguely pleasant. I had time to reflect on all those years that my heavy head was bearing down on those cushiony neck discs and the relief traction was bringing.

More Flexibility

Two conditions besides my woodchopping pain also cleared during the weeks of traction. For several years I had not been able to turn my head to the right as far as I could turn it to the left. There was no pain, but I had noticed that when sitting by a window on the right side of an airplane, I had difficulty turning to look out. After a couple of weeks of traction, I could turn my head easily in both directions.

My other unexpected benefit of traction was the disappearance of some finger tingling. People with a cervical disc problem often feel pain in the shoulder area, like mine, and a tingling in the fingers. Once I read this fact in the medical literature, I recalled that I had had such a sensation in my right hand, but, like the neck stiffness, it cleared up after several weeks of traction.

Other Pains Respond to Traction

There is a good possibility that pressure on cervical discs can also be the cause of headache, particularly the persistent kind. That theory was put forth by Murray M. Braaf, M.D., and Samuel Rosner, M.D., in the *Journal of Trauma* (May, 1975). In it, they described their work with over 6,000 cases of chronic headache, a large proportion of which they could trace to cervical spine injury.

Dr. Braaf, in a recent phone conversation, told me that people with strong necks have less of a problem with headache from that cause but that a wide variety of injuries can lead to persistent headache problems. Sometimes the injury occurs many years before the headache problem starts.

Dr. Braaf and Dr. Rosner feel that headaches which originate in neck strain are caused by a more complex

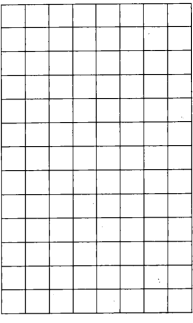

People with a cervical disc problem often feel shoulder pain and tingling in the fingers. It may also be the cause of persistent headaches.

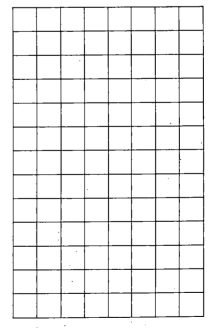

series of events than the pinching of a nerve, the common explanation for the problem. They point out that compression of the vertebral artery, "even on an intermittent basis," can cause partial restriction of blood flow to the head. That can cause pain and other symptoms, especially dizziness. Another possibility is that a pinching of the nerves in the neck somehow affects the nerves serving the head.

Whatever their causes, the usefulness of traction in relieving these problems is clear. Except in very serious cases, the affected nerves are not actually damaged. They are merely pressed. So, pulling on the head in a regular and systematic way gradually separates the vertebrae slightly and relieves the pressure. However, traction treatment is not a permanent cure for the problem in most people. Dr. Dickson told me, "Don't forget where you put your apparatus after you're finished with it. You may need it again in a year or two." Apparently, a compressed disc never returns to its original shape and strength.

Take Your Traction Lying Down

There is some controversy about which method of applying traction is best. Dr. Braaf says cervical traction, to be effective, must be carried out with the patient lying down on his or her back. He feels that traction applied when a person is sitting up "doesn't pull in the right direction." The sitting position is less comfortable, he says, and the patient can't tolerate appropriate amounts of pull in it. However, Dr. Braaf recommends just 5 to 15 pounds of pull, and my experience with traction proves that a patient can accept a good deal more pull while seated.

People who want to take their traction lying down can do so at home, but it is cheaper and easier to use the upright, over-the-door method I tried. As I said before, the discomfort was tolerable, especially considering the relief from pain which traction provided me.

Can the kind of neck problems I've been describing be prevented? I asked that question of Dr. Dickson.

"There is no way to prevent them that I know about," he told me. But at the same time he gave me an instruction sheet listing exercises that are useful in cases of cervical strain and some "helpful hints for a healthy neck." They included instructions to sit straight in your chair instead of slouching, not sleeping on your stomach, and using a thin

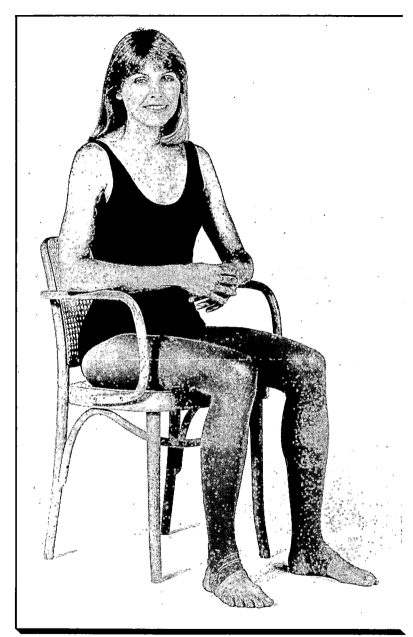

The correct sitting position – back straight, feet flat on the floor.

pillow placed under your neck instead of your head. Special pillows are sold that support the neck instead of the head, but Dr. Dickson was less than enthusiastic about them.

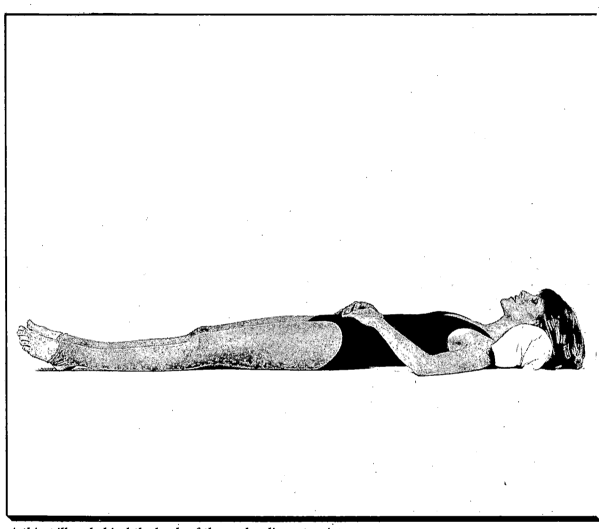

A thin pillow behind the back of the neck relieves tension.

A Three-Step Program

One doctor who feels that it is possible to prevent and greatly reduce cervical disc problems is James Greenwood, Jr., M.D., chief of neurosurgery at Methodist Hospital in Houston. He has a three-step program. The first is mild exercise, which builds neck strength; swimming is a good example. Dr. Greenwood also believes that gentle exercise helps to get the nutrients needed to prevent degeneration and aid self-repair to the joints and discs. Supplementary amounts of vitamin C in the range of two to three grams daily are a part of his program. Finally, he recommends weight control, which is certainly a good idea in any case.

STRETCHING

Do you remember a time when you had to reach out and *stretch* to get things done? We're not talking about major tasks; we mean the little things. The push lawn mower is long gone, of course, but until recently you still had to bend over and pull the cord to start the gas models. Now an electric starter up on the handle eliminates even that minimal effort.

You once had to roll car windows up and down by hand, but that's not always the case any longer. One switch at the driver's armrest closes all four windows at once, and another locks the doors. At one time it was impossible to watch TV without actually walking to the set, bending over and flicking it on.

Everyone knows that exercise is vital for healthy living. The push-button age not only discourages major efforts like running but eliminates less strenuous, though just as important, exercise as well. Even the smallest stretching movement can be avoided today. Without regular stretching of tight, tense muscles, real fitness is impossible.

Most of the things we regard as exercise primarily involve muscle contraction. The muscles manipulated in most sports are repeatedly tensed up, pulled shorter, by the activity. That's exactly what you have to do to muscles if your intent is to make them stronger.

But if you want to maintain the muscle flexibility you need, not just to run marathons but to stay active and comfortable into your later years, you have to *stretch* muscles as well as contract them. Most people are not even aware how flexible their joints can be, because their muscles are not loose enough to allow them the fullest possible range of movement.

If you want to maintain the muscle flexibility you need to stay active and comfortable into your later years, you have to stretch muscles as well as contract them.

Flexible Muscles Influence Arthritic Stiffness

Joint stiffness, an affliction common to aging, is probably more a problem of muscles and connective tissues than of the joints themselves. Experiments at Johns Hopkins Medical School with the wrists of cats found that the most important factors in flexibility are the muscles, the tendons and the capsule of tissue enclosing the joint. The scientists found that the friction generated by the rubbing at the joint itself was a minor factor limiting movement of the wrist. *That was true even in joints afflicted with arthritis.*

So, to increase the flexibility of the joints, you have to work mainly with the muscles and connective tissue. Pliable muscles, tendons and ligaments would make for flexible joints.

But ligaments, the tissues which hold bones together, and tendons, which attach muscles to bones, are both inflexible, inelastic tissues. A ligament or tendon stretched beyond its rather meager limits will not return to its original length. It doesn't bounce back as it should. The joint it holds together becomes too loose and prone to injury.

That leaves the muscles. Muscles are much more elastic than tendons and ligaments. A muscle repeatedly and properly stretched continues to bounce back, but it bounces back to a longer resting shape. Since the muscle is meant to move the frame rather than to hold it together, this is all for the good. A properly stretched set of muscles means maximum freedom of movement.

There are other benefits. Many scientists believe that aging muscles, or muscles deprived of exercise, go through a progressive shortening. It's not simply a matter of unstretched muscles staying too short. The muscles *actually* grow shorter the longer they are neglected. *As the muscles grow shorter, they put more and more pressure on the nerves running through the muscle sheaths.* That, some scientists think, may be behind the mysterious muscle aches and pains that commonly afflict older people.

The Splinting Reflex

It becomes a vicious circle. Whenever muscle pain occurs, it sets off a "splinting reflex" in the muscle. The splinting reflex causes the muscle to stiffen for protection. The muscle forms a rigid, natural splint, for the same reasons a doctor uses a splint on a broken leg.

When shortened, muscles set off the splinting reflex, however, the contraction of the muscles tightens pinched nerves even more, and the pain increases. The contraction of the muscles increases until they are knotted up in an uncontrollable spasm people experience with lower back pain.

Herbert A. deVries, Ph.D., of the University of Southern California, describes tests he made of this phenomenon in his book *Vigor Regained* (Prentice-Hall, 1974). Dr. deVries and his colleagues measured the electrical activity present in the muscles of injured athletes. A normal muscle, completely relaxed, shows no electrical activity, while a muscle in spasm, or tensed with pain, does.

Dr. deVries put his injured athletes through a program of special stretching exercises. In almost all cases, the stretching produced a sharp drop in the electrical activity of the muscle as well as partial to complete relief of the muscle pain. Stretching seemed to break the cycle of pain, muscle contraction, and still more pain.

Stretching for muscle flexibility, Dr. deVries believes, is invaluable for older people. "It appears to me," he writes, "that the best insurance (probably the only insurance) against the aches and pains that so often accompany the aging process . . . is that of maintaining an optimum level of physical fitness with appropriate emphasis on improvement of joint mobility."

Stretching is also important for people suffering from arthritis. Stretching muscles at arthritic joints several times a day has been shown to be very helpful in preventing permanent stiffness.

Stretch Gently—Don't Bounce

Many people think that they're stretching their muscles when they go through the bouncy, calisthenic exercises like touching your toes. You bounce down quickly to touch your toes, then pop back up into a standing position. But that bounce is what causes problems. Whenever a muscle is stretched too quickly or with too much force, the splinting reflex is set off.

You meet the same kind of resistance when you stretch in a standing position. Muscles in your legs hold your body up by contracting. Stretching leg muscles in a standing position is not as effective as stretching while lying down or sitting, because you're again working against contracted muscles.

Ben E. Benjamin, Ph.D., author of the book *Sports Without Pain* (Summit Books, 1979), emphasizes that the best way to stretch is to ease yourself into the stretch position. Stretching is a gentle, conditioning exercise. Relaxation is very important. Once you have extended your muscles as far as they want to go, *don't force them any farther.* Just keep breathing normally and hold the position for 10 to 15 seconds. Next time you might stretch farther and hold the position longer.

"You must be able to tell where the action is happening," Dr. Benjamin writes. "Pay attention to precisely where the pulling sensation is. You should feel the pull in the meaty part of the muscle. If the sensation is felt near a joint only, you are stretching the ligament or tendon. Always try to do the exercise so that you feel it throughout the bulk of the muscle."

Dr. Benjamin says that the best time to stretch is after a warm-up. Warm muscles, surging with blood, are more pliable than cold muscles. A common mistake, Dr. Benjamin told us, is that "people confuse warming up with stretching. They do stretching exercises to warm up when they should be doing it the other way around. Stretching is not really a good way to warm up. It's good for cooling down after exercise." Both Dr. Benjamin and Dr. deVries recommend that stretching be done at the end of an exercise routine.

The muscles which probably need the most stretching are those in the lower part of the body. Muscles in the legs and lower back are almost constantly in use during the day, holding us erect. Because of that constant contraction, they are more susceptible to shortening and tightness.

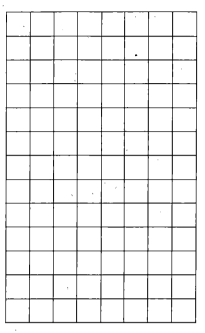

The best time to stretch is after a warm-up. Warm muscles, surging with blood, are more pliable than cold muscles.

Stay in Touch with Your Body

According to Bob Anderson, a stretching expert who has tutored professional sports teams on the art of stretching and has authored the book *Stretching* (Shelter Publications, 1980), you should "learn to stretch by *feeling*. Be aware of the daily fluctuations in muscle tension and tightness so you can adjust your stretches to meet your body's changing state. Some days you will be more limber than others, but as long as you work by feel you will be able to enjoy the process.

"You can stretch to varying degrees, ranging from comfortable to easy to developmental. The length of time you hold a stretch will vary, too, from 5 to 60 seconds. A comfortable, painless stretch should be held long enough for the muscle tissues to adapt naturally to the slightly elongated positions.

"In an easy stretch, you feel just a slight tension. Hold this easy stretch for 5 to 30 seconds, depending on which stretch exercise you are doing. If the feeling of tension

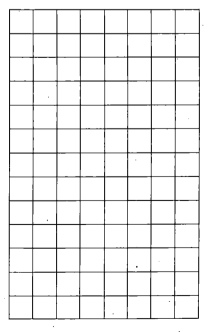

increases or becomes painful, you are overstretching. Ease off slightly until you are more comfortable. Hold only the stretch tensions that feel good to you. Easy stretching reduces unwanted muscle tension and readies the tissues for the developmental stretch.

"After holding the easy stretch, move a fraction of an inch further into a developmental stretch. Hold this stretch for 5 to 30 seconds. Again, if there is any pain, ease off until you feel comfortable. This developmental stretch reduces muscle tension, safely increases flexibility and improves circulation."

We have selected the following exercises because they generally stretch lower body muscles and because they can be done with relative ease, even in your office after a midday workout:

- **Calf stretch**—Sitting on the floor, with your feet about a foot apart, place a towel around the ball of your foot. Without locking your knee, but holding it straight and steady, pull the towel toward you by leaning back. When you feel the stretch in the calf muscle, hold it for about 15 seconds. If it hurts, let up, or don't hold it as long. Alternate feet for two to four stretches. Gradually work up to 30-second stretches.
- **Wall lean**—Move on to the wall lean for further stretching of the calves after you have mastered the calf stretch. With your feet two to three inches apart, stand three to five feet from the wall. Put your hands on the wall directly in front of you, and bend your elbows until your forearms are resting against the wall. Your feet should be positioned as far as possible from the wall with your heels on the floor and your legs straight. After holding the position for 10 or 15 seconds, walk toward the wall and relax. The wall lean is fairly tough, so repeat it only three or four times. Over time you may build up to stretches as long as a minute.
- **Side stretch**—Sit in a chair with your feet about a foot apart, and bend your body to the right, imagining as you do so that you are lifting upward against the bend. Don't hold this stretch; just repeat on the left side, then go back to the right. Bend five times on each side. As the stretch becomes easier, add more weight to it by holding your hands behind your head as you bend. For even more weight later on, hold your hands up above your head as you bend.

(continued on page 442)

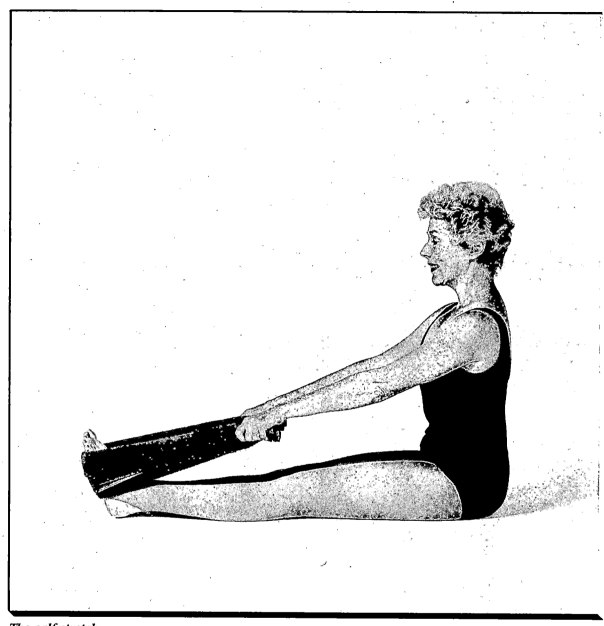

The calf stretch.

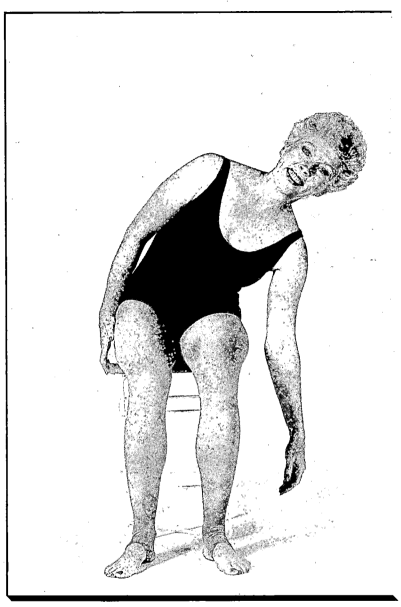

The side stretch.

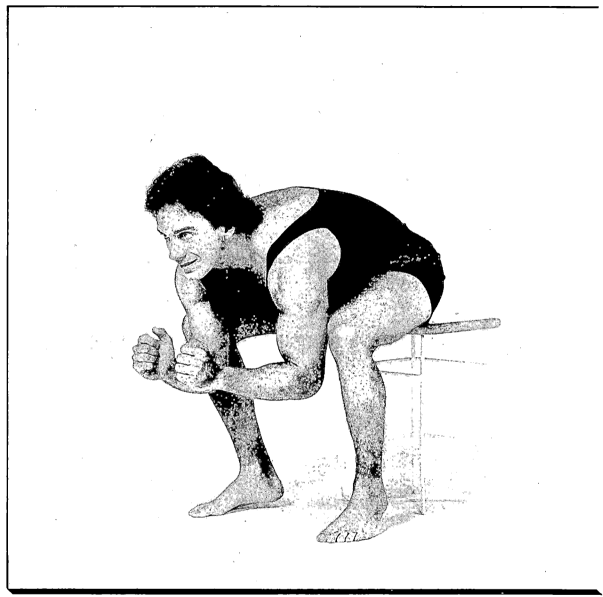

The back stretch.

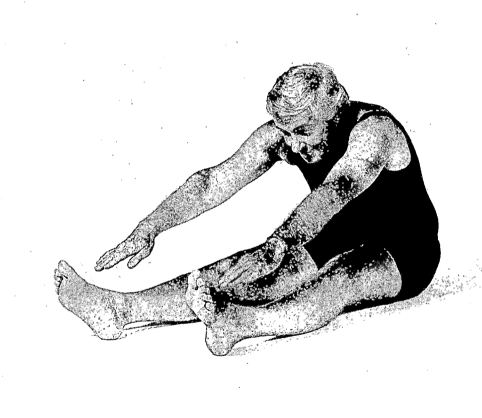

Touching the toes.

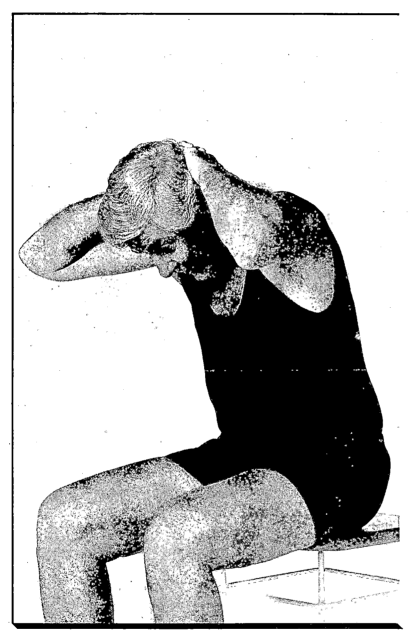

The neck stretch.

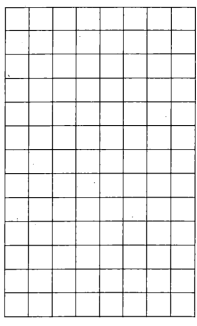

You should learn to stretch by feeling. Some days you will be more limber than others.

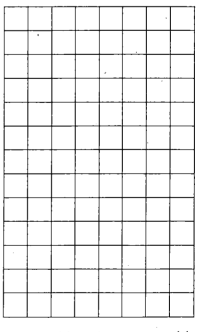

- **Back stretch**—Sit in the same position in an armless chair. Bend forward, bringing your arms and shoulders between your knees. Lean forward as if you were going to put your elbows on the floor. Repeat the stretch several times, and gradually build up your holding time.
- **Bath stretch**—One relaxing way to stretch tired legs is in a bathtub full of warm water. Sitting in the tub with your legs straight, bend forward slowly until you feel the stretch in the muscles at the back of your legs. Relax, keep breathing normally, and hold the stretch for at least 50 or 60 seconds.
- **Inner thigh stretch**—For this stretch, you need an empty wall about six feet wide. Lie on your back with your legs stretched against the wall, at a 90-degree angle to your body. Your buttocks and heels should be touching the wall. With your knees slightly bent, open your legs as far as they will go.

SWIMMING

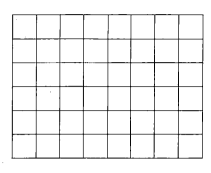

P once de Leon hoped to live forever by finding the Fountain of Youth. Of course, he never located that age-erasing pool. But even if he had, he might have been better off *swimming* in it than drinking from it. "Swimming," says Paul Hutinger, Ph.D., "is the closest thing we have to an antiaging formula."

Swimming is the closest thing we have to an antiaging formula, says Dr. Hutinger.

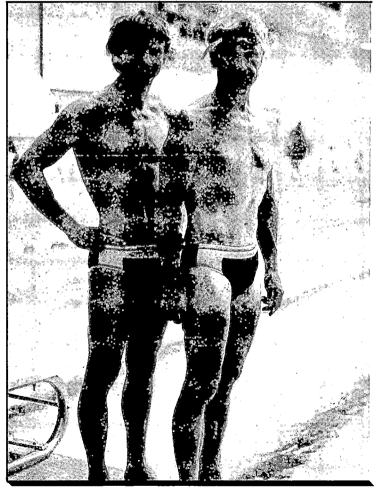

Dr. Paul Hutinger and his son—lifetime swimmers.

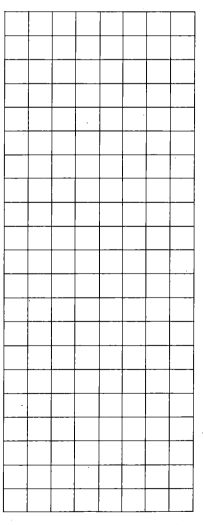

Dr. Hutinger, a professor at Western Illinois University, should know. He's an avid swimmer who logs miles a week in the pool, and he claims that, at 57, his body is as well conditioned as that of most 20-year-olds. But you don't have to take his word for it. A study conducted at the University of Maryland's Human Performance Laboratory showed that two women swimmers, both in their seventies, had a percentage of body fat similar to that of women 19 to 25 years old! Regular physical training such as swimming, said the lab researchers, "may delay the accumulation of excess fat that accompanies inactivity during aging, and may also offset the age-related decline in aerobic power" (*The Physician and Sportsmedicine,* December, 1981).

Aerobic power: the strength of your heart and lungs. Aerobic power is so central to your health that scientists have found they can actually *predict* how long a person may live by measuring the strength of his lungs (a measurement called "vital lung capacity"). Swimming stops the deterioration of lung capacity – or restores what age and disuse have taken away.

"When you swim regularly and blow out air against the water's resistance, you maintain lung capacity," says Dr. Hutinger. And, he told us, swimming can put back to work parts of the lung that have shut down because of neglect, such as some of the alveoli, the small sacs that transfer oxygen from the lungs to the bloodstream.

Less Wear and Tear on Your Body

While being good for your body, swimming is also easy on it. When you swim you don't have to worry about blisters, tennis elbow or runner's knee.

"No other physical activity offers such an unlimited possibility of exercise without the . . . joint, bone and muscle problems that plague runners and people who play racquet sports such as tennis," says the President's Council on Physical Fitness and Sports.

However, it's not the swimming itself but the water that's kind to your muscles and bones. Stand in water up to your neck, and you're suddenly 90 percent lighter. That means a person weighing 150 pounds would weigh only 15 pounds in the water. And the body's lightness in water gives swimming a "superior advantage over other sports," says Allen Richardson, M.D., chairman of the USA Swimming Sports Medicine Committee. "Swimming is what is called a 'non-weight-bearing' sport," he told us. "This is great for the joints, especially for people with ankle, shoulder or back problems. It doesn't put stress on the joints."

And that's great for anybody with arthritis. "People with painful joints . . . will usually find it possible and comfortable to move in the water," says the President's Council. But James Counsilman, Ph.D., swimming coach at Indiana University, believes that any older person (he's 60) will find swimming the best exercise.

"Swimming seems to be the standard exercise for older people," he points out, "because these are the people who, like me, can't jog because of some ache or another."

And if you're overweight, the fact that swimming is non-weight-bearing means you won't have to fight gravity at every step to exercise those pounds away. Swimming burns 350 to 400 calories an hour – without burning you out.

And the last (but not the least) reason swimming may be the best exercise is that it gets you fit fast. Scientific studies show that you can get into good shape by swimming only twice a week for 15 minutes each time. Of course, "swimming" doesn't mean splashing around in the pool. But it doesn't mean wearing yourself out, either. Swim a lap (about 25 yards or meters) every minute, and you're doing as much for your heart and lungs (and much more for your arms, back and stomach) as any jogger.

Breathe Easy

All those benefits sound great, but perhaps you're hesitant about swimming regularly because you never learned how to swim *right*. It may be hard for you to breathe in time with your strokes, and the strokes themselves may not seem too proficient, either. Well, to learn how to breathe correctly, you don't even need to get near a pool. "You can learn breathing techniques at home using a basin filled with water," says Jane Katz, Ed.D., professor of health and physical education at Bronx Community College of the City University of New York.

"Using a basin, you can practice blowing bubbles in the water, and inhaling as you turn your head out of the water" (see photo).

According to Dr. Katz, author of *Swimming for Total Fitness: A Progressive Aerobic Program* (Doubleday, 1981), "Too many swimmers never bother to learn the fundamen-

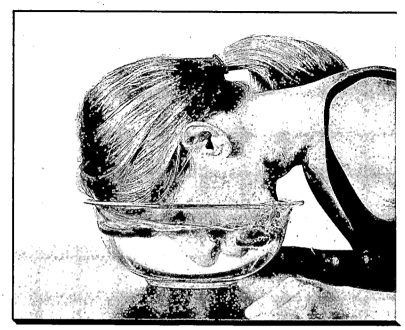

Blowing bubbles in a basin of water can develop your breathing technique for swimming.

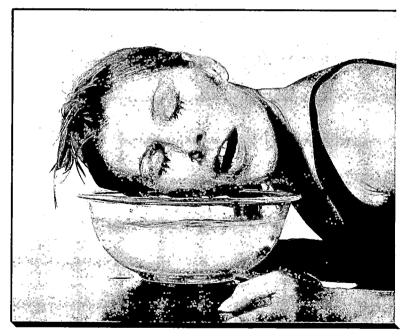

Alternate sides when you turn your head to inhale.

tals of their sport. They neglect things like breathing techniques. Instead of breathing out into the water, many swimmers simply hold their breath.

Another problem many swimmers have, says Dr. Katz, is "overkicking."

"When you're doing the crawl, most of your effort really should be put into arm pull. That should represent up to 70 percent of your effort. And your arms should do an 'S' pull. They shouldn't pull straight back. The motion of the right arm should form the shape of a question mark in the water. The left arm should perform a reverse question mark."

"To get the most out of swimming laps," says Dr. Katz, "you should start easy and end easy. Don't use maximum effort when you do your first laps. Warm up first. And your laps at the end should be a cool-down."

Of course, swimming laps is not the only kind of exercise you can do in the water. "For some people," says Dr. Katz, "treading water is a complete exercise in itself. And some people burn up more calories treading water than they do when they're swimming."

And there are a flood of other possibilities for aquatic exercise. Just ask Gretchen Schreiber, a swimming instructor in Kansas.

Splashing Away Medical Problems

"I was teaching swimming at the YMCA in Johnson County, Kansas, and I'd have the people jog through the water to warm up, since the water was cold," Ms. Schreiber says. "The people liked that, so I gradually built that up into a whole exercise program. After I had been teaching the exercise class for a while, people began telling me that it was helping their arthritis and back problems. We found that specific exercises helped specific problems."

Like the swimming experts we quoted earlier in the chapter, Ms. Schreiber believes that exercise in the water has two unique qualities that result in special benefits for the body. The buoyancy of the water makes exercise seem easier, she says, while the water's resistance to movement forces the body to work harder.

"When you exercise in water," Ms. Schreiber told us, "your body floats, and it's easier, or at least it feels easier, than exercising on land. When you do arm exercises on land and you put your arms out, gravity pulls down on them. When you're in the water, the water holds them up.

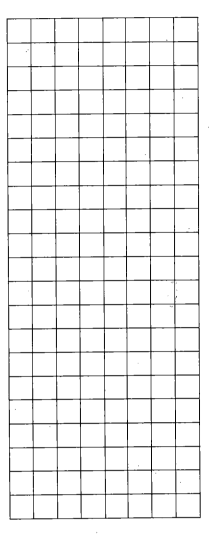

When you exercise in water, your body floats. This is good for people who are overweight or pregnant or have back problems, because it supports the spine where there might be a strain.

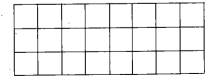

Slimming Exercises

"This is good for people who are overweight or pregnant, or people with back problems, because it supports the spine in areas where there might be a strain.

"At the same time, the water resistance makes it kind of an isokinetic exercise, where you have to push against a resistance."

In her book *Swim-Lite, Body Shaping Water Exercises* (Loggerhead, 1979), Ms. Schreiber sums up the effect nicely: "The buoyancy of your body in the water makes you feel light and graceful as you move, yet the resistance of the water makes each of the exercises doubly effective."

Ms. Schreiber's book lays out six water exercise routines incorporating a number of different exercises. Each of the routines begins with three to five minutes of warm-up exercises, just as Ms. Schreiber begins her swimming classes. The routines end with cooling-down exercises. Ms. Schreiber, a physical education major in college, stresses the importance of warming up first and cooling down afterward.

The routines themselves are a carefully balanced combination of different exercises for different parts of the body. The arms and legs are toned up simply by using them to draw big circles and numbers under the water. Once you've mastered that, you move on to writing your name.

An exercise called the "ballet stretch" strengthens the back. You stand at a right angle to the poolside with one arm holding onto the edge, just as a ballet dancer stands at the exercise bar. You bring your free arm out to the side and raise your leg up through the water to meet it, then bring the leg down straight as you swing your arm over your head and bend to touch poolside. It's a graceful, swaying movement.

Another movement, although a little less classy looking, is good for your shoulders, chest and back. Standing with your arms extended straight in front of you, you pull them back through the water at shoulder level until your hands meet behind you, then pull them back to the front again. The exercise produces just the kind of arching and stretching your back muscles need to stay in shape.

A number of exercises in Ms. Schreiber's book are designed with the weight-conscious in mind. Those movements are meant to firm muscles in the waist, hips and thighs. The "waterwheel" is a simple, vigorous exercise that is good for working the waist and building up endurance.

Standing with your legs astraddle and your arms stretched out straight to the sides, twist to the right and left as far as possible, pulling your arms through the water as you do so.

Several of the slimming exercises make use of the side of the pool. "Double tuck kicks," which give your abdomen and hips a thorough workout, begin with your hands holding onto the edge, your knees tucked up under your chin and your feet propped against the pool wall. You take your feet off the pool wall and thrust them back straight behind you into the water, then return to the original position. Double tuck kicks are good for developing endurance.

The "wall bounce," as the name implies, involves holding the pool's edge with your feet straddled against the wall and bouncing to a straight-legged position with your feet in front of you (on the wall), then bouncing back again. It's great for firming up the thighs.

For swimmers who have advanced beyond clinging to the side of the pool, Ms. Schreiber has come up with a number of exercises that can be performed in deep water with flotation boards or by treading water. A typical exercise, the "helicopter," is particularly good for toning the waist, hips and thighs. From a basic position with flotation boards tucked under each arm, your arms out to the sides and your legs extended below, rotate your entire lower body.

Another exercise involves riding an imaginary bicycle in the water as you float in place.

And what kind of results do such exercises produce? Take a look at some of the testimonials from Ms. Schreiber's students.

"Last January I was bothered with some arthritis in my knees and tendinitis in my shoulder," says one student. "I visited the doctor to see what we could do to remedy the situation. I was told that if I would take off some weight, the joints would last ten years longer.

"I joined an exercise program, and the weight dropped off at an astonishing rate. Meanwhile, the county parks and recreation department was offering a water exercise class to be taught by Gretchen Schreiber. Not having swum in years, I approached the first class with hopes that maybe it had been canceled, what with my varicose veins and flabby skin.

"It wasn't canceled, the other members of the class looked just like I did, and thanks to Gretchen, we had a simply marvelous time. I began to feel better, much more agile. The tendinitis was gone! The arthritis in the knee was gone! Nothing else has changed – it had to be the water exercises."

Another student experienced a marked improvement in her circulatory problems. "My circulation has definitely improved. Both my thighs from my knees upward toward my hips were numb when I started class in June. This problem has all but completely cleared up, with practically no numbness left. The exercises really helped my circulatory system."

A student who lives on a lake found Ms. Schreiber's winter classes the ideal way to keep in shape year-round. "I swim almost daily from May through September. This is the first winter I have sought and found a way to keep on swimming regularly throughout the winter months."

Ms. Schreiber's classes are open to nonswimmers. "Often people start out holding onto the side of the pool throughout the class, but after a couple of sessions, they're using kickboards to kick their way across the pool. Many of them go on to take swimming classes."

For the Timid, a Bathtub

Even if you're too scared to go close to a swimming pool, or unable to get to an indoor one in the winter months, Ms. Schreiber has found ways to keep you wet and exercising all year long. A section at the back of her book turns the shower and bathtub into a veritable health spa. The benefits of combining water and exercise, Ms. Schreiber believes, apply even when the water is streaming out of a shower head or lying six inches deep in the bottom of a tub. "The warm water relaxes your muscles," she writes, "and lets you stretch and relieve tension and fatigue. This type of exercise is especially beneficial to those with arthritis or stiff muscles."

Most of the tub exercises are stretching routines that use the confines of the tub to best advantage. For example, in one torso toner the shoulders and feet are braced against opposite ends of the tub, and the hips are raised and held to a count of ten. Another exercise, designed to stretch the muscles of the lower back, is simply a matter of putting your feet against the faucet end of the tub, straightening your legs and leaning forward to grab the tub's front edge. It's kind of like touching your toes, but in this case, you're in the comfort of a warm bath rather than on the hardwood floor of a drafty gym.

But whether you exercise in the tub or in an Olympic-size pool, your health will be "in the swim."

VACATIONS

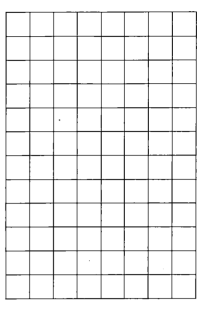

We're into proverbial wisdom around here, we guess, because old things that have lasted *must* have a thing or three going for them, *must* have appealed to a person or two along the way. It impresses us that the way we eat – a way that seems strange to many fast-food folks – used to be the standard way of eating; it was and is a *natural* way of eating. And it is impressive, too, that many homes – built 50 or 60 years ago – were placed facing the warming sun and sheltered from wintry blasts by trees and shrubs. Those old carpenters didn't know the terms "passive solar" or "protective landscaping," but they sure knew the techniques.

Of course, you do have to be a bit careful with proverbial wisdom. Since there are so many different kinds of people, and since different gems of advice appeal to each group, gilt-edged items of time-tested truth sometimes conflict with one another. Consider, for instance, that "a penny saved is a penny earned." But that being "penny-wise" is considered "pound-foolish" in some quarters. And that, to still others, "Spend, and God will send" is a truism. Yet, there is one homely saw that most folks agree on – that it's good every now and then to "get away from it all," "it all" being the daily grind of work and bills and kids and tension and stress; you know, normal life. Part of the reason that vacations and travel (if that's your idea of a vacation) are good is that they do relieve us of our usual and habitual pressures. But it's also true that it's refreshing to temporarily substitute one set of duties for another, to get outside our own skin (so to speak) and get into someone else's – that is, "when in Rome, do as the Romans do."

We all know, then, that a vacation is important, especially when it's been a long time since the last one. But the question is, *how* important is it? Important enough to spend time and trouble and money on? *Yes!* Whether you're taking off for the Alps or a mountain lake 30 miles from home, the pink beaches of some tropical island or the back porch of your cousin's cottage at the shore, your vacation is going to contribute to your health in a lot of ways. At least 15.

When you take a vacation, you escape the humdrum of daily life. You recharge your batteries and return to everyday life refreshed and renewed.

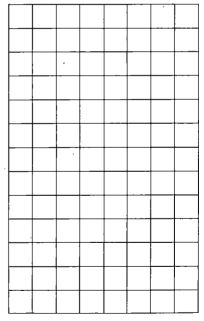

451

15 Reasons for Taking a Vacation

1. **Relaxation.** "Just the act of getting away from your daily frustrations will relax you," says Richard I. Curtis, author of *Taking Off* (Harmony Books, 1981). "Even if you come up against some new problems on your trip, you can treat these like a game. They're temporary. The important thing is, you are getting out of your day-to-day rut."

   Edward Heath, Ph.D., professor in the department of recreation and parks of Texas A & M University, agrees: "When you take a vacation, you escape the humdrum of daily life. You leave your troubles behind you. Even if all you do is sit on the edge of the river and watch a rock move, it's a valuable change of pace. You're going to recharge your batteries. You'll return to everyday life refreshed and renewed."

2. **Stimulation of new sights.** Mr. Curtis told us, "Almost any travel is good. Staying at home for too long tends to crimp our awareness. We need the exposure to new sights and experiences. Think of the first time you saw mountains, or the sea, or the desert, or the Grand Canyon – I don't mean pictures. I mean actually being there, in a place which is totally different from anything you're used to."

New Sights Bring New Insights

New sights of things around us can give us new *insights,* too, according to Dr. Heath. "You can get a broader view, a new perspective on your own world, if you visit a different place. For example, if you live at the mouth of the Mississippi, or the Hudson, or some other great river, you may understand your own region better after visiting the headwaters of the river. You may learn something about yourself, too; namely, that you might like to move to that new area. Lots of people take advantage of their vacations to look over other regions they might like to move to someday."

3. **Meet new people.** "We're very social animals," Dr. Heath says. "A vacation gives us the opportunity to form new friendships – or just to satisfy our curiosity about how other people live. This gives us a broader perspective on our own lives."

Mr. Curtis agrees. "The more people you know, the more eyes you can borrow to look on the world," he says. "And the further those eyes are from your own world, the better."

4. **Fellowship and camaraderie.** According to Dr. Heath, "Sharing an adventure with other people allows us to share their enthusiasm, too. That's good. It's positive reinforcement for our own enthusiasm about life. But it doesn't necessarily have to be easy going. Shared *hardships* also form bonds of love and friendship and give us something to look back on with pride and pleasure.

"Every year thousands of people meet at one spot in Canada and form a caravan with their recreational vehicles and eat each other's dust all the way to Alaska. Then they're back again the next year.

"Twenty years from now, you'll remember and talk about the canoe trip where the weather suddenly changed and you spent two days huddled over a campfire, shivering.

"There's also a benefit in associating with like-minded people in some competitive event. People travel thousands of miles to cheer their team in the Super Bowl or the playoffs or the college championships. Marathon runners travel halfway across the world to run in a race and be surrounded by thousands of other runners."

The Educational Pluses of Travel

5. **Education.** "You may need or want to learn new skills on your vacation," Dr. Heath says. "You may decide to learn a new language before traveling to a foreign country. Or you may learn as you go along in order to communicate with people there. You may decide to learn snorkeling, or tennis, or golf, or skiing, or mountain climbing, or hang gliding, or any new skill."

6. **Adventure.** "Travel returns a sense of adventure to your life," says Mr. Curtis. "Pulling yourself off your native turf is going to make demands on your resourcefulness – to find suitable lodging and food. But you're also allowed to *experiment* with your personality and lifestyle without having to live with the consequences. If you're usually too shy to say hello and smile at strangers, you may allow yourself the adventure of

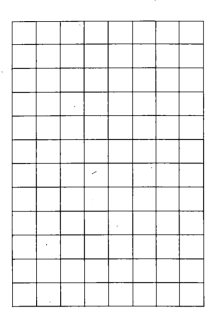

Happy people are those who give full attention to what's going on at that moment, not what happened before or what might happen later.

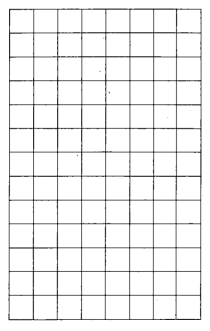

doing just that on your vacation in a new place. It may then become a habit you can bring home with you."

The element of *risk* is also a part of many vacation adventures, according to Dr. Heath. "Most travel involves accepting and meeting challenges. You test yourself against a new environment. You can improve your self-esteem by taking on challenges that everyday life doesn't offer. Of course, sometimes everyday life may involve greater risk. Water skiing, mountain climbing, skydiving – all seem quite scary. But though they may be more thrilling, they actually are safer than driving on the freeway."

Expect the Unexpected

7. **Surprise.** "It is the unexpected in life that we learn from," says Mr. Curtis. "We gain the most when we put ourselves on the line and remain open to new experiences. On a trip, you have to adapt very quickly. You bring much of that enhanced adaptability home with you." Not to mention the stories of all your surprises, which you'll remember and tell over and over for many years.

8. **Beauty.** "When you're standing in the middle of a beautiful environment, and you open your eyes to it, you start to feel in tune with it. You can actually begin to feel beautiful *yourself*. You share in some of the beauty and power," Dr. Heath told us. "You may have such a peak experience in a natural setting, like the Grand Canyon; or your awe might be inspired by the beauty of some man-made edifice such as the Vatican, a bridge or a whole city. These experiences we never forget are very important to our enjoyment of life."

9. **Anticipation.** Have we got you itchin' to hit the road for action and adventure and new people, places and things? Are you so excited you can't wait to plan your vacation? Good, because that's part of the benefit of a vacation. "Your vacation," according to Dr. Heath, "is more than the actual time spent away from home. The planning and preparation are also good for you. Many vacations are actually year-long projects. A person may prepare for a fishing trip, for example, by tying flies. You might prepare for a sight-

seeing journey by reading all you can about the places you're going to visit. The anticipation is pleasurable. The trip is, too, because you reap the rewards of extensive preparation."

10. **Memories.** "Your life is enriched before, during and after a vacation," Dr. Heath says. "You'll always have the joy of reflecting on pleasant memories."

11. **Appreciation of things taken for granted.** "You'll be surprised at the things for which you become homesick," Mr. Curtis says. "You'll crave the simple pleasure of finding someone who speaks your language. I have felt almost sick for the sight of a lilac, for a maple tree, for ice cream sodas, for a long, hot shower and even – I hate to admit it – for American fast food. I once ran alongside an American's car for three blocks in Yugoslavia – just to hear an old Simon and Garfunkel song on his tape player.

    "When you get home, you will get more from life. You'll see the miracles where you live."

12. **Self-discovery.** "A vacation can be a great opportunity for sorting out life's experiences," Dr. Heath says. "You can shut off the sensory overload that may be your everyday life and get away to a deserted beach or a mountain stream. You can let your soul talk to itself. You need it to develop your creativity and your inner peace and harmony."

Travel on the Road to Freedom

13. **Freedom.** "A vacation gives us the freedom to do what we want to do," says Dr. Heath.

    "Our bodies have the remarkable ability to recognize a deficiency and try to compensate for it," notes Mr. Curtis. "For instance, North American Indians who lived in northern regions when sources of vitamin C were rare compensated by eating pine needles. The mind seems to have a myriad of ways to deal with psychological problems, too, without necessarily consulting the brain's owner. Our desire for change occurs regularly. Even if you are generally satisfied with your life and work, you may still feel the need for something more. You may feel closed in. Take a vacation, and you will realize your own freedom. You'll see that the mundane world can be transcended at will. It can be left behind. You're not a prisoner if you choose not to be."

14. **Time stands still.** "If you're really enjoying yourself," Dr. Heath says, "time does not progress in equal units. You stop thinking about everything else but what you're doing then and there. You get lost in the activity of the moment. You may be catching fish, or trying to keep dry while canoeing through the rapids, or looking for pretty shells along the beach. Time is standing still for you, and that's good. There's evidence that happy people are those who can give full attention to what's going on at *that moment,* not what happened before or what might happen later."

15. **Happiness.** We save the most important reason for last: "The major goal of a vacation is happiness," says Dr. Heath. "Your leisure time should make you happier. A vacation is not a necessary evil you endure to enable you to work harder when you get back. Your leisure makes up a large segment of your life, and it can and should be a valuable force for good.

VARICOSE VEINS

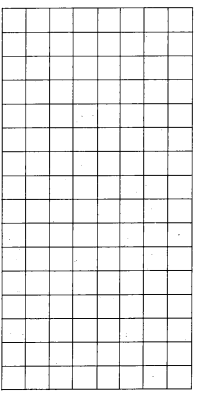

T he patient, a robust woman in her fifties, couldn't quite fathom what went wrong in paradise. Wearing a new puka shell necklace and a flawless tan, she'd just flown into New York after three weeks in Hawaii. Of course, everything had been fabulous, from the Polynesian repasts at the Kahala Hilton to the languid sunbathing at the pool. What, then, could possibly account for the painfully inflamed veins she developed her first day home? "I can't understand it," she complained to her physician. "It was such a wonderful trip."

No doubt it was, agreed her doctor, Howard C. Baron, M.D., an attending vascular surgeon at the Cabrini Medical Center in New York City. The culprit, however, wasn't the vacation itself, but the tedious, uncomfortable eight-hour jet ride home. Perhaps if the woman had suspected a predisposition for varicose veins, she'd have occasionally flexed her calf muscles and left her cramped seat every hour to stroll up and down the aisle.

Obviously, the patient didn't know that "movers and shakers," as Dr. Baron dubs fitness enthusiasts, are the best candidates for healthy legs. For that reason, he singles out exercise and diet in his book *Varicose Veins: A Commonsense Approach to Their Management* (William Morrow, 1979) as the key preventive measures against the symptoms and complications of those bulging bluish cords down the leg.

It's no secret that those gnarled and swollen leg veins afflicting one in four American women and one in ten American men aren't very pretty. They're malformed, defective blood vessels that are no longer elastic. Stretched out of shape, they appear enlarged, twisted and discolored. That appearance stems from problems with the delicate valves within the leg veins that provide a pathway for used blood to be carried back to the heart from everywhere in the body. To ease the arduous task of forcing blood up the leg against the gravitational pull, the tiny, one-way valves close between heartbeats to prevent a backflow of the pumped blood.

Normally, that action occurs millions of times throughout life without a hitch. But the process may be disrupted.

Exercise is a key preventive measure against varicose veins. "Movers and shakers" are the best candidates for healthy legs.

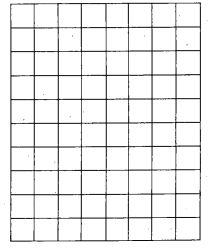

457

Pressure on the leg veins may interfere with the circulatory system and prevent the valves from shutting properly. When this happens, or if vein valves are inadequate, defective or malfunctioning, blood seeps back and pools in the legs, further dilating the veins. After a few years, the vessels begin to lose their flexibility. They sag and push toward the surface, shifting the entire burden to the larger, deeper veins.

Early Signs Ignored

Many people dismiss the early warning signals of varicose veins – the slight tingle of impaired blood flow followed by the eruption of small bluish veins near the skin's surface – and don't take action until the veins pose a cosmetic problem. But that may be a big mistake. Dr. Baron and other physicians believe that early detection and treatment can prevent more serious symptoms and complications from occurring.

Unfortunately, millions don't stop varicose veins in time, and they typically experience a dull, aching heaviness and fatigue in the legs. Ankles may swell, particularly in warm weather; painful calf cramps may develop at night; legs may itch or burn. More serious complications such as leg ulcers, phlebitis (inflamed veins, a condition that plagued former president Nixon), blood clots and hemorrhage may occur. Disfigurement, emphasizes Dr. Baron, is the most blatant sign of the disorder. He describes the appearance of the troublesome vein as "bunched, twisted, lumped and contorted into an angry blue rope with grapelike bulges."

But even though varicose veins lead to so much trouble, physicians are divided on their precise cause. Many experts blame one's ancestors for the affliction. "It's a degenerative process that runs in families, and when the cause is due to heredity, it can't be prevented," maintains James A. DeWeese, M.D., a renowned vascular surgeon at the University of Rochester Medical School.

Robert A. Nabatoff, M.D., a clinical professor of vascular surgery, also indicts genetics as the major contributing factor to varicose veins. "The vast majority of patients have inherited their condition, and the veins usually first appear in the late teens or early twenties," says Dr. Nabatoff, who teaches at Mount Sinai School of Medicine in Manhattan.

Too Little Fiber?

Nonetheless, the notion of varicosities as a disorder caused by *lifestyle* is gaining credence among a number of physicians. One of them is Denis P. Burkitt, M.D., who believes highly developed and industrialized cultures pay a severe price for progress with heart disease, ulcers, obesity and varicose veins. The prominent British surgeon contends that inflamed vessels are rare among people living on fiber-rich diets but common in Western nations where meals are low in roughage. A fiber-depleted diet, he explains, necessitates abdominal straining to evacuate small, hard stools, putting enormous pressure on leg veins. Prolonged toilet-sitting, he says, further aggravates the problem by cutting off circulation along the back of the legs.

Other forms of inactivity, such as standing or sitting too long in one place, may also worsen varicosities. Because the malady results from impaired circulation, authorities speculate that chair-sitting may especially wreak havoc on one's legs. "The chair," states Dr. Baron, "is a terrible invention of civilization. While it makes sitting comfortable, it increases the pressure on the leg veins, and it also leads to a damaging habit – crossing your legs."

Although the problem is far more prevalent in women, Dr. Baron notes that pregnancy does *not* cause varicose veins. Instead, it's generally thought today that female *hormones,* especially those released during pregnancy, play a role in producing varicose veins in susceptible women. Frequently, inflamed veins may be the first sign of pregnancy, even before a missed menstrual period, but they often recede after delivery. Because the unsightly blue cords pop out before the veins come under increased pressure, this suggests the weight of the fetus may be less a factor than hormones.

If you already have varicose veins, there's no need to despair. Dr. Baron believes minor adjustments in daily routines may help diminish the number and even the size of the snakelike embarrassments. Some tips for preventing and "pampering" varicose veins as well as precluding future complications include the following:

- Avoid, whenever possible, long periods of sitting or standing. If you must sit or stand, make a conscious effort to flex your leg muscles. Wiggle your toes frequently, and slowly raise and lower yourself on the balls of your feet. Don't cross your legs. Break up lengthy trips by walking several minutes every hour or two. On long plane or train rides, pace up and down the aisle at least once an hour.

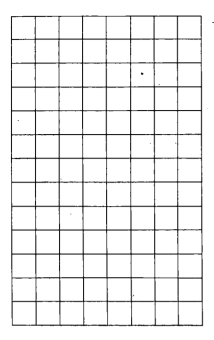

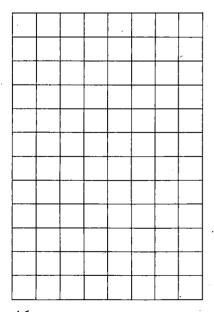

Going barefoot at home exercises the foot muscles and improves venous blood flow. Brisk walks several times a day are also good for your veins.

Brisk Walks Can Help

- Get sufficient exercise through walking, jogging, running, cycling or swimming. Walking, note Eric P. Lofgren, M.D., and Karl A. Lofgren, M.D., both of the Mayo Clinic in Rochester, Minnesota, lowers the venous pressure to about a third of the standing pressure under normal conditions (*Geriatrics,* September, 1975). Dr. Robert May, a specialist in surgery and circulatory problems at the University of Innsbruck in Austria, advises brisk walks for 15 minutes, four times a day. He also advocates going barefoot at home to help exercise the foot muscles and improve venous blood flow (*Medical Tribune,* February 27, 1980).

- Adopt a high-fiber diet. A lack of roughage hardens stools and puts pressure on the pelvic veins. Dr. May recommends patients eat salad daily, along with potatoes in their skins and other vegetables, and take two to three tablespoons of wheat germ. Another expert suggests increasing the daily intake of fiber fivefold, using foods such as whole grains, bran and fresh fruits.

- Shun tight garments such as calf-length boots, panty hose too snug at the groin, girdles, corsets and binding belts. Any clothing that tends to constrict the venous blood flow just beneath the skin can be hazardous to your health.

- Elevate your feet, whenever possible. Lean back, kick off your shoes and put your feet up on your desk. Placing the legs 12 to 24 inches above heart level reduces the pressure in the veins to nearly zero.

- Stop reading on the toilet. The shape of the hard wood or plastic seat puts undue pressure on the abdominal veins, which, in turn, put pressure on leg veins, notes Dr. Baron.

- Avoid bathing in a tubful of hot water, warns Dr. May, who recommends showers in the morning and at night. He also suggests a final spray of cold water on the legs.

- Wear elastic support stockings throughout pregnancy, and support hose at other times if you must stand a lot.

For uncomplicated varicose veins, either bandages or well-fitted elastic stockings can be used to relieve symptoms by acting like muscles to facilitate blood flow. Because the fit is so critical, however, Dr. Baron cautions about the stockings' main drawback: they stretch out gradually, and support may disappear.

Should those fail to provide sufficient relief, a treatment popular in England involves injecting a chemical into the veins to close them off. Called sclerotherapy, it is seldom used anymore by American specialists because of its high failure rate, permanent brown pigment stains left in the skin and serious side effects.

Experts agree that complete surgical removal of the malfunctioning veins has proved to be the best approach for correcting significant varicosities.

The most common method involves tying off and removing the troublesome veins – also known as "stripping" them. Once the defective vessels are removed, other healthy ones assume their function without harming normal circulation.

Even though the procedure is deemed safe and often yields permanent results, the treatment and cure of varicose veins in a sense are always failures – of prevention.

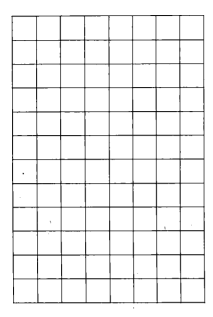

Even though walking is easier than running, it's still an excellent way to improve your aerobic capacity and get into good physical shape.

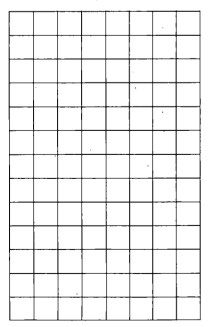

WALKING

W alking was probably invented to convince the *last* holdout to exercise. There's no such thing as the perfect exercise, but if there were, walking would be it. If you think about it, that's not too surprising.

What other exercise is adaptable to so many different physiques, so many exercise needs, and can still be done without a $200 athletic club membership? No matter where you stand on the fitness scale, from lean and hungry athlete to jelly roll, walking is good for you and feels good. As a matter of fact, some doctors prescribe walking for emotional problems, claiming that walking reduces neuromuscular tension better than a standard dose of tranquilizers. Consider the experience of one of our authors, who used to commute to New York City, where he worked at a high-pressure desk job: selling advertising over the phone.

> While I was living on Long Island, the Long Island Railroad mounted an ad campaign designed to entice commuters to take the bus to the train station and leave their cars at home. Its key slogan was: "When it's too far to walk and too expensive to drive." I agreed that it was too expensive to drive. But I also felt that – for my own mental and physical well-being – it was too expensive *not* to walk.
>
> I lived a mile from the railroad station. That mile walk, briefcase in hand, was my safety valve, my defense against the pressure-cooker environment of a working day spent sitting behind a desk, my ear glued to the phone receiver, trying to sell advertising space to those who didn't want it.
>
> In the morning, walking replaced coffee as a wake-up stimulant. Strolling briskly, watching the sun come up, I could feel my mental and physical powers being revitalized. On cold winter mornings, I'd arrive at the station feeling pleasantly warm, my coat open (or draped over one arm), and watch my fellow commuters huddled in their coats, teeth chattering, sipping coffee out of Styrofoam cups. In the evening, the walk back home helped me work out the tensions and frustrations of my day in the Big Apple.

Before I started walking, I was a much harder person to live with – just ask my wife. I'm not saying that I was all sweetness and light once I started walking, but I left a lot of my bad feelings out on that mile of sidewalk between the train station and the house. By walking instead of taking the bus or subway, I saved $2 a day. I became a familiar figure at the shoe repair shop getting my shoes fixed. But I figured that was money well spent when I compared the wear and tear on my soles to the wear and tear I had saved on my soul, not to mention my heart.

I tend toward being overweight and hypertensive. If I'm not careful about my diet, I'll easily put on ten pounds around the waistline. As long as I kept up my walking, I could worry less about what I was eating (of course, I couldn't neglect it entirely) and still maintain a low weight. As for my high blood pressure – ten years ago I was 4F from military service because of it. But when I had a physical recently, the examining physician couldn't believe that I was ever hypertensive. (His exact words were, "You *never* had high blood pressure!")

A Sustained Activity

Almost no one is disqualified from walking. Maybe you won't be able to walk very far or very fast, but some degree of walking is almost always possible.

Walking seems relatively easy to do compared to running or cross-country skiing, but don't think that its aerobic benefits and its potential for getting you into good physical shape are inconsequential.

According to a study at the Heller Institute of Medical Research at the Tel Aviv University Medical School, "It is possible to improve substantially aerobic physical fitness in three weeks by walking daily with a light backpack load." In the study, those people who were in the *worst* physical shape (attention all you soft-limbed armchair quarterbacks out there) showed the quickest improvement in physical condition. The subjects in the Israeli study walked at a speed of about three miles an hour for 30 minutes a day, five times a week, and carried backpacks weighing only about 6½ pounds.

After three weeks, the participants in the study showed an average improvement in aerobic capacity of 15 percent. After four weeks, they improved 18 percent. When the load they were carrying was doubled during the fourth week, the average total improvement was 30 percent.

If you decide to start a walking program, a briefcase or shopping bag could be substituted for the pack, and your physical fitness gain would be just as fast.

Besides improving your aerobic fitness, walking can also change your body chemistry for the better. According to Dan Streja, M.D., a California endocrinologist, "Metabolically speaking, walking is as good as jogging. To favorably alter cholesterol, to lower sugar, insulin and triglycerides, and to lose weight, walking will do it. I expect it would lower blood pressure as well."

Along with David Mymin, M.D., of the University of Manitoba in Canada, Dr. Streja has published results of a study in which 32 men, all of whom were 35 to 68 years old and had heart disease, were put on a program of walking, working up to slow jogging if they could manage it. But, in fact, the average speed of the participants was less than 4 miles per hour at the beginning of the 13-week program and just slightly over 4 miles per hour at the conclusion. In other words, the average speed was no faster than a businesslike walking gait, about as fast as you'd normally be walking on a cold day. There was only an average of three sessions per week, and the average distance walked at each session was slightly less than 1¾ miles. Yet, despite this relatively modest degree of effort, some very impressive results were obtained.

Most important, perhaps, there was a very promising change in cholesterol. Specifically, there was an increase in the fraction of cholesterol known as high-density lipoprotein (HDL), a substance that helps prevent cholesterol and fat accumulation within artery walls. The higher the HDL, the less chance there is of a heart attack. And there *was* a significant increase in the HDL count of this group of walkers. Previously, it had been known that long-distance runners and other extremely active types had elevated HDL counts, but this was one of the first times anyone had demonstrated the beneficial effect resulting only from walking.

Besides the increase in HDL, there was a *decrease* in circulating insulin levels. Now most of us don't think about insulin outside the context of diabetes, but the fact is that many Americans have too much of this hormone (which is secreted by the pancreas to aid in the metabolism of sugar) drifting through their system. To make a long story very short, high insulin levels can help bring on both diabetes *and* heart disease. Pretty serious stuff. Yet the walkers in this program enjoyed a very significant (an average of 20 percent) decrease in plasma insulin. Altogether, it seems, everything that happened to these walkers did nothing but good for their hearts (*Journal of the American Medical Association,* November 16, 1979).

Walking for Stronger Bones

Ever hear of osteoporosis? It's the medical name for the bone fragility that's so common among older people, particularly women. Some 350,000 bone fractures are blamed on osteoporosis each year, as is a considerable amount of back pain. And it's all because of the lack of calcium. Or lack of walking. While taking about 1,000 milligrams of extra calcium a day will help stop or even reverse the process of osteoporosis, walking will do much the same thing. In one interesting study reported by K. H. Sidney, Ph.D., and colleagues from the University of Toronto, a group of people in a preretirement conditioning program exercised an average of four hours a week. Concentrating on brisk walking, they lost no calcium at all from their bones over the course of a year. That was the average, but actually the people in the program who walked the least often lost some calcium from their bones. These results are very impressive, because they show that a simple thing like walking can halt a chronic and progressive disease like osteoporosis in its tracks.

Where to Start

Okay, you may be thinking, walking is good for the body and mind, but how, where and when should one start? Can you just make it a casual part of your life, walk a couple of blocks here and there, now and then, and still get healthier and happier? The answer is that you need a program and the incentive – that is, a method of making walking part of your daily or weekly routine. A little walking can go a long way, but only as part of a regimen incorporated into your life.

The "walking experts" differ on how much walking per week will produce a significant training effect. Simon J. Wikler, M.D., in his book *Walk, Don't Run* (Windward Publishing, 1980), defines "walking" as a 15-minute mile, four days a week. "Some like their walks after dinner, others before retiring, others on getting up in the morning when the streets are deserted. It really doesn't matter too much when you do it – *as long as you don't leave it to chance,"* says Dr. Wikler.

On the other hand, Fred A. Stutman, M.D., in *The Doctor's Walking Book* (written with Lillian Africano, Ballantine, 1980), argues that a 15-minute mile (walking at four miles per hour) is "too demanding and exhausting for most people, [and] . . . is not suitable for a lifetime program." He recommends walking regularly for 45 to 60 minutes at least three times per week. Dr. Stutman feels that the pace isn't as important as the regularity of the exercise. "It isn't important which pace you choose, as long as you're comfortable." Two miles an hour (slow) or three miles (moderate) is acceptable. Dr. Stutman goes on to add that the time spent walking does not have to be continuous. For instance, you can divide your 45 minutes of walking in a day into three sessions of 15 minutes each. "For best aerobic benefits, however, try not to make any session shorter than 15 minutes."

Whatever program you start with, be sure to start slowly, especially if your main exercise the past year has been getting up to change the TV channel. Even in walking, the sports cliché, "Train, don't strain," still applies. If you are very unsure about your physical fitness, you can consult your doctor about how much exercise is safe for you.

There are several tips you should keep in mind, especially at the beginning stages of your walking program. First, don't go for a vigorous walk after a large meal. This could put too much strain on your heart and circulatory system. Avoid extreme forms of weather. Don't go out in very cold, hot, humid or windy conditions. Be comfortable. Wear clothes suitable for the temperature. Wear shoes that fit and have low heels.

Walking Correctly

Contrary to popular opinion, proper walking does not come naturally to all people. To prove this, all you have to do is stand on a big-city sidewalk someday and watch the 1,001 examples of poor walking technique. Some people shuffle along with their chins folded into their chests. Others use a ducklike waddle with their feet pointed awkwardly outward. Many of them don't look as if they're enjoying their walk very much. Their bad habits have stifled and limited many of the rewards they could be getting from their walking.

One of the most important aspects of good walking is posture. For many people who have been indulging in bad posture for years, trying to achieve good positioning of the trunk and spine is difficult and requires a great deal of practice before it feels as if it comes "naturally."

In *Walk, Don't Run,* Dr. Wikler recommends keeping "your head high, with chin parallel to the ground, shoulders squared backward, abdomen sucked in a little keeping the small of the back straighter, feet pointing straight ahead."

Walking correctly puts less strain on your neck and back muscles and increases your sense of what is going on around you. It also improves the image that you present to other people. There are few things more unattractive than someone walking around with his nose on his shoelaces.

The proper foot motion involves pointing the feet straight ahead with a heel-to-toe gait. Unlike running, where both feet fall along the same line, in walking the feet follow two parallel lines. This parallel motion will carry you the farthest distance with the least amount of fatigue. Each foot should come down in front of the heel and produce a long stride through the entire foot in a rolling motion through the foot and ending in a push-off from the space between the big toe and the little toe. This fluid motion distributes stress through the foot rather than concentrating it in a staccato footfall. The foot contacts the ground in a wave motion from heel to toes. As the heel of the lead foot contacts the ground, the rear foot pushes off between the first and second toes.

Another important point to remember when walking is to keep your muscles relaxed and fluid. Tightening them unnecessarily will only cause you to tire more easily. Tension in your muscles will also make you more prone to injury, since a tightened muscle has much less "give" to it. When stressed during activity, this lack of "give" puts pressure on the connective tissue around the muscle, heightening the chances of a tear.

When it comes to buying shoes for walking, you may find yourself sacrificing fashion for comfort. The worst thing you can do to your feet is to buy shoes that are attractive but do not fit properly. Wearing poor-fitting shoes can do extensive and sometimes irreparable damage to your feet and body.

Many walkers purchase running shoes. For comfort and protection, the consensus among walkers is that running shoes are probably your best choice of footwear. Designed

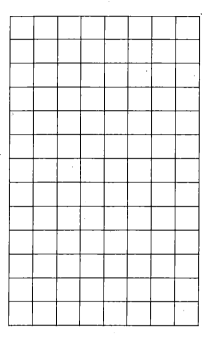

A simple thing like walking can halt a chronic and progressive disease like osteoporosis in its tracks.

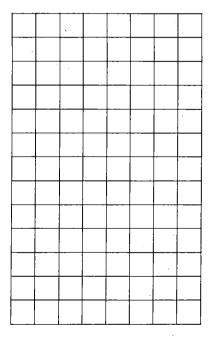

to protect the foot against the forces involved in running, they do an excellent job of sheltering the foot against the stresses produced during walking.

No matter what kind of shoe you buy, the first thing to remember is to buy footwear large enough for your feet! Fashion pushes people into shoes that don't fit and are harmful. Somehow, during the past hundred years, the notion has become popular that large feet are unattractive. Therefore, millions of people are constantly trying to squeeze their feet into shoes that scrunch their toes and make mush of their insteps.

Many people find that one of their feet is larger than the other. You should buy shoes that fit the larger foot. It will be easier to make the small foot fit the larger shoe (by means of pads or heavy socks) than it will be to fit the larger foot into a shoe that is too small for it.

When you buy shoes, make sure that your toes have ample room; there should be at least one-quarter inch of space between the end of your longest toe and the front of the shoe. The best way to measure the space in the toe box of the shoe is to stand up in the shoes, wiggle your toes and feel where they are with your fingers. There better be ample wiggle room, or your walks in those shoes will be painfully difficult from the blisters forming on your toes.

There you have it – the easiest road to fitness ever invented. So shoe up and shove off!

WATER THERAPY

O f all the branches of physical therapy, water therapy, also known as hydrotherapy, is one of the most useful. Water is present in abundance around the world and is nearly always available for application in therapy. It is one of the most economical substances known. Taken internally, water is not irritating, and it can also be used freely on the skin; its only limits are individual tolerances for certain extremes of temperature.

The application of heat (through warm water) to the skin produces a local dilation (expansion) of the blood vessels that increases the speed of the blood's flow. Local applications of heat also increase capillary pressure, causing an increased flow of fluid into the lymph spaces and back to the heart through these channels. In addition, local application of heat increases perspiration. When prolonged, this sweating can become general. One of the outstanding effects of all forms of heat therapy is the relief of pain.

When cold water is applied to the skin for a brief time, the skin becomes reddened with an increase of blood. This is particularly true when the cold stimulus is accompanied by the friction of rubbing and massage. Nerves in the blood vessels are stimulated, and a type of "vascular gymnastics" takes place; in other words, the blood vessels pump vigorously, alternating between dilation and contraction. Extra amounts of oxygen are delivered to the skin through these maneuvers.

Most people have experienced the relief of muscular fatigue that comes from a warm bath. Normal rest and sleep are promoted by its relaxing influence. On the other hand, if a warm bath is followed by a vigorous application of cold, as from a shower or the friction of a cold mitten, the body acquires new energy. The brain becomes more alert, the extremities warmer, and more work can be accomplished – all without the injurious aftereffects of stimulants such as caffeine.

One must remember that these general treatments affect the entire body, including the nervous system, the liver and its chemistry, and the muscles. They enhance the conver-

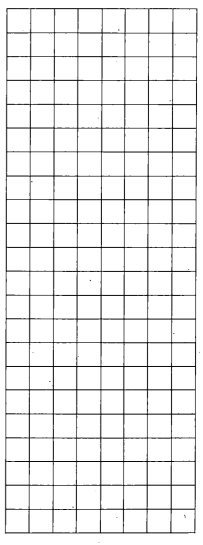

If a warm bath is followed by a vigorous application of cold, as from a shower, the body acquires new energy. The brain becomes more alert.

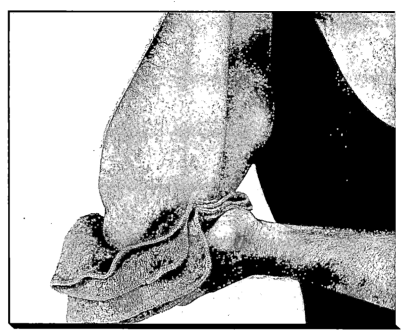

A hot compress is soothing.

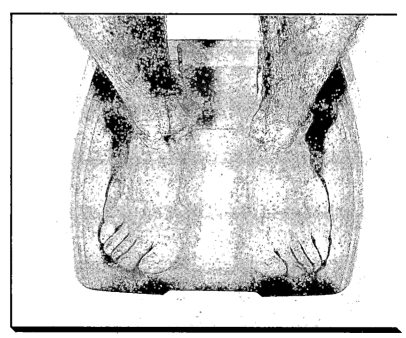

Treat tired feet with a tub of hot water.

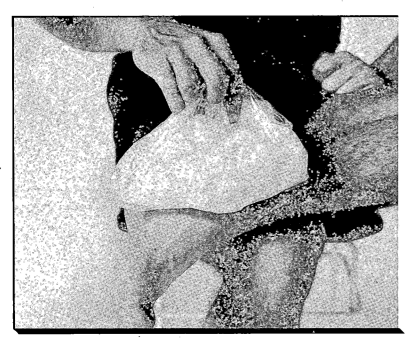

Put ice on a sore ankle.

sion of lactic acid from fatigued muscles back into useful sources of energy, and they improve oxygen delivery, allowing the muscles to work effectively again. Digestion is enhanced, the muscles "come alive," and sensations from the skin are more accurately perceived.

The ability to react in these ways is limited in the extremes of life. Neither infants nor aged persons bear cold treatments well. Certain disease states also produce a profound weakness and sensitivity to cold. Anemia and emaciation as well as some nervous conditions require the modification of cold/hot contrast. In these cases, it may be best to apply heat alone, by means of sunshine or electric heating pads, to secure the stimulating effect. In cases of extreme exhaustion, no cold treatment at all should be given, since the body's reactive powers have been taxed to their utmost.

Techniques of Therapy

Fomentations. A fomentation consists of the application of moist heat to the body's surface. A fomentation cloth is

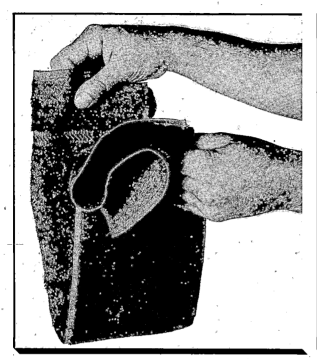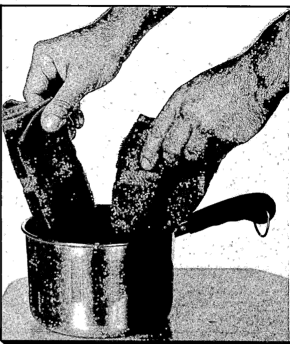

1. To make a fomentation cloth, first fold the towel in thirds. 2. Dip towel in hot water.

usually made of blanket material, 50 percent wool to retain heat and 50 percent cotton to retain moisture and provide greater durability. A kettle for boiling water, such as those used for home canning, can usually provide enough water for most treatments. At least four fomentation cloths should be used, along with a few Turkish towels. A basin of ice water and a foot tub complete the setup.

First, start the water boiling. Fold a fomentation cloth into three thicknesses. Grasp the ends and partially twist the cloth, submerging all but the ends in the boiling water until the material is thoroughly soaked. Then stretch or pull the fomentation cloth to wring it dry. Untwist the wet "fomie" quickly and wrap it in a dry cloth. Fold both double crosswise and roll them to hold the heat. Unfold the cloths at the bedside and place a dry towel over the area to be treated. Cover the whole thing with another towel.

If the fomentation cloth is very hot, rub the skin underneath until it can be tolerated. The additional towel under the fomentation prevents burning and absorbs lost mois-

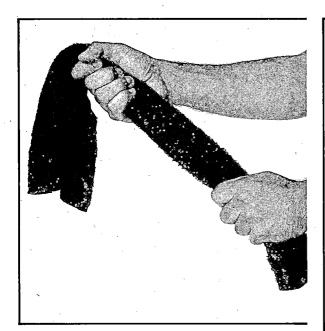

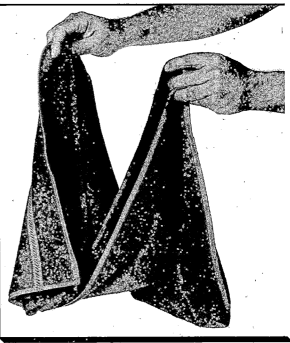

5. Fold the two towels like this.

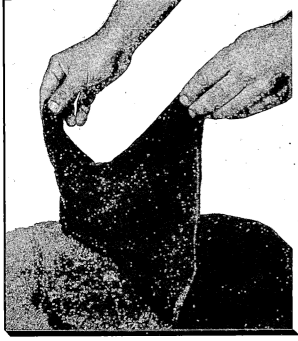

3. Wring the towel. 4. Fold hot towel into a dry towel.

ture. Each application should be left on from three to five minutes. Three applications are usually best. When the last fomentation is removed, cool the area with a cold wash-cloth, and dry the skin thoroughly. All changes of these fomentations should be made quickly, and the area treated should never be left exposed. During the treatment, it is usually necessary to keep a cold cloth on the forehead or neck of the patient to keep his head cool.

Fomentations are very useful in relieving the congestion of chest colds, coughs, bronchitis and influenza. Fomentations can ease the pain of neuralgia, arthritis and other inflammations. They may also stimulate, when alternated with cold, or sedate in nervous conditions. For sedation, apply cloths to the spine; they should be warm, not hot, and the application should be prolonged. Elimination is enhanced by sweating when the fomentations are applied properly. *Take great care to avoid burning the patient,* particularly when there is paralysis, anesthesia, atherosclerosis, diabetes, edema or recent surgery. Protect the bony areas especially, lifting the fomentation frequently to allow steam to escape, or padding them with an additional towel.

Hot footbath. As one would expect, a hot footbath is the submerging of the feet and ankles in water ranging in temperature from 100° to 115° F. This therapy is used to increase the blood flow locally and indirectly from the feet to the entire skin surface. In a derivative way, the hot footbath promotes decongestion in the internal pelvic organs and the head. For this reason, it is often used to relieve congestion in the head and chest and to treat headaches. Even a nosebleed can be stopped by this simple treatment when used in combination with ice packs over the face.

When prolonged, these baths will induce sweating and may help to prevent or abort a common cold. Relaxation and comfort are produced, and, of course, local inflammation of the feet may be relieved by this simple measure.

A metal foot tub or plastic container large and deep enough to contain the feet and ankles should be used. Even a five-gallon can or a plastic wastebasket will do. If a thermometer is not available, test the water temperature with your elbow. Protect the bed or floor from spilled water. Any prolonged treatment to the feet should be combined with a cold compress to the head to increase the derivative effect and avoid headaches.

After testing the water temperature, lower the feet slowly and carefully to avoid burning. If there is vascular disease in the extremities or conditions (such as diabetes) in which sensation is reduced, this treatment is not advisable. Frostbite may be treated with a *warm* footbath, but no hot applications should be used. Except for cases of vascular disease, the water temperature is usually started at about 103° F. Hot water is then added from time to time, increasing the temperature to the patient's level of tolerance. The treatment is continued for 10 to 15 minutes, changing the cold compress on the head frequently. When the bath is finished, lift the feet out of the water, pour cold water over them and dry them thoroughly.

A Bracing Rubdown

Cold mitten friction. One of the finest hydrotherapy measures for stimulating blood flow in the skin is cold mitten friction. Increased circulation benefits the entire body, and as a tonic, it is better than anything downed with gin. This treatment is also useful for closing the pores and toning the skin after fomentations. And it can heighten nerve and muscle tone and skin sensitivity. Heat production is increased, as is tissue oxidation. Reflex effects in the internal organs stimulate muscular-glandular and metabolic activities. The friction increases antibody production, thus helping to fight infections and fevers. It builds up general body resistance and is good for those suffering frequent colds. This treatment is also invaluable for people suffering from a lack of energy, particularly when they are cutting out coffee or tobacco.

Although a washcloth can be used to deliver cold mitten friction, it is more effective done with Turkish toweling sewn into the shape of a mitten. The mitten is dipped into ice water, wrung out lightly and rubbed briskly on the skin, up and down, two or three times. The upper extremities are usually treated first, beginning with the fingers and moving up the arm to the shoulders. Each side is dried and covered before the next limb is treated. The chest and abdomen are also rubbed briskly with the friction mitt and then dried and covered. The lower extremities get the same, and then the back. Friction is applied as vigorously as the patient can tolerate and continued until the skin is pink. This type of physical "tonic" is so simple that it can routinely be used after a shower as a morning "pickup."

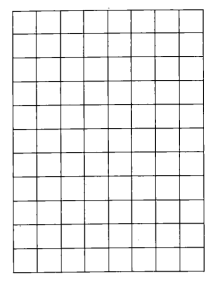

Cold mitten friction stimulates blood flow and increases muscle tone and skin sensitivity.

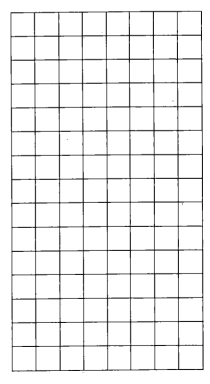

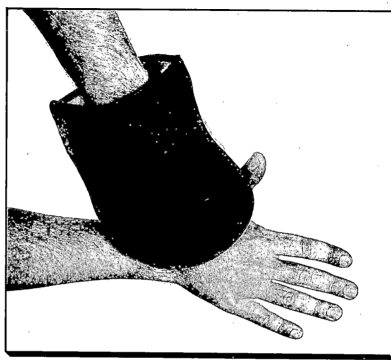

Cold mitten friction is stimulating.

Sitz bath. One of the oldest water therapy procedures is the sitz, or sitting bath. Many abdominal and pelvic conditions were treated in this way by the Austrian practitioner Vincenz Priessnitz, who used water extensively as a curative remedy.

The modern sitz tub is made of metal or porcelain and is fashioned so that a patient may sit in comfort in it while his feet are placed outside in a footbath. A washtub or plastic basin may be used at home; however, it must be slightly tipped and made stationary with blocks of wood. A similar tub or basin can be used for the accompanying footbath. An ordinary bathtub becomes a makeshift sitz bath when the knees are drawn up, leaving only the feet and pelvic organs submerged. Or one can substitute a hot *half*-bath with just enough water to reach the navel.

The temperature of the water may be varied, depending upon the effect desired. Cold sitz baths (55° to 75° F) are useful in the treatment of constipation and *chronic* pelvic inflammation. Hot sitz baths (105° to 110° F) are used to treat pelvic pain during the menstrual cycle and in *acute*

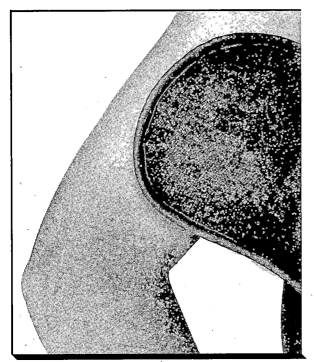

When you massage yourself, slowly move up the leg.

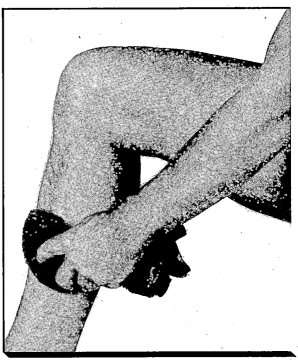

An ice-cold cloth gives a stimulating massage.

pelvic inflammatory conditions. They are also used to treat patients who have trouble urinating. Alternating hot and cold sitz baths is very valuable therapy for both hemorrhoid and prostate trouble and following surgery of the perineum or rectum.

The patient should be protected from contact with the basin by towels placed behind his back and under his knees. He should be covered with a blanket. The water should cover his hips and reach the abdomen. The temperature of the accompanying footbath should be several degrees hotter than the temperature in the sitz tub. Friction may be used with a cold sitz bath if the patient feels chilly or if it is desirable to intensify the effects of the bath. Hot sitz baths should be concluded by cooling the water to neutral or by pouring cold water over the patient's hips and thighs. A cold sitz should be concluded by rubbing his hips and thighs with warm alcohol. Cold compresses to the head and neck should also be used with a hot sitz bath. Watch closely for feelings of faintness.

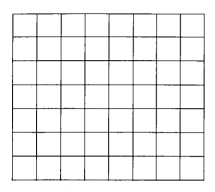

Contrast baths can help poor circulation as well as arthritis.

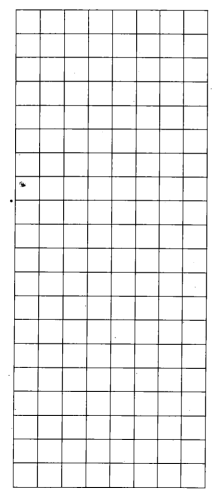

After all such treatments, the patient should rest for 20 to 30 minutes.

First Hot, Then Cold

Contrast baths. As the name implies, a contrast bath consists of alternate applications of hot and cold water to an area of the body. The resulting contraction and dilation of the blood vessels improves the circulation and the elimination of muscle waste products from the area. The increased blood flow delivers the oxygen and nutrients necessary for natural healing processes plus the white blood cells that defend the body against infection.

Two containers large enough to allow water to cover the limb involved are used. Plastic or metal pails are suitable; even a double kitchen sink is okay. Because it is very important to keep the hot water at the correct temperature, a thermometer should be used.

The limbs to be treated are submerged in the hot water, at 105° to 110° F, for three to four minutes, then plunged into cold tap water or ice water for 30 to 60 seconds. One should always start with hot water and end with cold, changing back and forth from three to six times. After the treatment, the limbs should be dried carefully and kept warm.

Contrast baths are used for several conditions. Poor circulation caused by blood vessel diseases can be helped, although, in such situations, temperatures above 105° F are not advisable. A cold water plunge should be no longer than 30 seconds, and a treatment should end in neutral or hot water. Arthritis also benefits from contrast baths, beginning with temperatures of about 110° F and switching to cool tap water on a four-minute and one-minute cycle. After four to six changes, closed with *hot* water, the treatment can be stopped, but it should be repeated at least twice daily.

Put an Injury on Ice

Ice packs. It was Mr. Priessnitz of Austria who first advocated the use of cold compresses after injury. Applications of cold are now given not only to stop the swelling of minor injuries but as anesthetics as well. In proper situations, applications of cold can be just as important as the use of heat later.

For a sprained ankle, ice or even cold water should be applied at the earliest possible moment. When combined with the elevation of the injured limb, the application of cold can prevent swelling and lessen the black-and-blue discoloration of blood vessel injury. The cold contracts blood vessels and keeps blood from oozing into torn tissues. If the injured joint is kept elevated and bandaged with an elastic support, healing will begin rapidly.

Any application of ice or extreme cold should be removed periodically to avoid upsetting the body's ability to react to temperature changes.

Cold can also be applied by immersing the sprained ankle in ice water or cold tap water for 30 minutes out of every two hours; this cycle should continue for at least eight hours. An ice bag or ice pack may be applied to the elevated limb if submersion is difficult.

Tub baths. A neutral tub bath with a temperature of 94° to 98° F can be a valuable sedative. Effective in treating exhaustion of the central nervous system, insomnia and nervous irritability, a tubbing is one of nature's finest tranquilizers and an aid to restful sleep. The tub should be filled with enough water to *cover* the patient to the neck. The room should be quiet, the light should be subdued, and a pillow or folded towel must be placed under the head. While the individual lies quietly in the water, the tub can be covered with a sheet to preserve both his privacy and the water's temperature. After the bath, the skin should be dried with gentle blotting. At least 30 minutes of undisturbed rest should follow the treatment.

WEIGHT TRAINING

Many people picture weightlifters as huge hulks in love with their bodies or as Olympic titans who heft barbells that would give King Kong a hard time. Well, if that's your image of weight training, you might want to change it. Lifting weights isn't just for weirdos and supermen – it's for *anyone.* That is, anyone who wants either to get in shape or to improve on the fitness he's already achieved.

Aerobic activities like running, of course, will give you endurance over the long run; they can help you work or play with more energy by teaching your body how to keep up moderate levels of activity over an extended stretch of time. But weight training teaches your body how to reach a greater short-term intensity. Building yourself up through strength development means you can cope with the sprints of daily life. And that applies to both men *and* women.

A woman shouldn't shrug off the idea of weight training because she's afraid that she'll end up looking like a female Arnold Schwarzenegger. The normal balance of female hormones doesn't allow women to acquire large hunks of muscle. A study of young women by University of Arizona exercise physiologist Jack Wilmore, Ph.D., covering ten weeks, had each woman lifting weights in basic exercises for 40 minutes, two times a week. Strength gains were reported for all women, ranging from 10 to 30 percent. The size of hips was reduced, while bust size increased slightly. No change, on the other hand, was reported in arm size or weight.

In other words, the women in that study didn't gain bulky muscle, but they did make their bodies look better. Flabby became firm, and fat was whittled away.

But maybe you're not interested in building the body beautiful. However, if you like the idea of being able to fetch supermarket bags out of the car trunk without huffing and puffing, weight training is going to be a help. Because not only will weight training give you the extra strength to easily grab that double-bagged sack of cans and bottles, it'll also reduce your chance of hurting yourself in the process.

Clyde Emrich, an Olympic world record holding weightlifter who is the strength coach of the National Football

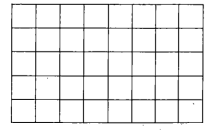

Women who lift weights don't gain bulky muscle, but they do make their bodies look better. Flabby becomes firm and fat is whittled away.

League's Chicago Bears, feels that strong muscles reduce the chance of injury and help in injury rehabilitation. "A strong muscle is easier to control than a weak one," he says. "That's the principle of weight work in general."

According to Rachel McLish, a female bodybuilder who has won the Miss Olympia title, achieving strength by weight training may be especially important for women. "The normal social conditioning for women prevents them from developing their arms and upper bodies, and as a result, they're much weaker than men," she told us. "While it's socially acceptable for men to do a lot of lifting and develop adequate muscles, women don't get the chance to do the same thing. With weight training, although women will never develop the muscles or strength level of men, they can make a big improvement."

Build Up Step by Step

When you start a weight training program, you have to start light. Otherwise, there's a real danger of hurting yourself, and a main objective in any fitness program is *not to get hurt*. You'll do yourself no good to make what seems like spectacular progress, lifting heavier and heavier weights each week, when in reality, you're just setting yourself up for a disastrous injury and a month or two of no exercise while you recuperate.

The idea is to start with light weights that you can easily handle, and progress gradually, adding extra pounds to increase your strength. You do a *slow progression*. That's why the experts call it "progressive" weight training.

The original progressive weight trainer was Milo of Crotona, who lived in the sixth century B.C. According to legend, Milo developed his muscles by lifting a growing calf every day. As the calf grew, so did Milo's biceps and triceps, until one day he could pick up the grown bull and stand with it on his shoulders.

What Milo probably didn't know was that he was using the principle of *overload*. "Once muscle becomes accustomed to a given load it stops gaining, so the load must continually increase," says John Jerome in *The Runner* (March, 1981). "To grow larger, muscle must meet with 'progressive resistance,' represented (in Milo's case) by the growth of the calf. Modern-day experimenters have replaced the baby bovine with the weight machine."

Circuit Weight Training—An Aerobic Tool

If Milo had *run* around the barnyard with the cow on his back, he might have also been able to lay claim to the invention of aerobic weight training, otherwise known as *circuit weight training.*

Circuit weight training is a way to get the best of both worlds – endurance and power. It combines sustained activity with the shorter work periods of strength development. It's a weightlifting routine that consists of 25- to 30-minute sessions of fairly constant effort, with very short breaks between lifts.

In a noncircuit weight training program, people are allowed rest time between exercises. In other words, during a workout, a lifter might plan to do six different kinds of lifts. When he finishes one kind of lift, such as curls, he takes a few minutes to catch his breath before moving on to the next lift. But that rest time slows down the development of aerobic, cardiovascular fitness, since the key to getting your heart and lungs to grow in their ability to deliver oxygen to the body is to keep them working for a prolonged period without stopping to catch your breath.

To aid your aerobic development, then, you should optimally take no time off between exercises. Since zero time between movements probably isn't possible to achieve, rest time should be limited to 15 seconds or less. This technique of exercising with weights is, as we said, circuit weight training.

Writing in *The Physician and Sportsmedicine* magazine, Larry R. Gettman, Ph.D., executive director of the Institute for Aerobics Research in Dallas, and Michael L. Pollock, Ph.D., director of the cardiovascular disease section of the department of medicine at the University of Wisconsin Medical School, say that CWT (circuit weight training) has three main uses. One is its use as an exercise program by those who, for a variety of reasons, want to exercise but don't want to run, swim or bicycle: "CWT may have value as a beginning exercise program if the intensity and musculoskeletal stress are kept at a minimum in the early stages of the program."

The second use is as a means for effectively reducing fat and increasing muscle. This will not necessarily result in weight loss, because you're replacing lost fat tissue with more muscle mass: "CWT can be used as a weight-control program, although compared with aerobic training programs, the change in total body weight may not be as apparent, because the increases in LBW (lean body weight, or muscle) and the losses in body fat may offset each other."

The third use of CWT is as a maintenance program for injured athletes. If you're a runner, for instance, and you hurt your leg, you could have a hard time trying to give your leg time to heal while keeping up your aerobic fitness. A CWT program could let you keep strain off your injury while still giving your heart and lungs a workout.

According to Dr. Pollack and Dr. Gettman, "Persons who suffer leg soreness or injury in a running program or sports activities requiring running could participate in a CWT program to help maintain cardiorespiratory fitness during convalescence. The ability to maintain cardiorespiratory fitness with CWT is probably related to the fact that once fitness is attained, it takes less effort to maintain it. Two studies showed that subjects who reduced their jogging mileage by as much as 50 percent still maintained their cardiorespiratory endurance for 5 to 15 weeks."

Weight training, then, can be adapted to fit many needs. At the beginning, remember, you should use light weights, no matter what your eventual goals. But as you progress, you can decide if you want to use weights to support your aerobic fitness or mainly to increase your strength. If you decide on the aerobic route, then your emphasis will always be on light weights and a lot of repetitions. You'll be pumping small amounts of iron for longer periods of time.

On the other hand, if you want to emphasize your strength development, then you'll try to move to heavier weights which you'll be lifting fewer times. Heavier lifts put maximum strain on the working muscle, resulting in the greatest gains of strength but not necessarily endurance. Your muscles will be able to move larger amounts of weight, but only for a short time before exhaustion.

Before You Lift, Stretch

Before you touch a weight, you should know something about stretching. Stretching is a slow motion designed to relax muscles and lessen their chance of injury. It used to be that athletes used calisthenics to warm up before doing vigorous exercise, but stretching has now largely replaced jumping jacks and push-ups as a means of getting muscles ready for work.

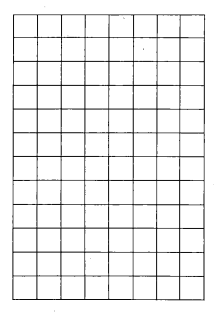

When you first start weight training, you should start with light weights that you can easily handle and progress gradually to heavier weights. Do a slow progression.

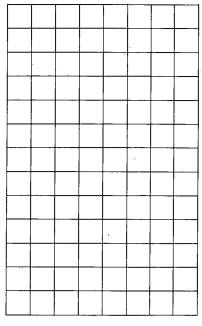

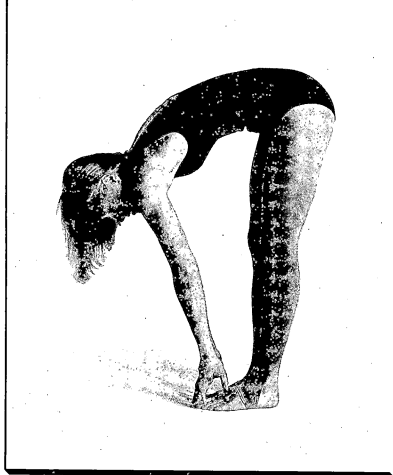

The toe touch.

You should do at least 7 to 15 minutes of stretching prior to a lifting session, and just as much afterward. The first stretch is a simple "toe touch" to loosen up the lower back, legs and hips. Staying relaxed, stand up with your feet slightly spread. Bend forward, and gently reach for your toes. (Don't force yourself; bend as far as you comfortably can, and don't worry if you can't make it all the way down to your toes.) Bob Anderson, in his book *Stretching* (Shelter Publications, 1980), recommends keeping your knees slightly bent as you reach down in order to avoid stressing the lower back.

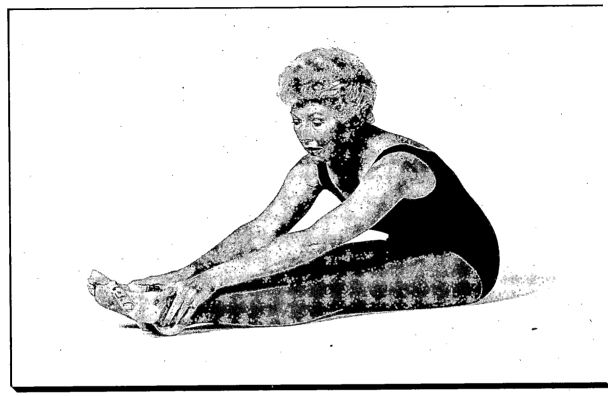

The ankle grab.

Do the toe touch for about 15 seconds. You'll probably feel most of the stretch in the back of your legs. After 15 seconds, relax for about 10 seconds. Repeat the stretch three or four times.

After the toe touch, move on to the "Achilles tendon stretch." The Achilles tendon is the long tissue connecting your heel to your calf. Lean against a wall, both feet pointing forward. Keeping your feet flat on the floor, move one foot back until you feel a pulling sensation in the back of your calf down toward your foot. Hold this position for 10 to 15 seconds, and then switch feet. Do this exercise for about two minutes.

The next stretch is the "ankle grab," done on the floor. Sit down with your legs straight out in front of you. Gently reach down and try to grasp your ankles without bending your knees. If you can't reach your ankles, grab your calves or whatever part of your leg you can comfortably reach. Hold this position for about 10 to 15 seconds.

Next, roll onto your back and bring your feet over your head. Without straining, try to bring your knees close to your ears while you are lying on your back. Hold this position for about ten seconds. Alternate the back stretch with the ankle grab for four or five repetitions.

On the last feet-over-the-head stretch, instead of putting your knees to your ears, hold your legs out straight, bringing your feet as close to the floor as possible, and try to grab your ankles. This is the yoga "plough position." Hold it for about 15 seconds. Eventually, if you develop your flexibility, you will be able to put your feet all the way down on the floor behind your head.

The last exercise is the "hamstring stretch." To do the hamstring stretch from a standing position, put your right leg out straight in front of you, resting the foot on a table or chair about three feet high. Keeping both legs straight, slowly lower your head toward your right knee while grasping your hands behind your right calf. Don't go too far! Stay comfortable, but create a slight pulling sensation in your upper thigh as you lean forward.

A slight variation of the hamstring stretch, which will

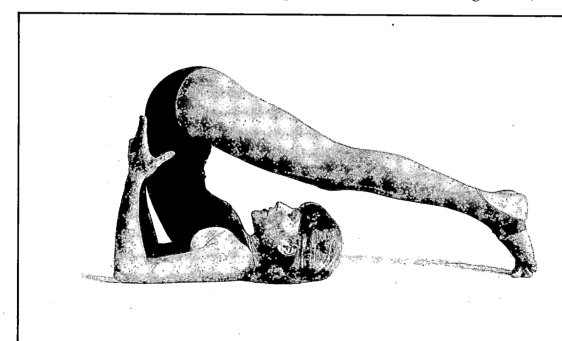

The plough.

loosen some additional muscles, is to reach for your ankle with alternate hands as you lean forward. In other words, first grab your ankle with your right hand and put your head toward your right knee and then grab the same ankle with the left hand. By switching hands instead of using both hands at the same time, you introduce a slight twist to the torso.

Weightlifting's Fundamental Tools

To lift weights, obviously, the first equipment you are going to need is a set of weights. According to experienced weightlifters, both pro and amateur, a set of barbells and dumbbells gives the best results.

A barbell is the big weight bar, the kind that you lift with two hands. Dumbbells are the small weights, the ones you can handle singlehandedly. By having both dumbbells and barbells, you'll be able to develop more muscles by doing more movements.

Olympic standard barbells are always seven feet long. The kind you'll probably buy will be five to six feet long. The central bar that holds the weights should have a loose-fitting sleeve that sits around the middle of the bar. Collars on each side of the bar secure the weights to the bar.

For the exercises, you'll need two dumbbells. These are usually about 18 inches long. Their construction is similar to the larger barbell.

In the book *Working Out with Weights* (Arco, 1978), Steve Jarrell, an experienced weightlifter, recommends having at least 90 pounds of plates. (Plates are the circular, weighted slabs that you attach to your bars.) Most sets available in stores are the 110-pound "basic set" that includes 90 pounds of plates. The most common plate sizes are 2½, 5, 10 and 25 pounds.

When you go to buy weights, you'll probably have a choice between metal plates and plastic plates filled with sand. The metal plates are more expensive and noisier when you lift them up and clang them down. Their advantage over the cheaper plastic weights is that they will last much longer. The cheaper plastic weights will eventually wear out.

The plastic weights usually cost about $35 to $40; the metal weights retail for about $70. When you think about it, much of this equipment is less expensive than many running shoes! And the weights, even if you use them every day, will outlast the shoes by a decade.

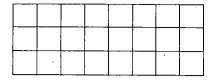

Always be conservative when you lift weights. Never lift on consecutive days. Your muscles need at least 48 hours to recover before another round of pumping iron.

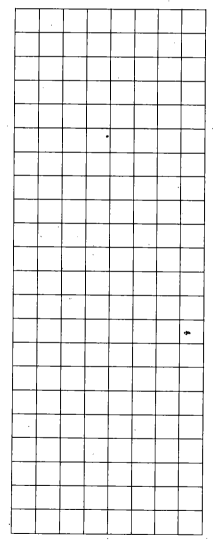

Start Out Lightly

No matter how strong you think you are, you should always be conservative in how much you try to lift. For at least the first month, stay with light weights until you feel comfortable doing the exercises. The exercises, for best results, should be done two or three times a week on alternate days – *never* on two consecutive days. The muscles used in weight training need at least 48 hours to recover before being subjected to the rigors of another round of pumping iron.

Some lifters do train on consecutive days by working different muscles on different days. That way, individual muscles get a 48-hour break even though workouts are 24 hours apart. For most people, however, workouts every other day are the best bet.

The first set of exercises is done with the barbell. Depending on your size and strength, you can probably start with a maximum of 40 pounds on the bar. Remember that, at first, it's better to start too light than too heavy.

For safety's sake, before you pick up a barbell with weights on it, make sure that the weights are securely attached. The collars that hold on the weighted plates should be screwed on as tight as possible. Otherwise, you run the risk of having them slide off the bar and land on you, your floor, your furniture or whatever else is nearby – with unpleasant results.

Another safety idea worth trying, if you can, is to do your lifting with a partner. That way, you have a "spotter" on hand to help out if you run into any trouble with your weights. A spotter is someone who watches you lift and stands nearby, ready to give aid in any kind of troublesome situation. If you restrict your lifting to moderate or light weights, you should have little difficulty and perhaps will never need a spotter. But just the same, having one can't hurt.

For instance, if you're on your back doing a bench press (described later in this chapter) and you feel that you might lose control of the weight, a spotter can take it out of your hands. Or, if you have a barbell across your shoulders and you're too tired to get it down to the floor easily, your spotter can assist you.

When you pick your barbell up off the floor, you should try to make sure that most of the lifting motion is carried out by your legs and arms. The *wrong way* to pick up a weight is by leaning forward, not bending your legs, and

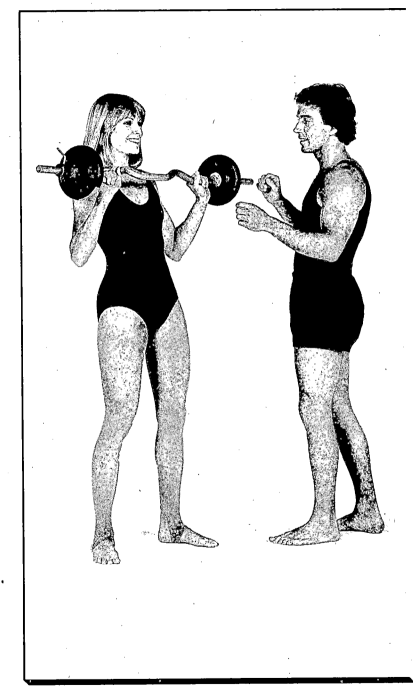

A spotter makes weightlifting safer.

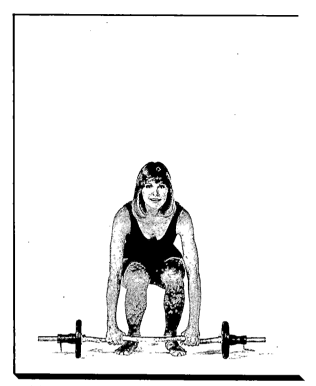 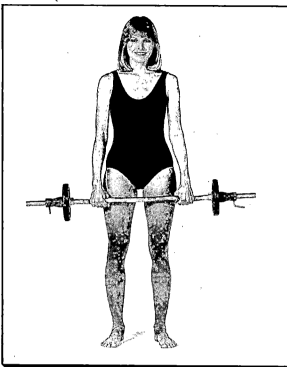

1. The military press requires a straight back. 2. Stand with weights at your thighs.

snatching it up to your chest. That kind of motion transfers all the stress of the lift to that narrow area of your back just above your buttocks. That's an easy way to hurt yourself and develop a chronic injury that will be tough to cure.

The *right way* is to bend your legs as you lift the barbell. Keeping your back as straight as possible, squat down in front of the weights with the barbell close to your ankles, the bar over your feet. With your arms straight, grasp the bar using an overhand grip (see photo).

You lift the bar by straightening your legs and standing, always keeping your back perpendicular to the ground. As the weights go past your knees, start tucking your elbows into your body and bring the barbell up to your shoulders using back and leg motion.

This is the starting motion for the "military press." With the weight down on your shoulders, push it over your head just using your arms until your elbows are locked and you've extended the weight as high as you can. Then lower the weight to your shoulders *slowly.*

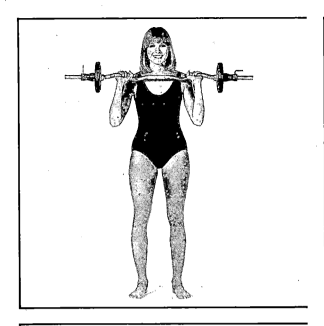

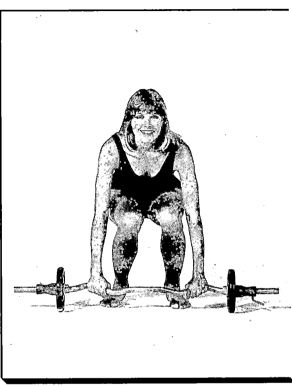

5. Put the weights down carefully at the end.

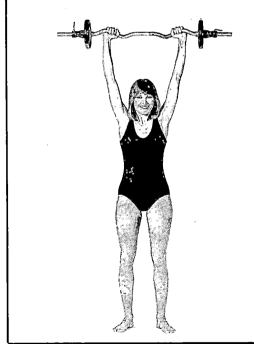

3. Bring bar up to your shoulders. 4. Lift weights over your head.

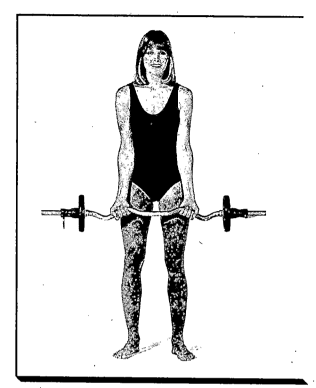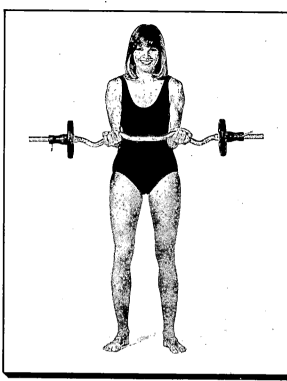

1. A curl is done with an underhand grip. 2. Bring the weights up using just your arms.

That last point is important for the military press and *all* the other exercises. If you let the weights down too fast, you'll miss some of the benefits of lifting. Lowering them slowly makes your muscles work more (in some cases even more than the lifting motion) by making them resist gravity.

The military press is a standard exercise for developing the shoulders. The muscles involved are primarily located there and in your arms and upper back. An alternative way to do the press is to lower the weight down to a position behind your head on your shoulders. That method will vary the motion you use and will give you a little extra workout.

Lifting the weight up from your shoulders and then back down is considered to be one repetition of the military press. You should do at least ten of them if you are trying to increase your aerobic endurance. If your goal is strength and you are lifting very heavy weights, you should aim for about half a dozen repetitions.

The "curl" is another good exercise for the upper body and the arms. It will develop your biceps and forearms.

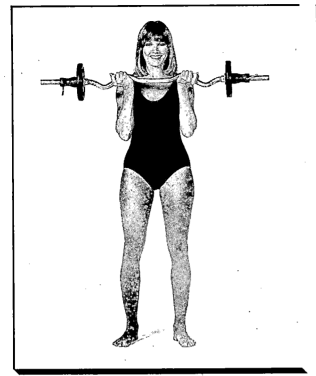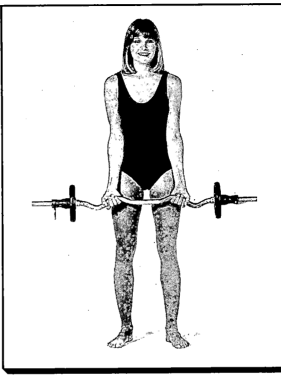

3. The bar comes up to your shoulders. 4. Then slowly lower the weights.

Curls can be done with either the barbell or the dumb-bells. Using the dumbbells will let you do the workout at different angles and make it possible, if you desire, to exercise one arm at a time.

To do the curl with the barbell, start with the barbell hanging from your arms, resting on your thighs using an underhand grip. Without moving your elbows or your upper body, use your forearms to lift the weights to your shoulders. If you move your back as you lift, your forearms and biceps won't get the full benefit of the exercise.

After you've raised the weight to your shoulders, lower it *slowly* to original position. During the curl, be sure to keep your elbows and arms close to the body.

Curls should be done at least ten times to build up your endurance. If you are working primarily on strength and you are using large weights, do at least five repetitions.

"Reverse curls" are done in the same manner as curls except that the bar in the starting position is held with an overhand grip. Usually, reverse curls have to be done with

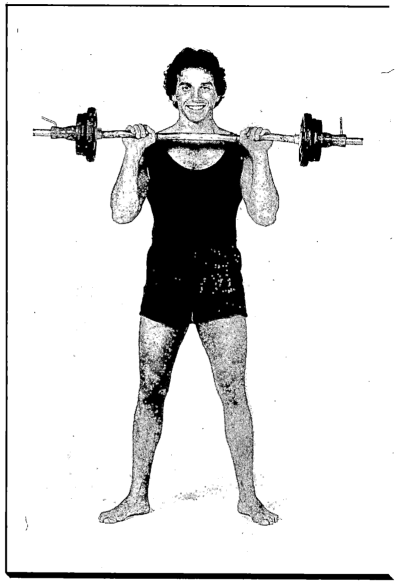

The reverse curl is done in an overhand position.

lighter weights (at least ten pounds lighter for a barbell reverse curl) than the regular curl because the muscles involved are not as strong as those involved with a regular curl.

"Rows" are variations of curls that allow you to move your arms and therefore develop a different combination of muscles than the other exercises.

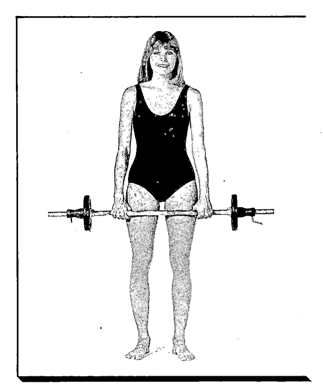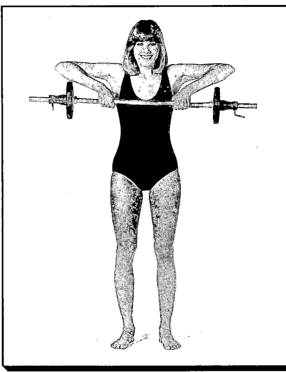

1. The upright row starts in an overhand position. 2. Lift, and bend your elbows.

The "upright row" starts in the same beginning position as the reverse curl. Keeping the barbell close to your body, raise it to your chin using your arms and letting your elbows flare out (see photo). Use only your arms for the lift, and don't let your body swing. After you raise the weight, *slowly* lower the weight to the starting position to complete one repetition. You should try to do ten repetitions of the upright row to build strength and endurance.

The "bent-over row" involves a similar rowing motion, but the weight is lifted from near the floor while you bend over it. To begin this exercise, you should bend from the waist, keeping your back straight and parallel to the floor and bending your knees slightly. Using an overhead position, lift the barbell until it touches your chest. Then lower the bar until it is near the ground but not touching it. Those two movements are one repetition. You should do 10 repetitions of this exercise for power development; do

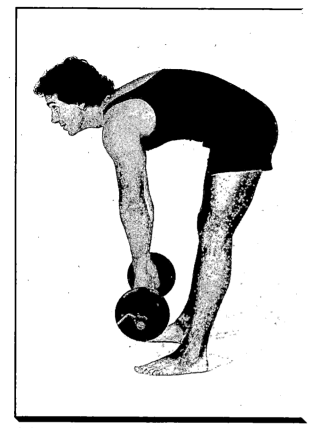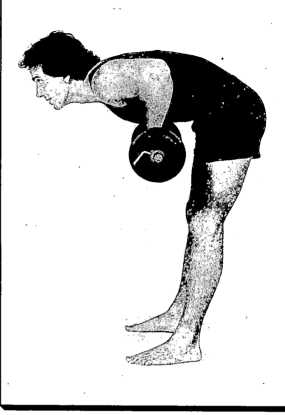

1. Extend your arms to start the bent-over row. 2. Then pull the weights to your chest.

as many as 20 to fully develop your aerobic endurance.

When you do the bent-over row, be sure to keep your body motionless except for your arms. Done that way, the exercise is very good for developing your upper back and forearm muscles.

The "bench press" is another good exercise for the upper body. It requires a bench to lie down on, as well as a stand for the weights (see photo) or a partner to assist you during the lift.

The lift starts with you lying on your back, the barbell gripped at about shoulder width at your chest. Raise the bar until your arms are fully extended, and then slowly lower it back to your chest. That motion is one repetition. For endurance purposes, the bench press should be done at least ten times. For developing power and strength, do it with heavier weights about six times.

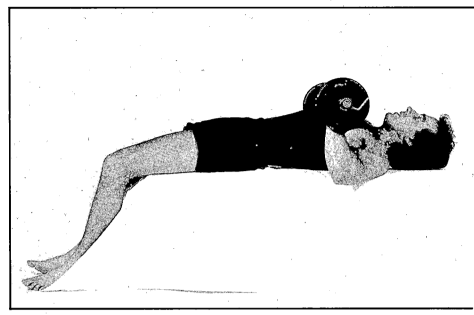

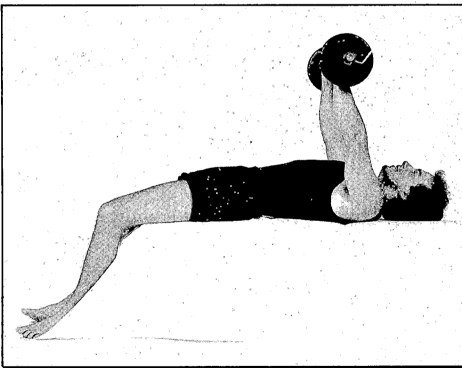

1. The bench press starting position. 2. The bench press, arms fully extended.

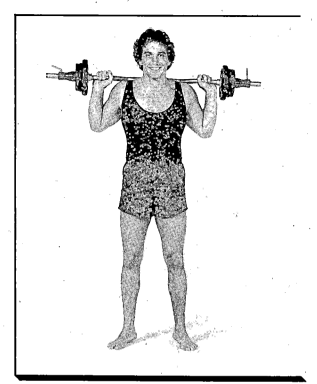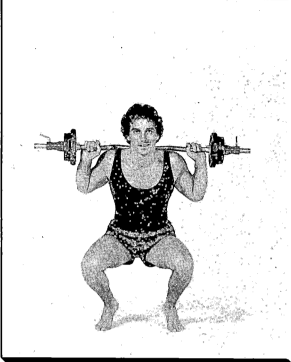

1. The squat starts with the bar across the shoulders. 2. Keep the back as straight as possible.

How to Have Slender, Strong Legs

Legs are important – both how they look and how they hold up (tired legs are no fun). A good exercise for developing lower body muscle is the "squat." Squats are very effective in tightening your thighs and buttocks as well as stomach muscles.

The squat begins with your feet a comfortable distance apart and the barbell on your shoulders. Point your toes slightly outward and grasp the bar with your hands midway between your shoulders and the weights (see photo). To do one "partial squat," you slowly bend your knees and squat one quarter of the way to the floor.

To do a "full squat," come down until your thighs are parallel to the floor. Your heels should be flat on the floor during the entire exercise. If you are not flexible enough to keep them down, put a board under your heels to give you extra support.

During the exercise, you should keep your back straight

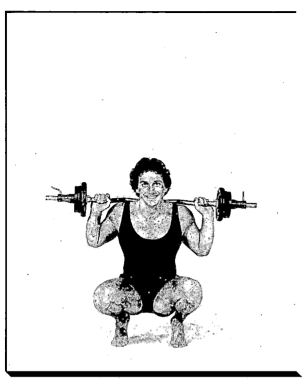

3. Full squat.

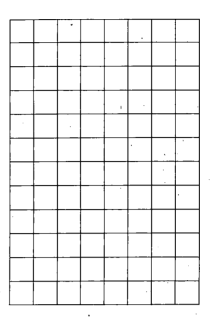

When you do squats, you should never bounce. Bouncing puts tremendous pressure on your knees and may cause joint problems.

and your head up. In his book *The Gold's Gym Book of Strength Training* (J. P. Tarcher, 1979), Ken Sprague recommends picking a focal point for your eyes during the exercise and keeping your eyes on that point the whole time. This will help keep your body in the proper upright position and put less stress on your lower back.

An important point to remember about squats is not to bounce on your way down. Bouncing puts tremendous pressure on your knees and may cause joint problems that will outweigh the exercise's benefits.

"Lunges" are also a good way to slim down leg and rear-end fat. They are similar to squats. The weights are held with the barbell across the shoulders, but the feet are separated, one foot forward and the other back (see photo on next page). You kneel forward, bringing the back leg toward the floor and the front leg bent at a 90-degree angle. Again, as you did during the squat, keep your head up (don't bend your neck down or bury your chin in your chest) and your back as straight as possible. To make the

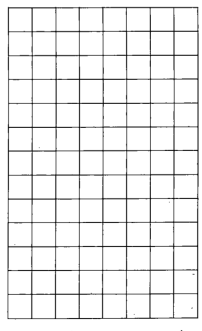

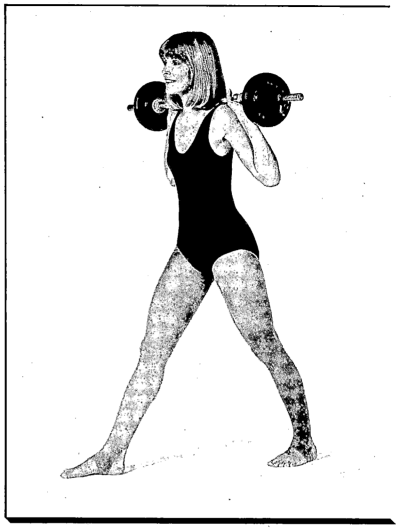

1. During the lunge, the bar is across your shoulders.

exercise develop as much of a range of motion – the move-ment of your joints – as possible, you should alternate foot positions every ten repetitions.

Squats and lunges should be done at least 20 times to develop your endurance, 10 times for power. If you do them for endurance, be careful when you get near the end of the exercise and are tired – resist the urge to bounce. This urge gets worse when fatigue sets in. During these and all lifts, you should always retain control of your body. Don't let yourself get overly tired.

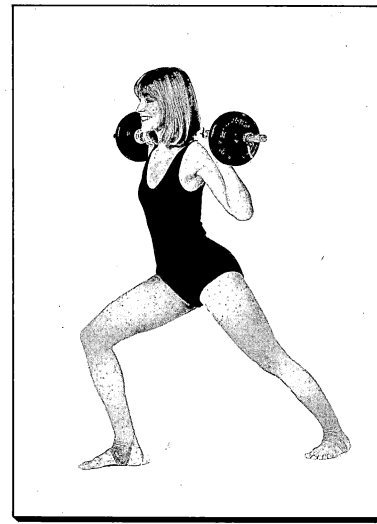

2. Don't lunge too violently or lose body control.

Bending Over with Dumbbells for Flexibility

Dumbbells are handier than the barbell for doing exercises that develop strength *and* flexibility. They allow you a greater range of motion than a barbell does; with a barbell, you're pretty much restricted to one plane of motion – straight up and down. Dumbbells, on the other hand, can be moved in arcs, and the angle of the lifts can be changed between repetitions of the same exercise.

The "stiff-legged dead lift" is done with a dumbbell in

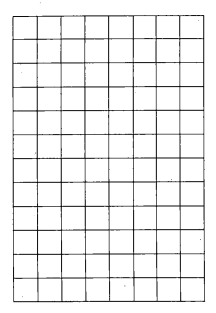

Dumbbells are handy for developing strength and flexibility. They allow a greater range of motion than a barbell does, and the angle of your lifts can be changed between repetitions of the same exercise.

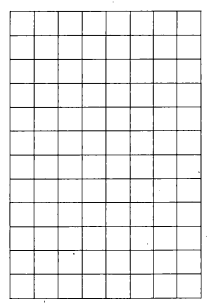

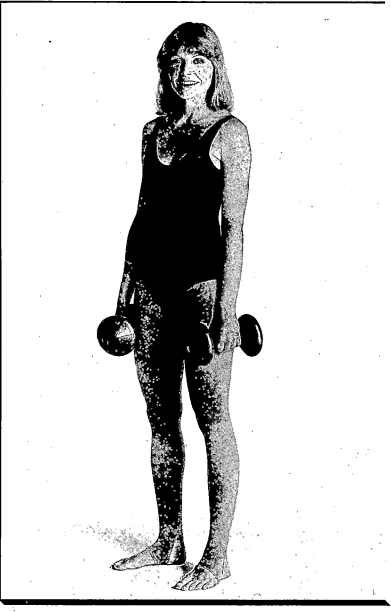

1. The stiff-legged dead lift starts with dumbbells at your sides.

each hand (see photo). You start out standing straight, your arms hanging at your sides. Keeping your legs straight, with the knees slightly flexed (to avoid back strain), *very slowly* lower the dumbbells to your toes as you bend over. Then stand back up in the original position.

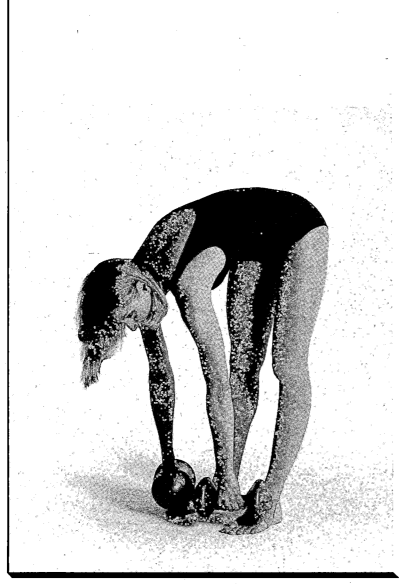

2. Second stage of the dead lift – lower weights to your toes.

Don't worry if you are unable to reach all the way down to your toes. If you do this exercise regularly for several months, you should be able to see some improvement in your flexibility. Don't do more than 20 of these exercises a day in the beginning, and start out with very

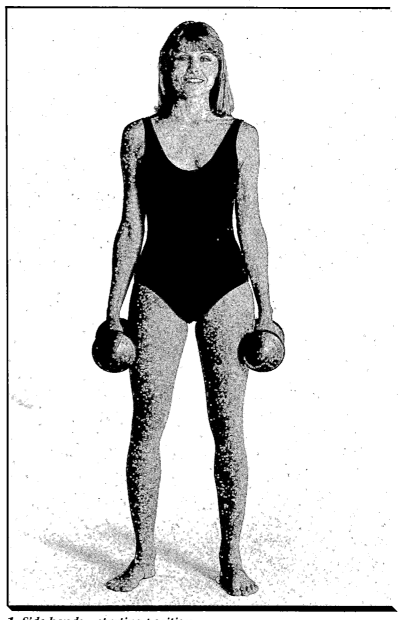

1. Side bends – starting position.

light weights. Eventually, as your flexibility improves, you can increase the amount of weight on the dumbbells.

"Side bends" will also promote the flexibility of your lower back. Side bends start out the same way as the stiff-legged dead lift, with the dumbbells in your hands hanging

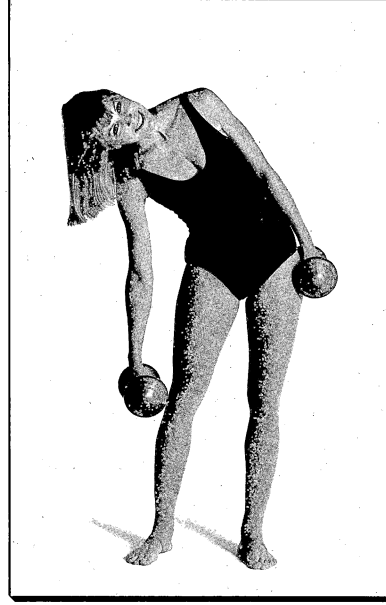

2. Bend from the waist to either side.

by your sides. To do the side bends, lean over to each side as far as you can ·go comfortably, alternating sides. The combination of a bend to each side is one repetition.

Charles Palmer, in the book *New Exercises for Runners* (World Publications, 1978), recommends doing at least

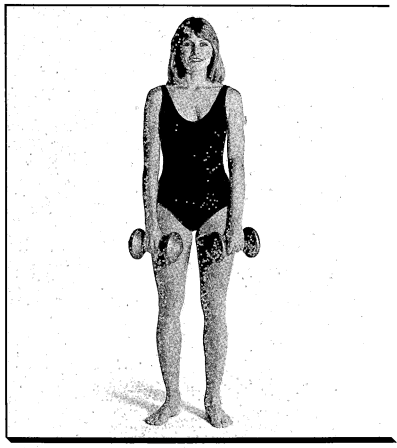

1. *The lateral raise begins with weights in front of your thighs.*

25 repetitions of bending exercises with dumbbells to promote flexibility. He also cautions lifters to limit the dumbbell weights to 30 pounds for these kinds of exercises. Once
you work your way up to the 30-pound level for this exercise, you should increase the number of repetitions you are
doing rather than increasing the amount of weight any further.

You can vary the side bends by bending forward and
sideways at various angles as you lean over. Remember to
keep your knees slightly flexed and your legs straight during
all of these bends.

"Lateral raises" are a good dumbbell exercise for developing shoulder strength. The exercise begins with the dumbbells held in an overhand grip in front of your thighs (see

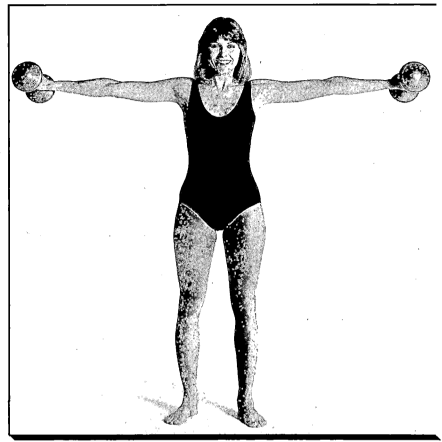

2. Keep your arms straight during the lateral raise.

photo). Keeping your arms straight at all times, very slowly lift the dumbbell outward to either side until they reach shoulder height. Then slowly bring them back down to your thighs, never swinging them and never losing control of the motion.

If you let the dumbbells swing during the lateral raises, you'll unnecessarily stress the ligaments and tendons in your arms and back. The swinging motion won't produce any benefits to the muscles involved in the exercise.

At the beginning, do the lateral raises 10 times with light weights to develop your form. For endurance, raise the number of repetitions you do gradually, up to around 20 to 25.

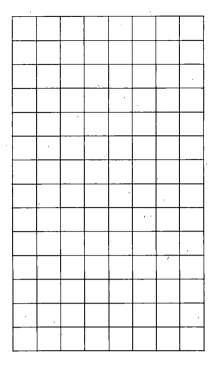

YOGA

At 5,000 plus years, yoga is one of the oldest forms of healing therapy. No longer regarded as the theatrics of Indian fakirs sitting on spikes, the amazing results of yoga are now being studied by scientists all over the world. Teams of doctors at the I. C. Yogic Health Centers in Bombay and Lonavala, India, keep detailed records of patients treated with yoga for diabetes, respiratory ailments, digestive complaints and obesity. In Krakow, Poland, Dr. Julian Aleksandrowicy, director of the Third Clinic of Medicine, has examined the effects of yoga postures on the composition and quality of the blood.

So, yoga is no longer thought to be a sideshow trick or the subject matter of exotic movies. It's a serious mental and physical discipline that many conventionally trained doctors think may help in both sickness and health. Fine. But what *exactly* is it? Basically, yoga teaches that a healthy person is a harmoniously integrated unit of body, mind and spirit. Therefore, good health requires a simple, natural diet, exercise in fresh air, a serene and untroubled mind and the awareness that man's deepest and highest self is identical with the spirit of God. As a result, to many devotees yoga becomes a philosophy that offers instruction and insight into every aspect of life: the spiritual, the mental *and* the physical. Of course, because it *is* all-encompassing, people who want to pick and choose from its smorgasbord can do so without being disappointed. Yoga is equally satisfying as a physical therapy alone.

Yoga teaches that a healthy person is a harmoniously integrated unit of body, mind and spirit.

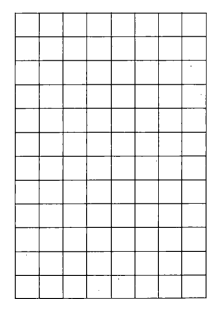

The Primacy of Relaxation

Yoga therapy begins with relaxation. Living in an age of anxiety, we are often unconscious of our tensions. With normal bodies, why are we depressed, tired, prey to disease? Because tension is invisibly draining away our health energies!

Ruth Rogers, M.D., of Daytona Beach, Florida, who has made a ten-year study of yoga therapy, says, "In understanding the healing process, relaxation is of supreme importance. You feel pain, and you don't want to move, so you tighten up. You're tense. Your muscles contract, constricting the blood flow. Swelling begins. More circulation is cut off, creating a vicious cycle. There's more pain, more tightening, more stiffness, more swelling. . . . This is also what happens in many back problems." She adds, "But if you can relax, fresh blood can circulate nourishment to the afflicted tissues and relieve pain-loaded nerve endings. Healing can begin."

Most yoga therapy – some experts would claim *all* successful treatments – involves a three-pronged attack. When you practice yoga postures, you are strengthening the body. When you control your breathing, you are creating a chemical and emotional balance. And when you concentrate your mind on affirmations, you are practicing the power of prayer. But when all three approaches are synthesized, you are entering the most powerful mystery of healing: the basic harmony of life.

"The benefits of the postures are greater," says Dr. Rogers, "if the patient concentrates the healing action where it is needed. In other words, you should mentally see the affected area as it receives fresh blood circulation, oxygen and physical massage. A diabetic should visualize the healing energies flowing into the pancreas, near the stomach. A rheumatic can concentrate on the release of synovial fluid. Synovial fluid is a lubricant and also disperses waste matter which can cause stiffness at joints."

An Indian Guide to the Healing Powers of Yoga

Most of the following common disorders, which are scientifically treated at the Yoga Research Laboratory at Lonavala, India, have also been treated successfully by Dr. Rogers. The performance of each posture should be preceded by relaxation and deep breathing. Directions for each posture are given later.

Asthma: *Corpse Pose, Mountain, Complete Breath.*
   Visualization: Lung expansion, renewed strength.
Backache: *Corpse Pose, Locust, Knee to Chest.*
   Visualization: Fresh circulation to nourish back muscles.
Bronchitis: *Mountain, Locust.*
Cold: *Lion.*
Constipation: *Bow, Corpse Pose, Knee to Chest* (reinvigorates liver, spleen, intestines), *Posterior Stretch, Uddiyana, Yoga Mudra.*

Visualization: Increased circulation to stimulate intestines.

Depression: *Yoga Mudra, Corpse Pose.*
Visualization: New energy from increased oxygen levels in the blood, pending new joyous activity.

Diabetes (not a cure!): *Corpse Pose, Kneeling Pose.*
Visualization: See healing energies of fresh circulation flow to pancreas.

Emphysema: *Complete Breath, Locust, Grip.*
Visualization: Healing circulation to lungs.

Eyestrain: *Neck and Eye Exercises.*
Visualization: Absorb invisible energy from the air ("prana") into the eyes.

Flatulence: *Knee to Chest.*

Headache: *Corpse Pose, Neck and Eye Exercises, Shoulder Roll.*
Visualization: A summer blue sky. No thoughts.

Indigestion: *Corpse Pose, Mountain, Locust, Posterior Stretch, Cobra, Uddiyana.*

Insomnia: *Corpse Pose, Mountain, Locust, Posterior Stretch, Cobra.*
Visualization: Blue sky. Enjoy the yoga. No thoughts.

Menstrual disorders: *Uddiyana, Cobra, Posterior Stretch.*

Neurasthenia: *Corpse Pose, Mountain, Posterior Stretch.*
Visualization: Energy-giving fresh circulation.

Obesity: *Locust, Posterior Stretch, Cobra, Yoga Mudra, Bow, Sun Salutation.*

Prostate troubles: *Kneeling Pose.*

Rheumatism: *Mountain, Knee to Chest, Posterior Stretch.*
Visualization: The dispersal of waste matter causing stiffness at the joints.

Sciatica: *Knee to Chest, Grip, Kneeling Pose.*

Sexual debility: *Uddiyana, Kneeling Pose, Complete Breath.*
Visualization: Youthful vigor from fresh blood circulation.

Sinus: *Neck and Eye Exercises, Corpse Pose.*

Skin diseases: *Sun Salutation.*
Visualization: A general physical tone-up, regulating and balancing any irregularity.

Sore throat: *Lion.*
Visualization: Constriction of blood vessels in the throat; the relaxation brings fresh circulation to sore area.

Wrinkles: *Yoga Mudra.*

The Next Step—A Yoga How-To

Now that you know what to do – that is, which yoga postures minister to your particular problem – you should know how to do it. Here is a simplified method for exercising with yoga each day and a step-by-step guide to executing the common therapeutic postures.

A Basic Daily Yoga Program

Daily yoga practice is a good investment in health. Twelve minutes a day will purchase a toning of the muscles and improved digestive, circulatory and respiratory systems. The following exercises will provide a well-balanced program, which should be supplemented, of course, by any other postures that are particularly good for your needs:

- First day: *Complete Breath, Knee to Chest, Cobra, Sun Salutation, Corpse Pose.*
- Second day: *Complete Breath, Sun Salutation, Corpse Pose.*
- Third day: *Complete Breath, Bow, Cobra, Posterior Stretch, Corpse Pose.*
- Fourth day and on: Repeat sequence.

A Posture Primer for Beginners

Before eating, in either the morning or the late afternoon, spread a blanket on the floor in a well-ventilated room. Wear loose clothing. As a general rule, backward-bending postures should be balanced by forward-bending poses.

Never force or strain in yoga. The postures should be performed slowly, even meditatively. Yoga postures are meant to be held in dynamic tension, and they should not be confused with vigorous calisthenics.

Bow Lie flat on your stomach, grasping the ankles. Inhale. Lifting legs, head and chest, arch the back into a bow. Retain breath, then exhale and lie flat. Repeat three or four times.

More advanced: While in the *Bow* position, rock back and forth, then from side to side. Slowly release and exhale.

Reported benefits: Massages abdominal muscles and organs. Good for gastrointestinal disorders, constipation, upset stomach, sluggish liver. Reduces abdominal fat.

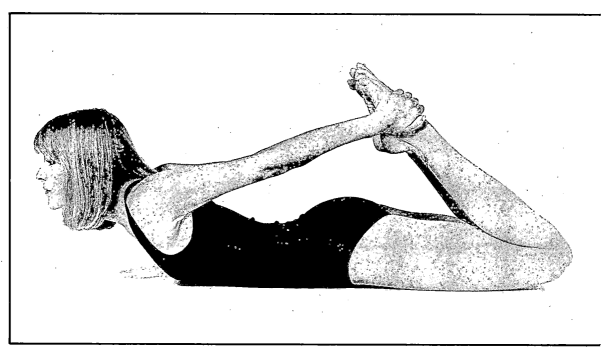

1. The Bow *begins in this position.*

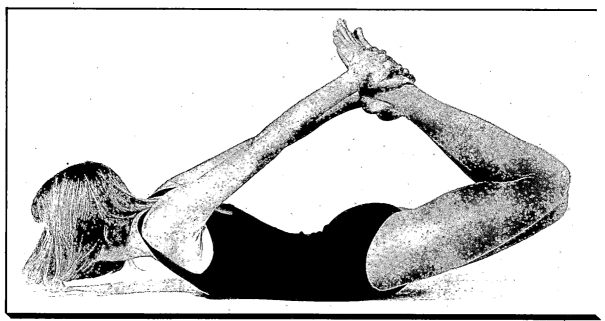

2. Rock forward.

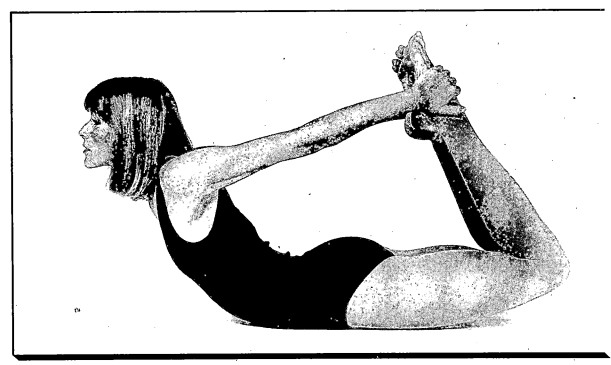

3. Then rock back.

Warning: Not for persons suffering from peptic ulcer, hernia, or cases of thyroid or endocrine gland disorders.

Cobra Lie on the stomach, toes extended. Place the hands, palms down, under the shoulders on the floor. Inhaling, without lifting the navel from the floor, raise the chest and head, arching the back. Retain the breath, then exhale while slowly lowering to the floor. Repeat one to six times.

Reported benefits: Tones ovaries, uterus and liver. Aids in relief and elimination of menstrual irregularities. Relieves constipation. Limbers spine. Excellent for slipped discs.

Warning: Not recommended for sufferers from peptic ulcer, hernia or hyperthyroid.

Complete Breath Crowded city living, air pollution and sedentary jobs are helping to increase respiratory ailments.

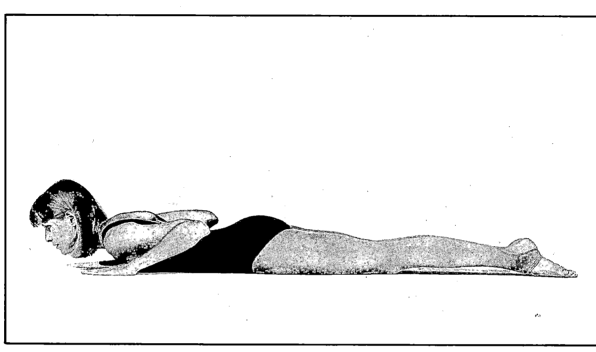

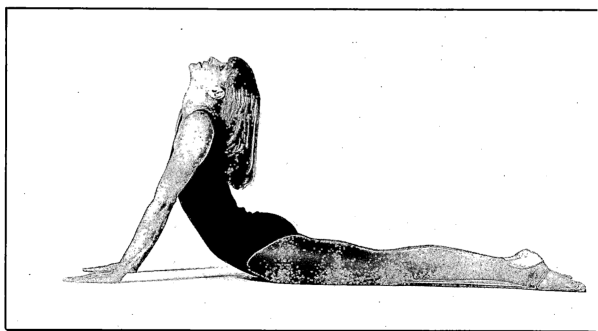

1. The Cobra *begins face down on the floor.* *2. Arch your back and look up to complete the* Cobra.

Tight clothes encourage shallow breathing and cramp the lungs. The purpose of the *Complete Breath* is to fully expand the air sacs of the lungs, thereby exposing the capillaries to the maximum exchange of carbon dioxide and oxygen.

1. Lie down. Loosen clothing. Place hands on the abdomen, and rest fingertips lightly on the navel. Breathing through the nose, inhale and expand only the abdomen. (The fingertips will meet.) Practice this *Abdominal Breath* slowly, without strain, ten times.
2. Place the hands on the rib cage and inhale, expanding only the diaphragm and the rib cage. (Watch the fingertips part.) Contract and slowly exhale. Practice this *Diaphragm Breath* ten times.
3. Placing the fingertips on the collarbones, inhale only in the upper chest. The fingers will rise, indicating a shallow breath. This is how we usually breathe. Notice the insufficiency. Now, raise the shoulders for more air. Exhale and practice this *Upper Breath* ten times.
4. Finally, placing the hands, palms up, beside the body, put these three breaths together. Inhale, expanding the abdomen, the diaphragm and the chest in a slow, wavelike movement. Hold. Exhale in the same order, contracting the abdomen, the diaphragm and the chest. Repeat these instructions to yourself as you adjust the *Complete Breath* to your own rhythm. Concentrate on what is happening: you are increasing the expansion of the terminal air sacs in the lungs. Notice how slow, deep breathing makes you calm, yet fills you with energy! Very logically, yoga traditionally links a long life with proper breathing.

Reported benefits: Increases vitality, soothes nerves, strengthens flabby intestinal and abdominal muscles.

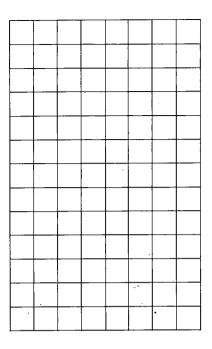

Yoga therapy begins with relaxation.

Corpse Pose Lie down on your back, in a quiet place. Place the arms beside the body, palms upturned. Keep heels slightly apart. Breathe slowly and deeply, feeling a sense of calm relaxation come over your whole body. Concentrate on loosening all tensions.

The following variation will increase your ability to relax:

1. Slowly inhale through the nostrils (always breathe through the nostrils during yoga, since the tiny hairs

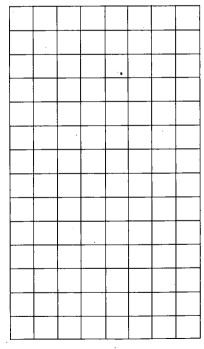

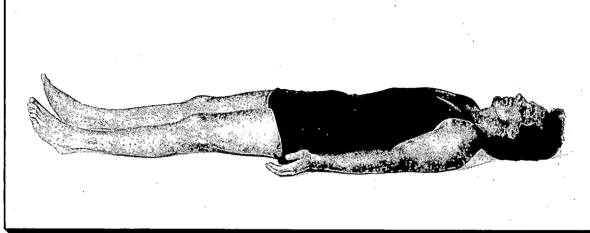

The Corpse Pose.

strain out impurities) and tense the ankles, feet and toes. Hold the breath while you tighten the muscles. Exhale and relax.

2. Slowly inhale and contract the kneecaps, calves, ankles, feet and toes. Hold and tighten. Exhale and relax.

3. Slowly inhale, contracting all the muscles of the abdomen, pelvic area, hips, thighs, kneecaps, calves, ankles, feet and toes. Hold the breath and tighten the muscles. Exhale and relax.

4. Inhale. Tense the neck, shoulders, arms and elbows, wrists, hands and fingers, chest muscles, down to the toes. Hold and tense. Exhale and relax.

5. Inhale and contract the scalp, the tiny muscles of the face, the forehead; squint the eyes, wrinkle the nose and mouth, tighten the tongue, constrict the throat and tighten the whole body. Hold and feel the terrible tension. Exhale and relax. Now, let the strain melt into the floor. Feel heavy. Enjoy the support of the floor. Sense the tingling of fresh circulation, the new muscle tone and emotional calm.

Reported benefits: Stimulates blood circulation and exercises inner organs. Alleviates fatigue, nervousness, neurasthenia (a general worn-out feeling), asthma, constipation, diabetes, indigestion, insomnia, lumbago. Teaches mental concentration.

Grip Sitting on the heels, raise the right hand. Bring it slowly behind the shoulder, touching the spine at the shoulder blades. Slowly bend the left arm behind the back from the bottom, and join the hands. Hold, then change arms and repeat.

Reported benefits: Proper execution develops the capacity of the thoracic cage, helps prevent tendinitis and the formation of calcium deposits at the shoulder joints. Helps alleviate emphysema and asthma.

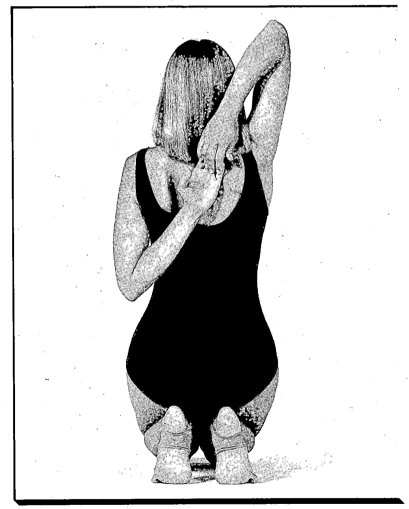

A rear view of the Grip.

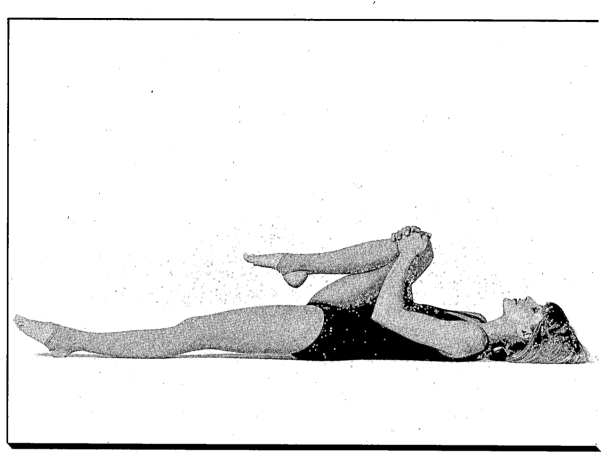

1. To do the second part of the Knee to Chest, *grasp one knee.*

Knee to Chest Lying on the back, bring the knees to the chest. Grasping the folded knees, rock gently back and forth. (This relaxes and massages the spine.) Lower the legs one at a time. Inhale and bend the right knee to the chest, pulling it into the chest with interlocked fingers. Retain the breath and raise the head, touching the knee with the nose. Hold for a count of ten. Exhale and lower the head almost to the floor. Repeat five times, then change legs. Exhale as the head is lowered to the floor. Straighten the right leg, and lower slowly to the floor. Repeat with the left leg. Now, draw up both legs, touch the nose to the knees. Hold with breath. Exhale and relax.

Reported benefits: Relieves stiffness and soreness of back and extremities, constipation, diabetes, flatulence.

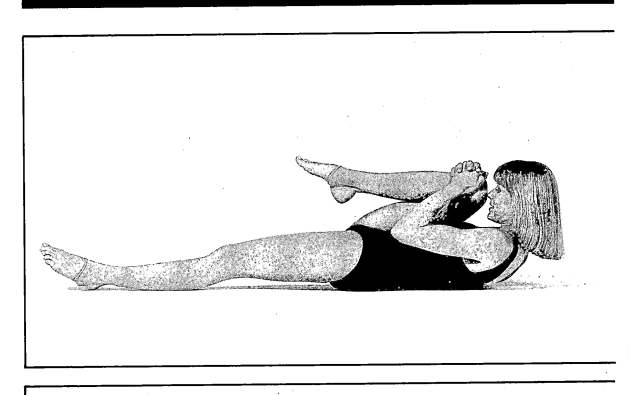

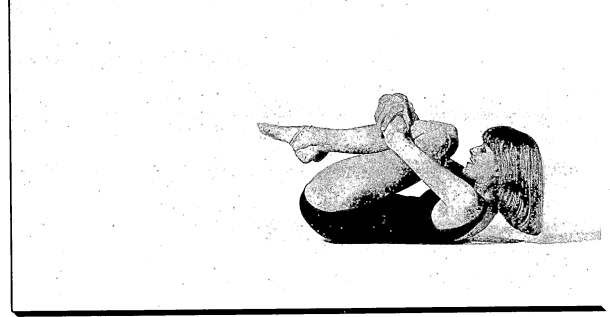

2. Bring your nose to your knee. 3. After alternating knees, bring both knees up.

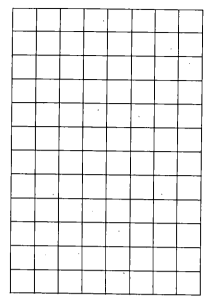

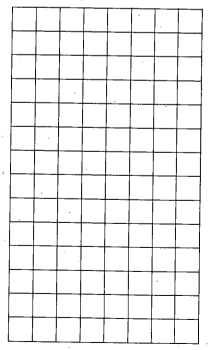

The benefits of yoga postures are greater if you focus your thoughts on where healing is needed, according to Dr. Rogers.

Kneeling Pose Sit on the heels, with a straight back. Relax. Separate the feet and slowly sink in between, letting the buttocks touch the floor, doing this slowly and carefully so as not to strain knee ligaments. Make sure feet are *not* turned out.

Reported benefits: Increased circulation to prostate gland or uterus.

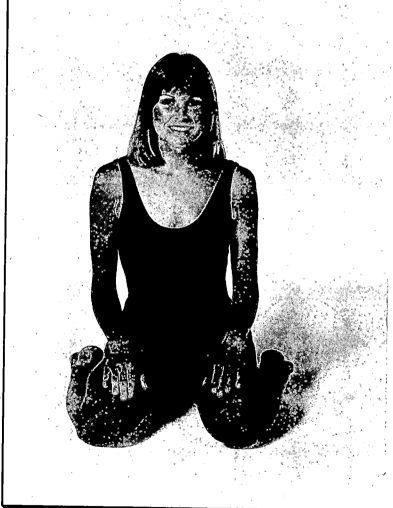

The Kneeling Pose.

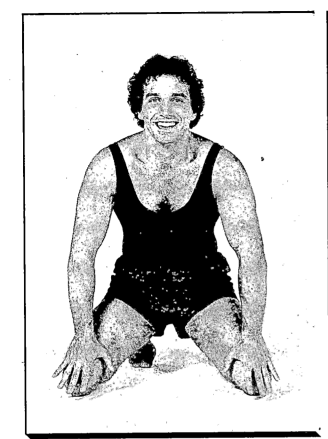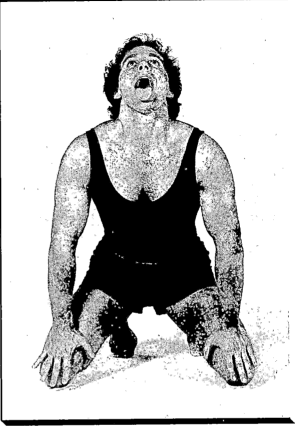

1. The Lion *exercises facial muscles. 2. Roaring out loud is not necessary.*

Lion Sitting on the heels, with palms on knees, stiffly fan out the fingers. Lean slightly forward over the hands. Protrude the tongue as far as possible, contract the throat muscles and roll the eyeballs upward. Completely exhale, saying, "Ahhhhhhh." Repeat four to six times.

Reported benefits: Helps to relieve sore throat. Stimulates circulation to throat and tongue.

Locust Lie face down. Clench the fists, keeping the arms on the floor at sides. Inhale. Using the lower back muscles, raise one leg toward the ceiling. Hold. Exhale and relax. Repeat with the other leg. Repeat two or three times, according to capacity.

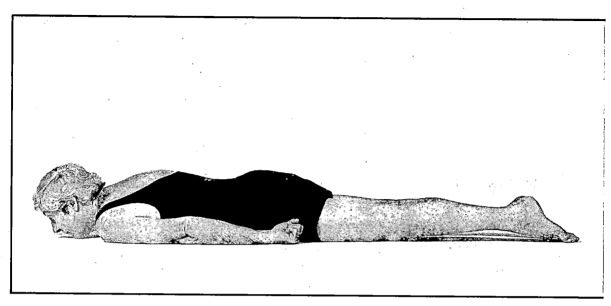

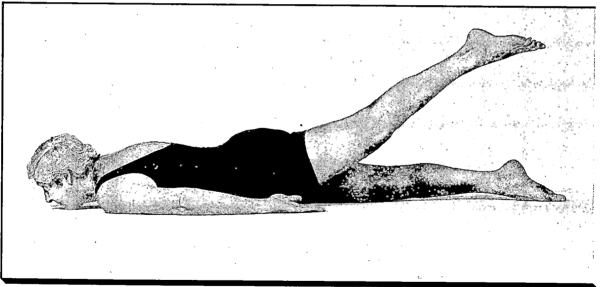

1. The Locust *is done lying flat. 2. Raise one leg, keeping it straight.*

More advanced: While in pose, raise both legs. A strenuous pose.

Reported benefits: Relieves problems of abdomen and lower back.

Warning: Not for those with hernia or back problem in acute stage.

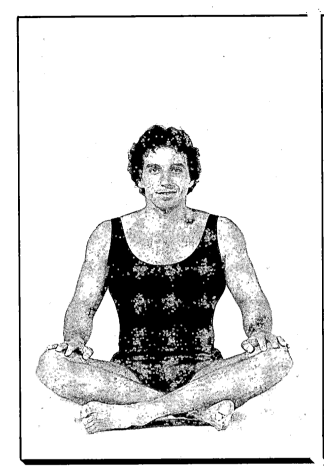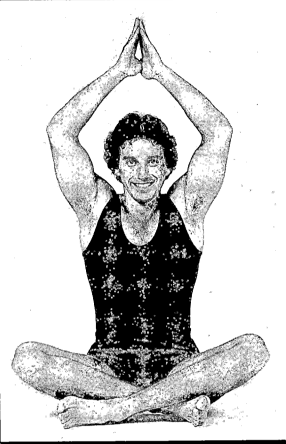

1. The Mountain *is done seated. 2. Then raise your hands.*

Mountain Sitting cross-legged, stretch both arms up toward the ceiling in a prayerlike pose, fingertips together. Stretch up and breathe deeply and slowly five to ten times. Exhale and lower arms.

Reported benefits: Strengthens lungs. Purifies bloodstream, improves digestive system, tones nervous system.

Neck and Eye Exercises Sitting upright, nod the head forward slowly three times. Nod to the left shoulder three times. Nod to the back three times, letting the mouth fall open. Nod to the right shoulder three times.

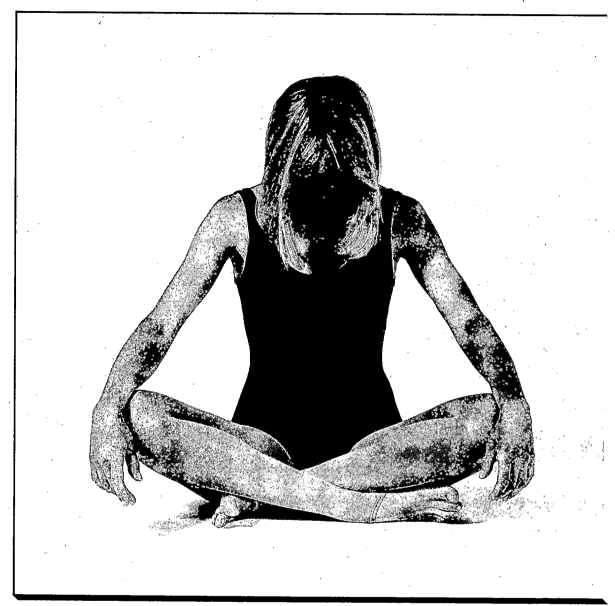

1. *In the* Neck and Eye Exercises, *you nod your head forward.*

Inhale. Shut the eyes tightly. Hold position with breath. Exhale, open the eyes wide and blink rapidly ten times.

Opening the eyes wide, look in a slow circle. Repeat in the opposite direction. Now, look diagonally. Next, look up and down ten times.

524   WHOLE BODY HEALING

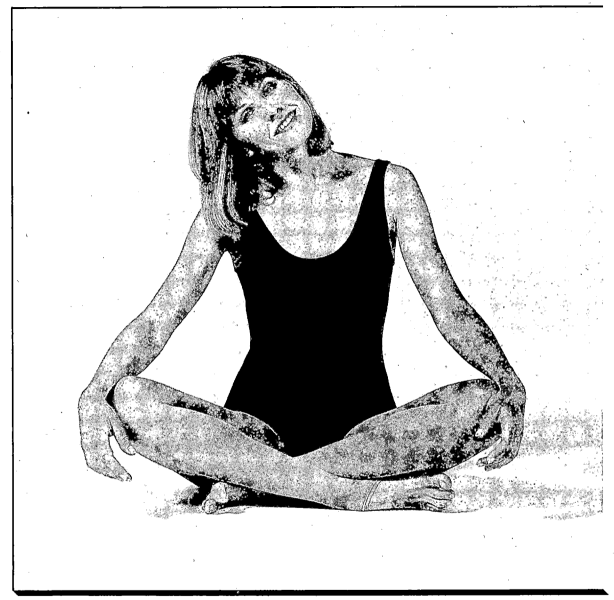

2. And then nod to your shoulders.

Rub the palms together vigorously. Close the eyes and cover with the palms. Take five very slow deep breaths, visualizing new energy and brightness into the eyes.
Reported benefits: Relieves headache and eyestrain; improves eyesight. Relaxes neck and shoulder tensions.

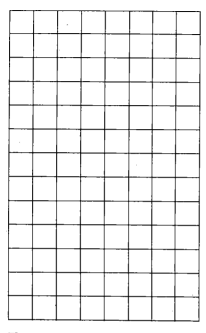

Three years ago I had all the classic symptoms of arthritis, says Ms. Bennett. But today, my arm is perfect, thanks to yoga.

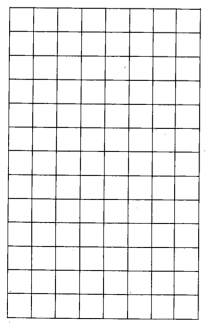

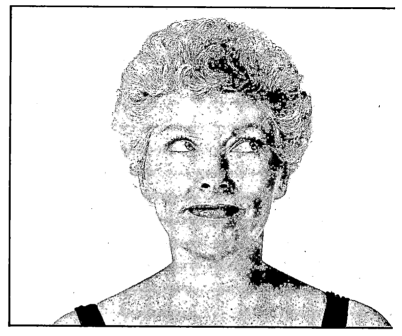

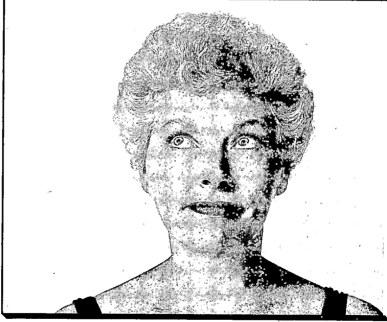

3. For the yoga eye exercise, move your eyes in a circle.
4. Then up, down, right and left.

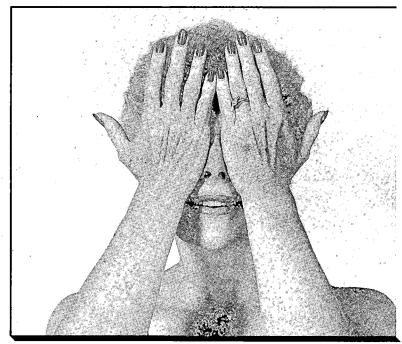

5. Rub your palms together before covering your eyes.

Posterior Stretch Sit on the floor, with the left leg outstretched, the right heel tucked into the crotch. Inhale and reach the arms overhead. Hold the breath, drop forward, reaching the arms toward the left ankle, the head to the knee. (If you can only grasp the calf, do that, and relax, breathing slowly.) Concentrate on the muscles as they slowly lengthen, and inch down lower. Close your eyes. Release any discomfort in a sensation of relaxation. Hold one minute. Inhale, raise up, arms overhead, and exhale as you lower the arms to the side. Repeat with the opposite leg. Repeat with both legs outstretched.

Reported benefits: A powerful massage to the abdominal organs. Improves digestion and elimination through the forward-bending movement: relaxes tensions in the back. Brings fresh circulation to face, firming tissue and improving color.

Warning: Not for those with slipped discs. It is important that the back is not rounded. All forward bends should be done from the hips.

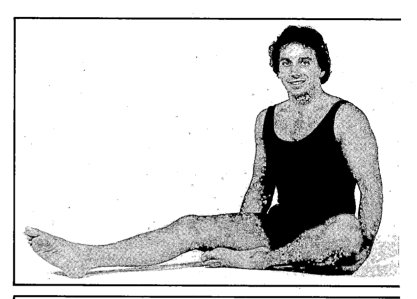

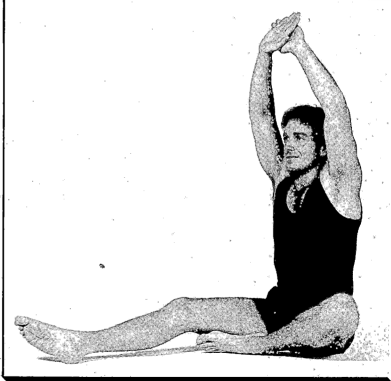

1. *The* Posterior Stretch *begins with one leg extended.*
2. *Reach up.*

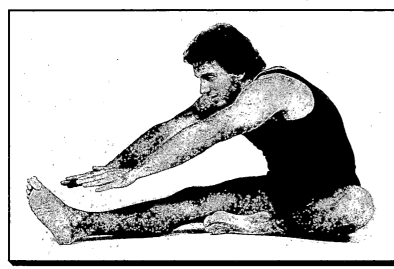

3. Then reach toward your toes.

Shoulder Roll Sitting or standing, roll shoulders loosely forward in a circular movement five times. Reverse.

For a bigger stretch, roll one shoulder at a time.

Reported benefits: Relieves headache, fatigue, tension, neckache.

Uddiyana Stand with feet apart, knees slightly bent. Lean forward, arching the back, hands on thighs. Exhale all air. Suck abdomen back toward the spine. Hold for several seconds. Relax and repeat, all within one exhalation. Work up to 20 repetitions with one exhalation.

Reported benefits: Alleviates constipation, indigestion and stomach problems. Good for combating obesity and diabetes.

Warning: Not to be practiced during pregnancy or by those with high blood pressure.

Yoga Mudra Sitting cross-legged, exhale and lean forward to touch the floor with the forehead. Place the arms behind the back, one hand grasping the opposite wrist. Hold the pose. Inhale and slowly return to sitting position. Practice up to 15 minutes.

Reported benefits: Gives energy, massages colon and intestines, relieves constipation. Good for complexion.

(continued on page 536)

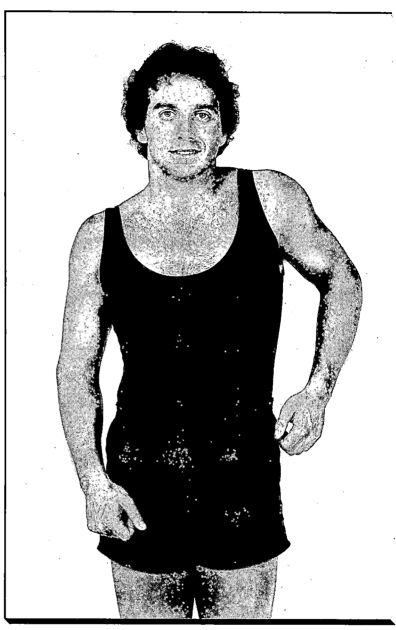

1. The Shoulder Roll *tones your muscles.*

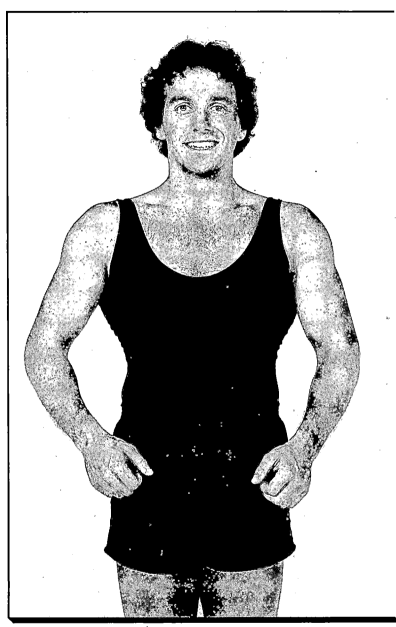

2. And relaxes them.

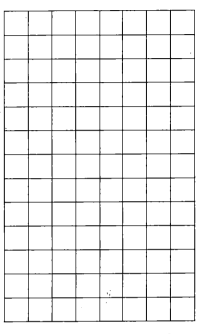

Yoga's easy stretches along with deep breathing exercises relieve the tension that binds up muscles. It's exercise and relaxation rolled into one.

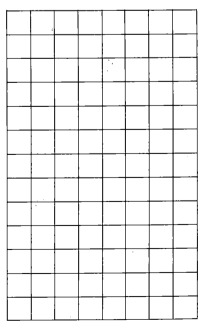

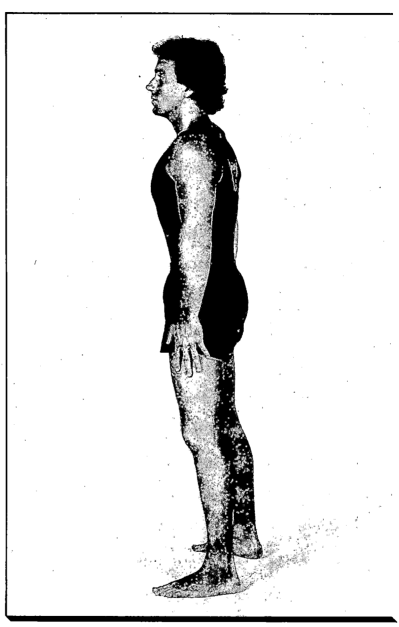

1. The Uddiyana *starts in this position.*

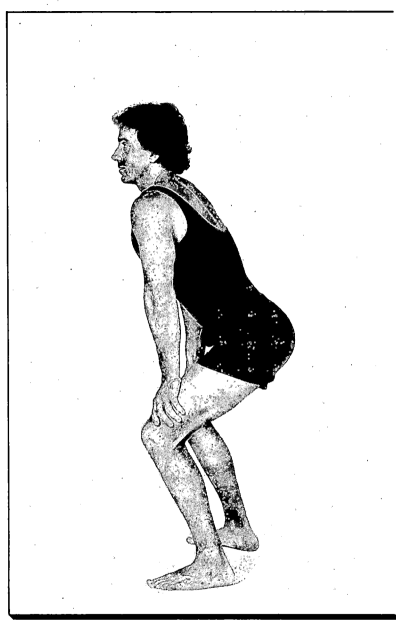

2. Then lean forward like this.

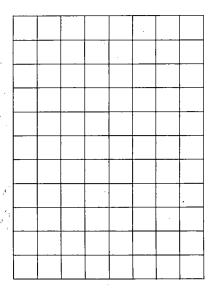

When the success of up-to-the-minute physiotherapy for severe breathing difficulties was compared with the effectiveness of a series of yoga exercises, yoga won—hands, legs and body down. Most of the patients who studied yoga learned to control their breathing problems.

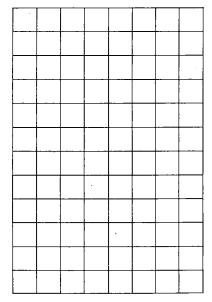

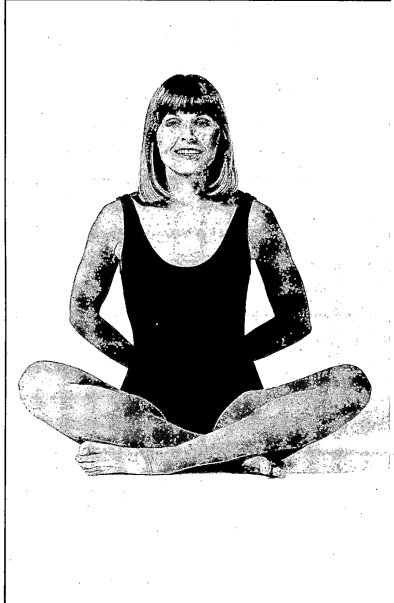

1. Exhale as you start the Yoga Mudra.

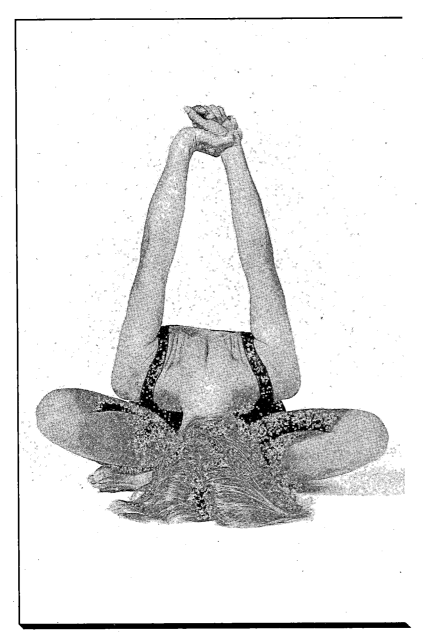

2. And try to touch the floor with your forehead.

Sun Salutation For people with limited time, the *Sun Salutation* exercises every muscle and joint and stimulates all major organs. The name itself means to give prostrations to the internal sun as well as to the external sun, the creative life-force of the universe which the yogis believe to radiate inside as well as outside the body.

1. Stand erect, feet together, palms prayerlike in front of the chest. Feel awareness of the whole body.
2. Inhale deeply, raise arms overhead, hands apart, leaning back.
3. Exhale, bending forward, legs straight. Touch the ground or try to, but don't strain.
4. Moving neither hands nor the left foot, bring the right leg back as far as possible, bending the left leg. Support weight on both hands, left foot, right knee, and toes of the right foot. Tilt the head back; look up. Inhale and retain breath.
5. Place the left foot next to the right and raise the abdomen, making the body a triangular arch. Place the head between the arms. Try to keep the feet flat. Exhale.
6. Hold breath. Lower the body to floor, keeping the abdomen and hips off the ground.
7. Inhale and raise the body in *Cobra* position, looking up.
8. Exhale, resume position 5.
9. Inhale, bring right foot forward and lower left knee as in position 4.
10. Exhale, resuming position 3.
11. Return to position 2, raising the hands while inhaling.
12. Exhale and return to position 1.

Reported benefits: Positions 1 and 12 – Establish state of concentration and calm. Positions 2 and 11 – Stretch abdominal and intestinal muscles, exercise arms and spinal cord. Positions 3 and 10 – Aid in prevention, relief of stomach ailments. Reduce abdominal fat. Improve digestion and circulation. Limber spine. Positions 4 and 9 – Tone abdomen, muscles of thighs and legs. Positions 5 and 8 – Strengthen nerves and muscles of arms and legs. Exercise spine. Positions 6 and 7 – Strengthen nerves and muscles of shoulders, arms and chest.

Some Convincing Case Histories

Okay. Those of you who were convinced of yoga's usefulness in your lives before we got going – and only wanted help in getting started – can stop reading now. Those of you who were intrigued by our description of the program but were *not* sure of its health benefits should read on. Here are three medically monitored applications of yoga exercises to common health problems whose success should help convince you.

Our first application isn't even a matter of illness or injury; it's exercise used to combat the effects of aging by a 70-year-old yoga instructor, Paulynne Bennett. Ms. Bennett feels that this particular form of activity is perfect for the older and not-necessarily-athletic group because the exercises are performed slowly and methodically. "You don't have to huff and puff to feel the benefits," the five-foot-three grandmother assured us. "As a result, your heart doesn't pound and your pulse doesn't race."

Furthermore, the slow, easy stretches do not deplete the body of energy; instead, they release trapped energy. According to Ms. Bennett, that trapped energy in the legs is a common cause of muscle cramps. So, if you're wakened frequently during the night by a charley horse, you've got one more reason to take up yoga.

Yoga also restores energy where it's needed. "Stretching is nature's way of eliminating fatigue," Ms. Bennett explains as she leads her students through a series of simple stretching exercises. "Just watch a cat when it's waking up from a snooze. It doesn't suddenly jump up. It gets up slowly and stretches its whole body. That's how all animals shake off fatigue.

No Straining Allowed

To Ms. Bennett, yoga is simply a systematic series of stretching movements. You stretch only as far as you are able to without strain – and no farther! For one person, that may be a few feet; for another, a mere fraction of an inch. It doesn't matter how far you go; you're still benefiting.

But no matter what the physical capacities of her students are, Ms. Bennett says, "I don't make a point of teaching the harder moves, because I don't want to discourage anyone. Besides, there's really no advantage in mastering the more advanced postures. They may require more coordination and balance, but when it comes to benefits, you're getting more in return for the simple exercises."

If you can get by with simple stretches, the question remains: why does yoga boast thousands of different positions? "Variety!" Ms. Bennett exclaims. "That's why you can

(continued on page 540)

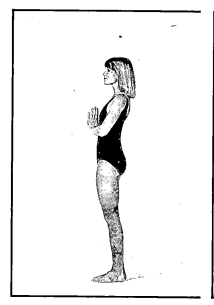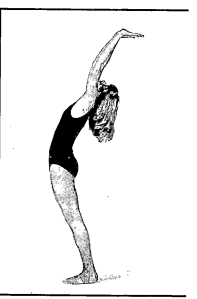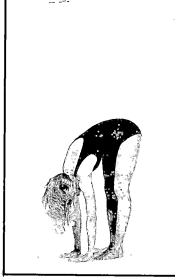

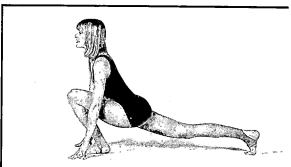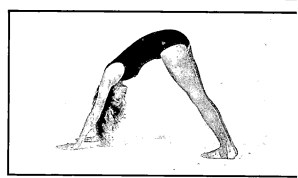

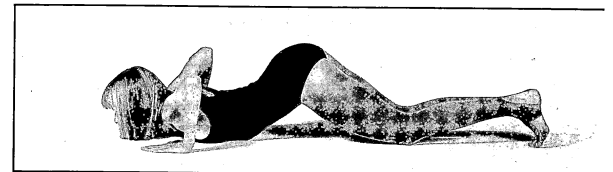

1. The Sun Salutation *starts in a prayerlike position. 2. Inhale as you lean back. 3. Keep your legs straight as you reach for the floor. 4. Bring the right leg back as far as possible. 5. Make a triangular arch. 6. Keep your stomach and hips off the ground.*

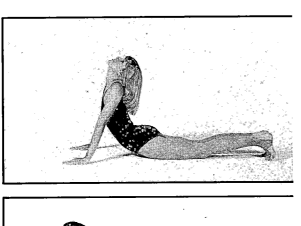

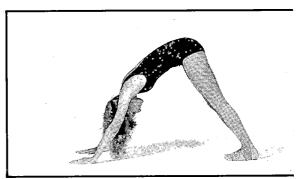

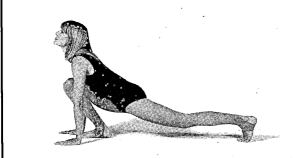

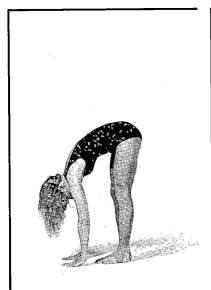

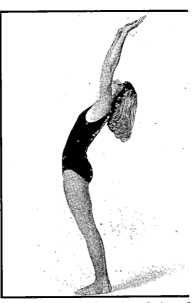

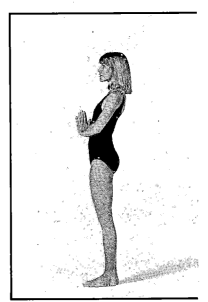

7. Assume the Cobra *position. 8. Do the arch. 9. This time bring the right knee forward.*
10. Keep the hands on or near the ground. 11. Reach back. 12. Finish with the prayer pose.

never get bored with yoga. There are so many variations to keep your interest. But that doesn't mean you have to try them all. My goodness, no. If you're happy with the simple stretches, then by all means stick to them."

Yoga is a very personal form of physical activity. It's not what you'd call a spectator sport or competitive sport of any kind. You do whatever stretches you like, and you progress at your own pace. There's only one universal law to keep in mind: never exceed your body's capabilities.

How to Tell Gain from Strain

"Learn to listen to your body," Ms. Bennett says. "It speaks to you. It will tell you where you really need a good stretch and when to stop. But be able to differentiate between discomfort and strain. Discomfort means you're benefiting; strain means you're pushing too hard."

And pushing too hard sometimes means that you've set your goals too high – another no-no, according to yoga philosophy. "You should never be desirous of 'making progress.' That kind of anxiety leads to tension, and that will defeat your purpose," warns Ms. Bennett. "The prime goal of yoga is to relieve the body of tension, not to create more of it by setting unreasonable goals."

Don't expect too much from yoga, either. "Some people take yoga because they think it will relieve all their aches and pains," she explains. "But yoga isn't a cure-all. My goodness, no . . . you can't expect to erase problems overnight that have taken years to develop. But if you do, well, that's a bonus.

"One woman said that yoga made it possible to go to sleep without a barbiturate, something she apparently hadn't done in some time," Ms. Bennett told us. "Another claimed that this was the first time in ages that she hadn't been bothered by a nagging backache. And someone else told me that yoga was the best thing she found for relieving her migraines."

Of course, tension is the underlying cause of many such problems. And since yoga, with its slow, stretching movements and regulated breathing, is ideal for releasing the tension that keeps our muscles bound up and mind bogged down, it's understandable that it can erase so many tension-related problems.

A former cigarette smoker, Ms. Bennett also insists that yoga is therapeutic for smokers. "Most people smoke because they are tense," she explains. "But if they become more peaceful, they can resist the urge to have a cigarette."

What about yoga for weight control? "I don't advocate weight watching," she snaps. "If you feel good, that's all that counts. I never weigh myself. In fact, I don't even own a scale. I don't need it. I can sense right away if I've let myself go, if I've put on some pounds or gotten flabby around the middle. You don't need a scale to tell you how you feel.

"Besides, losing pounds isn't really the issue," she insists. "Firming flab is. And that's where yoga is tops. Chances are the only way you'll lose weight with yoga is if you cut down on eating. With yoga, you may even gain a little weight as you lose inches because your muscles are becoming more firm, and firm flesh weighs more than flabby flesh."

Nevertheless, in homes where figure control is a concern, yoga is becoming a household word.

"One woman in my class went hog-wild over Christmas. She ate too much and neglected her yoga. Her body really showed it! Her weight skyrocketed to 170 pounds, and her muscle tone took a real nose dive," Ms. Bennett recalls. "Later, after she pulled herself together, she told me that her husband was instrumental in her getting back into shape. Whenever she'd start complaining about how awful she felt, he'd reply, 'Well, you know what Paulynne tells you to do.' That would remind her to get on with her yoga routine.

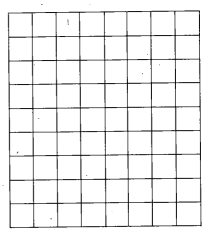

In homes where figure control is a concern, yoga is becoming a household word.

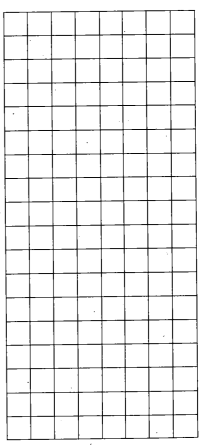

Yoga Slows Down the Aging Process

"According to yoga philosophy," says Ms. Bennett, "it's the flexibility of the spine, not the number of years, that determines a person's age. Yoga slows down the aging process by giving elasticity to the spine, firming up the skin, removing tension from the body, strengthening the abdominal muscles, eliminating the possibility of a double chin, improving the tone of flabby arm muscles, correcting poor posture, preventing dowager's hump and so on.

"It's like trading in characteristics of old age for characteristics of youth," says Ms. Bennett. "And who's not interested in that!"

So, if you're in reasonably good health and need only to tone up, slim down and stir up some sputtering energy fires, you needn't, according to Paulynne Bennett, make a systematic assault on the ancient wisdom that is yoga. You might simply follow this daily program designed by Ms. Bennett.

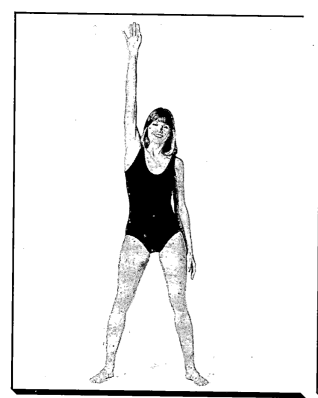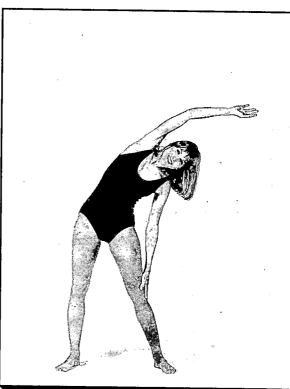

1. Reach up with your arm. 2. Then bend from the waist to the side.

Our Daily Yoga

1. On your feet, legs spread comfortably, reach up with your left arm.

   Slowly bend from the waist toward the right, letting your right hand slide down the right leg toward your ankle. Hold for 15 seconds, then come up slowly to the starting position. Repeat, bending toward the left.
2. To give your back a good spiral twist, stand with your feet together and stretch your arms upward.

   Twist your torso so that your chest will face left but your hips will remain facing forward.

   Now bend from the waist as far as you can. If you can touch your palms on the floor, terrific. If not, no sweat. Once you've held that position for 15 seconds, come gracefully up, twist back to the forward position and slowly let your arms come down at your sides. Now, repeat the spiral twist toward the right.

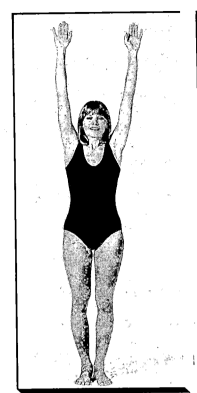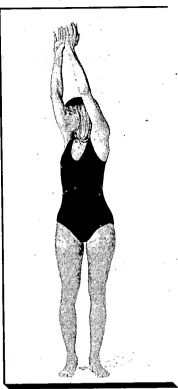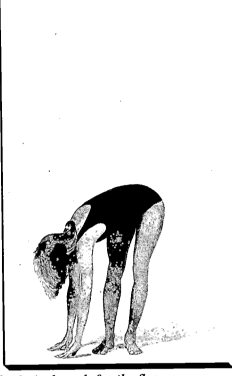

1. The spiral twist starts with both arms up. 2. Twist to the side. 3. And reach for the floor.

3. Start the chest expansion stretch by standing erect with your left foot slightly forward. Place the back of your hands on your chest, fingers touching.

   Circle your arms back until you can clasp hands and interlock fingers behind you. Straighten your arms, and bring them upward as you bend backward. Hold for five seconds.

   To counteract that strong concave stretch to the spine, bend forward as far as possible in the direction of your left knee. Hold for about ten seconds. Come slowly up. Repeat with your right foot in the forward position.

4. In a sitting position with your legs extended straight in front of you, raise your arms above your head. Lean back slightly and hold for five seconds. Bend forward and grasp the furthermost point on your leg that you can without strain. With elbows extending outward, very slowly pull yourself down to your knees – or in

that general direction. Hold whatever position you can attain for 30 seconds.

5. Still seated on the floor, spread your legs in a straddle position.

Bend forward as far as you can comfortably, grasping your legs to help maintain that position. Hold for 30 seconds.

6. In the same position, bend your knees and put the soles of your feet together. Clasp your hands around your feet to hold them together, and pull them toward your body as far as you can. Now slowly push your knees downward to do the push and reach. Don't worry if you can't touch your knees to the floor. Push as far as you can without strain, and hold for 15 seconds.

7. Lying flat on the floor, slowly raise your legs about 6 to 12 inches off the floor. Simultaneously, raise your shoulders off the floor so that your head and feet are at the same level. Hold about 15 seconds.

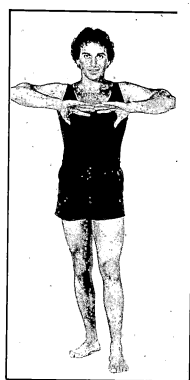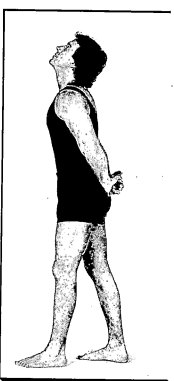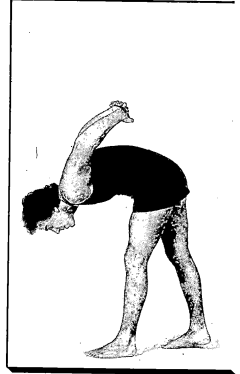

1. The chest stretch. 2. Clasp hands behind you. 3. Lean forward.

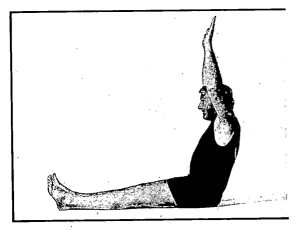

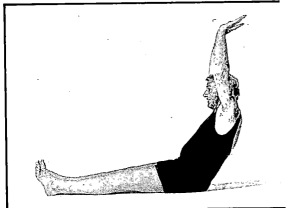

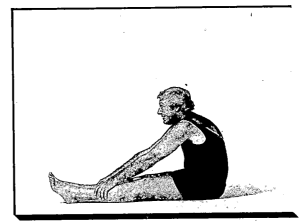

1. For the sitting stretch, first reach up. 2. Then reach back. 3. Then reach toward the toes.

Yoga and Arthritis

Now it's time to take a step up on the seriousness scale and enter a disease state – arthritis. Fortunately, we don't have to leave Ms. Bennett's capable and reassuring hands, because she has long treated her own condition with a specially tailored addition to the program we've just talked about.

"I had all the classic symptoms of arthritis – pain and stiffness in my joints, and tingling sensations, like electric currents, radiating down the entire length of my arm," says Ms. Bennett. "It got so bad that I couldn't do anything comfortably, not even rest my arm on a pillow.

"But that was three years ago. Look at me today," she smiles while swinging her "bad" arm back and forth like a pendulum. "My arm is perfect, thanks to yoga."

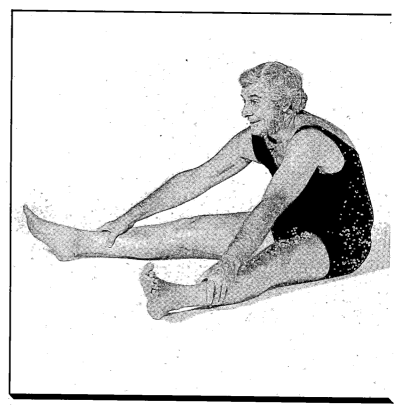

The straddle reach.

Before putting her efforts into yoga, however, Ms. Bennett went the usual arthritis route. She visited her doctor and had X-rays taken that confirmed she had osteoarthritis of the left arm and degeneration of the spinal column. Then she embarked on a prescribed course of therapy, which included taking aspirin to relieve the pain and reduce the inflammation.

"The only problem was, I ended up taking at least six aspirin a day," she sighs. "And some days were so bad I took 10 or 12."

Like so many others plagued by arthritis misery, Ms. Bennett eventually realized she couldn't find the answer in an aspirin bottle. But she had an excellent alternative right in her living room – an exercise mat.

"I had been teaching yoga at the time of my illness," she explains. "But with all my talking and instructing and

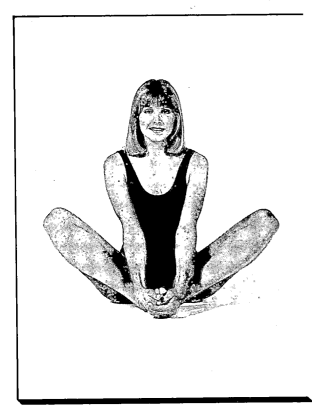
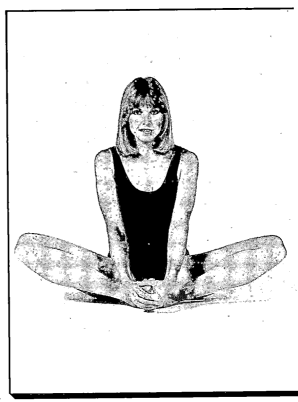

1. Pull your feet toward your body to start the push and reach. 2. Lower your knees as much as you can.

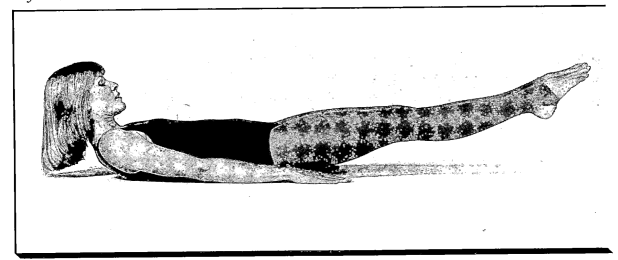

For the floor push, push hands down. Lift legs up.

worrying about other people's yoga needs, I was neglecting my own.

"It wasn't until the arthritis flared up that I took stock of my own well-being. I started a personal yoga program and concentrated on loosening up the joints in my left arm and improving the flexibility of my spine. Now my joints are as flexible as they were ten years ago. It's a miracle!"

Indeed, anyone who's fighting the uphill battle against arthritis would agree that her recovery was quite a feat. But, on the other hand, why should it be so surprising that yoga struck the winning blow? After all, it is an excellent form of exercise.

Exercise, an Old Foe of Arthritis

"Exercise has been recommended as treatment for arthritis for a long, long time – about 75 years," says Morris A. Bowie, M.D., a rheumatologist at Bryn Mawr Hospital in Pennsylvania. "People were exercising their arthritic joints before yoga was ever introduced into this country."

And, apparently, they were on the right track. "Exercise is very important to try to reestablish a complete range of motion," Dr. Bowie told us. "Of course, that doesn't mean you should induce a long continual strain. We encourage a moderate amount of nonstrenuous, non-weight-bearing exercises tailored to the individual's needs. Some yoga postures are not tolerated well, particularly by those past 50."

Louise Mollinger, a physical therapist at St. Margaret Memorial Hospital in Pittsburgh, Pennsylvania, agrees. "Getting the joints mobile is our main purpose," Ms. Mollinger told us. "We know that complete rest will further stiffen the joints and that overexertion will make them sore. So we feel that a balance of rest and simple range-of-motion exercises is best."

Therein lies one of yoga's benefits. Its slow-motion movements and gentle pressures reach deep into troubled joints. In addition, the easy stretches in conjunction with deep-breathing exercises relieve the tension that binds up the muscles and further tightens the joints. Yoga is exercise and relaxation rolled into one – the perfect antiarthritis formula.

And that brings us another reason why arthritis victims improve so markedly with yoga. It seems that a major problem in prescribing exercise is in getting the patient to follow through. If an exercise program is painful and too strenuous, it isn't likely to be continued. Chances are an arthritis sufferer winces at the mere mention of the word "exercise." Yoga can break into this vicious cycle. It eases you into exercise without causing strain or undue pain. Even if you are only able to move an inch and hold a position for five seconds, you are already enhancing your body's flexibility.

Some physicians have long recognized the advantages of yogalike exercises. Dr. Bowie recommends the pendulum, an arm-swinging exercise "devised by an orthopedic surgeon" for bursitis and shoulder stiffness. He also favors deep-breathing exercising for ankylosing spondylitis, an arthritis-related condition affecting the joints of the spine.

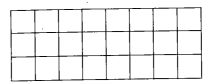

Yoga eases you into exercise without causing strain or undue pain. Even if you are only able to move an inch and hold a position for five seconds, you are already enhancing your body's flexibility.

"Don't Rush It"

With yoga, a little effort usually goes a long way. "Don't rush it, either," Ms. Bennett warns. Begin by moving only a few inches in any exercise – until you feel discomfort. Then hold for a count of five. Try to repeat the same movement two or three times. Each day, try to move only an inch or so farther and hold for a second longer.

You'll have to gauge yourself. Start with a few of the simple stretches we mentioned earlier. The simple leg pull, the chest expansion exercise, and the knee and thigh stretch are especially beneficial to the joints. If your arthritis is severe, settle for a modified version of these.

Then try some slow rotation exercises. Head circles performed in the yoga fashion – that is, slowly, with pauses in the forward, side and back positions – will help loosen up a stiff neck. Similarly, ankle rotation will improve arthritis conditions in those joints.

The *Flower* is a great yoga exercise for arthritic fingers. Whenever you think of it, make a tight fist and hold for five seconds. Then release and stretch your hand open as far as you can for an additional five seconds.

Ready to concentrate on those major problem areas? If your arthritis has come to rest in your spine, limber up that area with the seated spiral twist, the cobra, and the neck and shoulder stretch. Got it in the hips? Then lie down in bed and try some hip rolls.

"Of course, there will be some days that you can't practice at all," Ms. Bennett admits. "Don't worry about it. If the pain is too intense, just skip your yoga sessions for a day or two. Resume again when you're feeling better. Bad spells are part of the system, and in the case of arthritis,

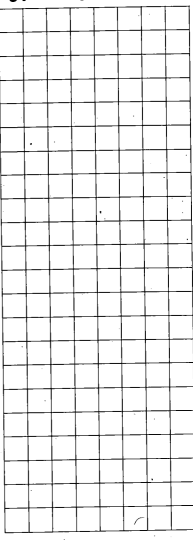

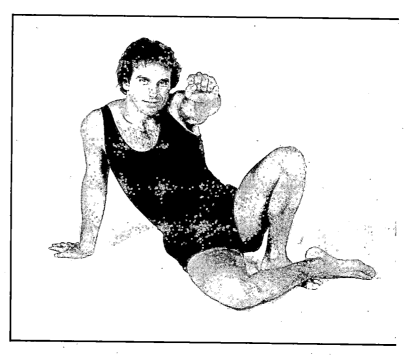

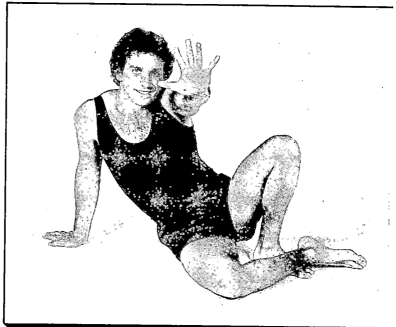

1. The Flower *starts with a fist. 2. Then the hand opens.*

progress is never in a straight line. It's usually a matter of taking a few steps forward and one backward. You're still moving ahead but at a slower pace."

Of course, on days that movement comes easy, don't overdo it. Overworked joints can be as painful as neglected ones. So, no matter how good the exercises feel, don't continue for more than a few minutes at a time. "For people with severe arthritis, it's usually better to divide the daily yoga routine into about three or four segments of about five minutes each," Ms. Bennett recommends. "Rest periods and deep-breathing exercises interspersed throughout the day's yoga sessions will help relax the muscles that tighten up joints."

A Rigorous Scientific Trial for Yoga

Finally, we have a very serious condition to look at in what is – fittingly – a most rigorous scientific testing of yoga's contribution to health. When the success of up-to-the-minute physiotherapy for severe breathing difficulties was compared with the effectiveness of a series of yoga exercises, yoga won – hands, legs and body down.

Dr. M. K. Tandon, of Repatriation General Hospital in Western Australia, worked with 22 male patients, aged 52 to 65, who suffered "severe airways obstruction" – chronic bronchitis, in some cases complicated by lung-deteriorating emphysema – that made normal breathing impossible.

For 11 of the men, the prescription was the standard one for this condition – physiotherapy, which included relaxation techniques, breathing exercises and general workouts to improve stamina.

The other 11 men were given a yoga teacher instead of a physiotherapist. He taught them techniques of yoga breathing, which encourage the use of all chest and abdominal muscles as well as ten yoga postures.

The patients practiced their particular exercises for nine months. Then they were reexamined at the hospital: a technician tested their lung function, a physician screened them closely to determine how their symptoms had changed, and a stationary exercise bicycle was used to measure their capacity for exercise.

The difference between the two groups was striking. The men who had practiced yoga showed a significant improvement in their ability to exercise, but the physiotherapy group did not. Even more important, perhaps, was the improvement in symptoms reported by the yoga group. Eight or more out of the 11 declared that they had definitely increased tolerance for exertion and that they recovered more quickly after exertion. The physiotherapy group reported no similar improvement.

Best of all, the patients who had studied yoga apparently gained the ability to control their breathing problems. A significantly greater number of patients reported that "with the help of yogic breathing exercises, they could control an attack of severe shortness of breath without having to seek medical help," according to the study.

Why did yoga seem to work better than physiotherapy in relieving respiratory problems? "After their training, the breathing pattern of the patients in the yoga group changed to a slower and deeper cycle, allowing them to tolerate higher work loads," reports Dr. Tandon. "On the other hand, patients in the physiotherapy group did not change their shallow rapid breathing pattern." (For a yogic breathing exercise, see the *Complete Breath* described earlier in this chapter.)

SPECIAL INDEX OF CONDITIONS AND DISEASES

Page numbers in boldface indicate photos.

553

yoga as therapy for, 510
    Cobra, 513, **514**
    Corpse Pose, 515-16, **516**
    Locust, 521-22, **522**
    Mountain, 523
    Posterior Stretch, 527, **528-29**
iron deficiency, 218-20
    mineral supplements, 218-20
irregular heartbeat, biofeedback for, 93
irritability, tub baths for, 479

J

jaw clenching, biofeedback for, 97
joint pain (chronic), vitamin and mineral
    supplements for, 327

K

kidney disease, danger with fasting, 211

L

leg ulcers, as complication of varicose
    veins, 458
liver (sluggish), yoga as therapy for, 511
liver disease, fat intake and, 324
lordosis, Alexander Technique for, 133
lower back pain
    acupressure for, 17
    acupuncture for, 27
    Alexander Technique for, 133
    biofeedback for, 97
    chiropractic treatment for, 180
    exercises as therapy for, 384
lumbago, yoga as therapy for, 515-16

M

menstrual cramping, Rolfing for, 360-61
menstrual irregularity
    yoga as therapy for, 510
        Cobra, 513, **514**
        Posterior Stretch, 527, **528-29**
menstrual pain, hot sitz bath for, 476
mental fatigue, acupressure for, 21
mid-back conditions, chiropractic
    treatment for, 180
migraine. *See also* headache
    acupressure for, 26
    biofeedback for, 97
    cause of, 101
    chiropractic treatment for, 174, 181
    hypnosis for, 268
    shiatsu for, 408-9
misaligned feet/limbs, Alexander
    Technique for, 133
motion sickness, acupressure for, 22
mouth ulcers, vitamin and mineral
    supplements for, 327
multiple sclerosis, acupressure for, 26
muscle disorders, biofeedback for, 105
muscle pain, vitamin and mineral
    supplements for, 327
muscular fatigue, water therapy for, 469
muscular soreness, heat therapy for, 244

N

nausea, as side effect of fasting, 211
neckache, yoga as therapy for, 529
neck fatigue, shiatsu for, 409

neck syndromes, chiropractic treatment
    for, 180
nerve damage, biofeedback for, 97
nervous disorders, chiropractic
    treatment for, 180
nervous indigestion, vitamin and mineral
    supplements for, 327
nervousness, yoga as therapy for, 515-16
nervous tension, chiropractic treatment
    for, 179
neuralgia, fomentations for, 474
neurasthenia
    yoga as therapy for, 510
        Corpse Pose, 515-16, **516**
        Mountain, 523
        Posterior Stretch, 527, **528-29**
neuritis, chiropractic treatment for, 181
neurological disease, chiropractic
    treatment for, 180
neuromuscular tension, walking as
    therapy for, 462
nosebleed, hot footbath for, 474

O

obesity
    diabetes and, 210
    heart attack and, 210
    as result of fiber shortage, 318
    precautions with rope skipping, 371
    yoga as therapy for, 508, 510
        Bow, 511, 513, **512-13**
        Cobra, 513, **514**
        Locust, 521-22, **522**
        Posterior Stretch, 527, **528-29**
        Sun Salutation, 536
        Yoga Mudra, 529, **534-35**
osteoarthritis
    acupuncture for, 27
    exercise as therapy for, 384
    sleeping bag as therapy for, 244-45
    yoga as therapy for, 546
osteoporosis, walking as therapy for, 465

P

paralysis
    biofeedback for, 105
    precautions with fomentations, 474
Parkinson's disease, biofeedback for, 97,
    105
pelvic pain, sitz bath for, 476-77
peptic ulcer, precautions with yoga,
    511-13
phlebitis, as complication of varicose
    veins, 458
phobias, biofeedback for, 102-3
pimples. *See* acne
plantar wart, running with, 221
plaque, formation of, 319
postural imbalance, Alexander
    Technique for, 133
pregnancy, varicose veins and, 459
pronation, as cause of knee pain, 397,
    398
prostate trouble
    sitz bath for, 477
    yoga as therapy for, 510
        Kneeling Pose, 520
psoriasis, ultrasound for, 246

R

Raynaud's disease, biofeedback for, 102
respiratory conditions
    chiropractic treatment for, 180
    response point therapy for, 25-26
    yoga as therapy for, 508
rheumatism
    Alexander Technique for, 133
    chiropractic treatment for, 180
    yoga as therapy for, 510
        Knee to Chest, 518, **518-19**
        Mountain, 523
        Posterior Stretch, 527, **528-29**
rheumatoid arthritis
    acupuncture for, 27
    heat therapy for, 244
    response point therapy for, 26
runner's knee
    cause of, 396
    exercises for, 398-99
    ice for, 399, **400**
    relief for, 397-99
running injuries, 395-404
    Achilles tendinitis, 402-4
        treatment of, 403
    knee pain, 396-99
        cause of, 396
        exercises for, 398-99
        ice for, 399, **400**
        precautions for, 397-99
        relief for, 397-99
    shin splints, 399-402
        cause of, 401
        treatment for, 401-2
    side stitch, 395-96, 399-402
        control for, 396
        treatment for, 401-2

S

sacroiliac strain, chiropractic
    treatment for, 180
schizophrenia
    fasting as therapy for, 210
    running as therapy for, 374
sciatica
    acupuncture for, 27
    chiropractic treatment for, 180-81
    yoga as therapy for, 510
        Grip, 517
        Kneeling Pose, 520
        Knee to Chest, 518, **518-19**
scoliosis, Alexander Technique for, 133
seizures, hypnosis for, 268
sexual debility
    yoga as therapy for, 510
        Complete Breath, 513, **515**
        Kneeling Pose, 520
        Uddiyana, 529, **532-33**
shin splints, 394, 399-402
    acupressure for, 7
    cause of, 401
    treatment for, 401-2
shoulder stiffness/soreness
    exercises to prevent, 79
    yoga as therapy for, 549
side stitch
    cause of, 401
    as running injury, 395-96, 399-402
    treatment for, 401-2

GENERAL INDEX

Page numbers in boldface indicate photos. For listing of conditions and diseases, please see previous index.

to reduce stress, 199
to release tension in children, **200**
for retarded, 198
DeBakey, Michael, M.D., on the heart, 232
depressant, alcohol as, 206-7
deVries, Herbert A., Ph.D., on stretching for muscle flexibility, 434-35
DeWeese, James A., M.D., on varicose veins and heredity, 458
diaphragmatic breathing, as basis of good health, 342
double tuck kicks, as swimming exercise, 449
drinking, hypnosis for, 272
dropped handlebars, on bicycles, 90, **91**
drugs and exercise, 206-9
 alcohol, 206-7
 amphetamines, 208
 antibiotics, 207-8
 aspirin, 208-9
 caffeine, 208
 high blood pressure and, 207
 penicillin, 207
 sedatives, 207
dumbbells, used in weight training, 487

E
eating, at bedtime, 108-9
eating habits
 arteriosclerosis and, 109-10
 impotence and, 110
effleurage, as form of massage, 298, 303, **304,** 305
elastic support stockings, for varicose veins, 460-61
electrical activity of nerve cells, measuring of, 98
electrical conductivity of skin, measuring of, 98
electro-acupuncture
 for dental problems, 3
 for headaches, 2
electrocardiogram
 for aerobic exercise, 38
 stress test and, 38
electrocardiograph (EKG), as biofeedback machine, 97-99
electroencephalograph (EEG)
 as biofeedback machine, 98
 epilepsy and, 104
electromyograph (EMG)
 biofeedback and, 94-95
 as biofeedback machine, 98, 105
electronic feedback, electromyograph for, 94-95
endorphins
 as antidote for depression, 375
 as pain inhibitors, 412
 secretion by body, 3-4
equipment
 for cross-country skiing, 190
 for weight training, 487
ergometer, recovering from heart attack and, 236
Erwin, Dabney M., M.D., on hypnosis, 268-69
exercise
 for arthritis, 548

for back pain, 342-45, 384
for back troubles, 56
combatting fatigue with, 384
cross-country skiing as, **189,** 190
dancing as, 30-52
drugs and, 206-9
dynamic, 421
for fit heart, 242
sex and, 405-7
static, 421
stretching as, 436-42, 484-87
swimming as, 447-50
for varicose veins, 460
warm-up, 163-68
exercise bicycles, developing aerobic capacity with, **214**

F
facet joint, worn, as backache cause, 54
fainting, acupressure for, 23
faintness, hot sitz baths and, 477
fasting, 210-12
 for depression, 210
 to detoxify body, 210
 heart attack and, 210
 liquid protein diets and, 211
 modified, 210
 rules for, 212
 side effects from, 211
 stomach cancer and, 211
 for weight loss, 210
fat
 buildup of, 322
 polyunsaturated, 322-23
 reducing intake of, 324-26
 saturated, 322-23
fatigue and stamina, 213-20
fat intake
 diabetes and, 324
 gallbladder problems and, 324
 heart attack and, 322-24
 hypertension and, 324
 liver disease and, 324
feet
 circulation of, 222
 footwear and, 221-26
 lower backache and, 221
 posture and, 221
 problems, 224-25
Feldenkrais Principles of Functional Integration, 137-51
 goal of exercise, 138-39
 movements of, **139-42**
 self-treatment, 147-48
 theory of physical therapy, 137-38
Fengchi point
 for headache, 16
 locating, 16
 pressing on, **17**
 for stiff neck, 16
fiber
 importance of, 317-18
 results of shortage, 318
fire hydrant exercise, 48, **49**
Fisher, Jeffrey, Ph.D., on hug therapy, 252
fitness, bicycling for, 86-92
floor push, as yoga exercise, **547**
Flower, as yoga exercise, 549-50, **550**
folate, for red blood cell creation, 220

folk cures. *See* biofeedback
fomentations, 471-74
 application of, **472-73**
 for arthritis, 474
 for bronchitis, 474
 for chest colds, 474
 cloth for, 471-72
 for congestion relief, 474
 for coughs, 474
 diabetes precautions with, 474
 edema precautions with, 474
 for neuralgia, 474
 for sedation, 474
 Turkish towels for, 472
food, absorption of, 208-9
 fructose in, 319
 heart attack and, 108-9
 stroke and, 108
footbath, hot, 474-75
 benefits of, 474
 for congestion, 474
 container for, 474
 for diabetes, 474-75
 for frostbite, 475
 for nosebleeds, 474
 water temperature of, 474
foot press, as runner's exercise, 390, **391**
footwear
 bunions and, 221, 224
 corns and, 221, 224
 for court sports, 226
 feet and, 221-26
 foot problems with, 221, 224-25
 nonporous man-made materials for, 225
 types of, 225-26
 for walking, 225, 466-68
forehead, massage for, **305**
Formica, Palma, M.D., on fatigue, 218
fracture pains, hypnosis for, 268
Frost, Elizabeth, M.D., on finding local acupuncturist, 28
frozen shoulder, from sprains, 76
fructose, in food, 319

G
galvanic skin resistance (GSR), and biofeedback, 98
gastrointestinal system, overloading of, 110
Gencheff, Todor, M.D., on acupressure, 9
getting out of bed, proper way of, 62, **63**
Gettman, Larry R., Ph.D., on weight training, 482-83
Goldberg, Herb, Ph.D., on expressing affection, 253
Golub, Benjamin S., M.D., on posture, 335, 342
Good Sources of Tryptophan (table), 5
Good Sources of Vitamin B_6 (table), 4
Good Sources of Vitamin B_{12} (table), 5
Gotto, Antonio, M.D., on the heart, 232
Greenwood, James, Jr., M.D., on prevention of cervical disc problems, 430-31

H
Halberg, Franz, M.D., on losing weight, 113-14